New Technologies in Dermatological Science and Practice

New Technologies in Dermatological Science and Practice

Editor: Racheal Hastings

AMERICAN
MEDICAL PUBLISHERS
www.americanmedicalpublishers.com

AMERICAN
MEDICAL PUBLISHERS
www.americanmedicalpublishers.com

Cataloging-in-Publication Data

New technologies in dermatological science and practice / edited by Racheal Hastings.
p. cm.
Includes bibliographical references and index.
ISBN 979-8-88740-337-3
1. Dermatology--Technological innovations. 2. Dermatology.
3. Skin--Diseases--Diagnosis--Technological innovations.
4. Skin--Diseases--Treatment--Technological innovations.
I. Hastings, Racheal.
RL72 .N49 2023

American Medical Publishers,
41 Flatbush Avenue,
1st Floor, New York,
NY 11217, USA

ISBN 979-8-88740-337-3 (Hardback)

Contents

Preface

I am honored to present to you this unique book which encompasses the most up-to-date data in the field. I was extremely pleased to get this opportunity of editing the work of experts from across the globe. I have also written papers in this field and researched the various aspects revolving around the progress of the discipline. I have tried to unify my knowledge along with that of stalwarts from every corner of the world, to produce a text which not only benefits the readers but also facilitates the growth of the field.

Dermatological science refers to a field that includes the study, research, diagnosis and treatment of any medical disease impacting the nails, skin, membranes and hair. Eczema, cold sores, acne, fungal infections, skin cancer, psoriasis, dermatitis and warts are some of the most common dermatologic conditions. There are various forms of dermatological therapies that can be used for the management of skin diseases, such as surgery, topical drugs, radiotherapy, photodynamic therapy, laser therapy, dermatohistopathology, immunotherapy and phototherapy. The most recent developments in medical and cosmetic dermatology comprises scientific discoveries for oral sun protection, breakthroughs in botanical blends for hair care, and new directions in red light photodynamic therapy (PDT). It also involves the development of new devices to treat superficial skin lesions and solar lentigines for improving aesthetics. This book is a valuable compilation of topics, ranging from the basic to the most complex advancements in the field of dermatology. It covers in detail some existent and innovative concepts revolving around this domain. This book will serve as a reference to a broad spectrum of readers.

Finally, I would like to thank all the contributing authors for their valuable time and contributions. This book would not have been possible without their efforts. I would also like to thank my friends and family for their constant support.

Editor

Social Media as a Platform for Information and Support for Melanoma Patients: Analysis of Melanoma Facebook Groups and Pages

Nishita Maganty, MPH; Muneeb Ilyas, BS; Zachary Ginsberg; Amit Sharma, MD

Department of Dermatology, Mayo Clinic Arizona, Scottsdale, AZ, United States

Corresponding Author:
Nishita Maganty, MPH
Department of Dermatology
Mayo Clinic Arizona
13400 E. Shea Boulevard
Scottsdale, AZ, 85259
United States

Email: nmaganty@email.arizona.edu

Abstract

Background: Social media is increasingly used as a source of health information and is useful for information exchange and patient support.

Objective: The aim of this study is to describe the Facebook groups and pages that are available for melanoma patients.

Methods: A systematic search of Facebook groups and pages was performed using the word "melanoma." The first 50 pages found in the search, sorted by most relevant, were analyzed for several characteristics, namely page name, category, verification status, number of likes, number of followers, visitor posts per week, page posts per week, ability to donate, date of inception, and for-profit or nonprofit. The first 50 groups found in the search, sorted by most relevant, were analyzed for name, category, number of members, and privacy setting.

Results: There were 669 pages and 568 groups related to melanoma found on Facebook. The first 50 pages had a combined total of 266,709 likes and 257,183 followers and, of these, 30% (15/50) were verified by Facebook. Within the analyzed Facebook pages, the average number of visitor posts per week was 0.48, the average number of posts by the page per week was 5.6, and the most common page categories were community and nonprofit. Of the 50 groups analyzed, 18 were public and 32 were private (closed). The total number of combined group members in all 50 groups was found to be 23,047 and 52% (26/50) of the groups were categorized as support.

Conclusions: Melanoma pages and groups on Facebook reach a large portion of the population. To provide resources for the population of patients diagnosed with malignant melanoma and ensure that proper information is distributed, physicians and health care organizations may consider using Facebook as a platform to support and educate patients with melanoma.

KEYWORDS

Facebook; melanoma; online health information; patient education; support; health promotion

Introduction

According to the Centers for Disease Control and Prevention, approximately 61% of US adults have searched for medical information online [1] and due to cost, convenience, and accessibility factors [2], patients search the internet for information regarding medical conditions more often than they communicate with their doctors [3]. In addition, some patients believe that the information on the internet is better than that provided by physicians [4].

In recent years, social media websites have emerged as an easily accessible source of health information [5,6] and social media is used by 39% of US adults to obtain health-related information [6]. Social media allows users to generate and share content with internet users across the world. Social networking sites have become a source of information on awareness, treatment, and updates regarding medical illnesses [7]. Furthermore, social networking websites allow for the creation of online support communities and create platforms to engage patients in discussion about medical conditions [7]. Facebook is one of the most popular social networking websites with nearly 2 billion active users [8]. Facebook allows users to create, share, post, and react to information. It is reported that Facebook is the fourth most popular source of health information in the United Kingdom [6]. A unique feature of Facebook is the "group" functionality, which has been defined as a space created by users to form a community of people to promote, share, and discuss a topic [9]. Another feature of Facebook is a "page" which is designed for brands, businesses, organizations, and public figures to create a presence on Facebook [10].

Skin cancer is the most common malignancy in the US and malignant melanoma is responsible for the most skin cancer related deaths [11]. The incidence of malignant melanoma is increasing worldwide and is associated with increasing health care costs [12]. Previous studies have evaluated the utility of Facebook groups in providing health education for hypertension and diabetes patients [9]; however, to date, there is no literature on the use of Facebook groups and pages by skin cancer patients, specifically those afflicted by melanoma. By gaining a better understanding of the use of Facebook for patient education, physicians, and health care organizations may be able to better utilize Facebook as a platform to support and educate patients diagnosed with malignant melanomas.

Methods

On May 23, 2017, a systematic search of Facebook in the groups and pages categories was performed using the word "melanoma." Groups and pages found in the search but were unrelated to malignant melanoma were excluded from this study. By default, Facebook provides search results by most relevant and the first 50 pages and 50 groups sorted by this method in the search results were selected for analysis in this study. The following information for each page was collected and analyzed: page name, category, verification status, number of likes, number of followers, visitor posts per week, page posts per week, ability to donate, date of inception, and for-profit or nonprofit. For each group, the following information was collected and analyzed: group name, category, number of members, and privacy setting.

Facebook pages and groups have categories identified by the relevant administers that define the main purpose of the page or group. The verification status of a page is determined by Facebook to let users know the page is authentic for a given public figure, organization, or brand. The "like" feature allows users to receive updates about a page and, if a user "likes" a page, this is displayed to their Facebook friends on their home page. The "follow" feature allows users to only receive updates from a page. The visitor posts used in this study were the posts designated under the visitor section on the Facebook pages analyzed between April 19, 2017 and April 26, 2017. The number of page posts defined in this study was the number of posts created by the page in the week of April 19, 2017and April 26, 2017. The "ability to donate" is a feature of a page that allows users to send money to the organization that created the page. The date of inception (defined as the date of inception of the organization if the page is representing an organization, or the date of inception of a page in the absence of an organization) and the type of organization (for-profit vs nonprofit) was determined by the start date and information listed on the pages' "About" sections. For the groups found in the search and analyzed, information about the number of members, privacy setting (either public or closed), and type of group was collected.

Results

Our search returned a total of 669 Facebook pages and 568 Facebook groups related to malignant melanomas. The first 50 pages had a combined total of 266,709 likes and 257,183 followers. Other features of the pages were analyzed, and Table 1 summarizes the general characteristics of the Facebook pages in this study. Of the 50 pages used in the study, 15 were verified by Facebook, 14 pages had the ability to donate feature enabled, and when the organization type was analyzed, it was found that there were 8 for-profit and 23 nonprofit pages, while the remaining 19 did not specify. For each page, the average number of visitor posts per week was 0.48 and the average number of posts by the page per week was 5.6. The categories of the pages (N=50) were classified as follows: personal blogs (n=4), community (n=12), health and wellness (n=3), nonprofit (n=11), charity organizations (n=5), medical research centers (n=2), legal companies (n=2), medical and health (n=2), medical center (n=1), mental health service (n=1), hospital (n=1), event (n=1), public figure (n=1), cause or awareness (n=1), health care administrator (n=1), organization (n=1), and medical company (n=1).

Of the 50 groups analyzed, 18 were public and 32 were private (closed) and the combined number of group members across all 50 groups was 23,047. The groups were classified according to type as follows (N=50): support (n=26), awareness (n=6), fundraising (n=6), personal blog (n=4), advocacy (n=1), and not listed (n=7).

Table 1. Number and Percentage of Characteristics of Melanoma Facebook Pages (N=50).

Characteristic	n (%)
Category	
Personal blog	4 (8%)
Community	12 (24%)
Health and Wellness Website	3 (6%)
Nonprofit	11 (22%)
Charity Organization	5 (10%)
Medical Research Center	2 (4%)
Legal Company	2 (4%)
Medical & Health	2 (4%)
Other	9 (18%)
Verification Status	
Verified	15 (30%)
Not-verified	35 (70%)
For-profit or nonprofit	
For-profit	8 (16%)
Nonprofit	23 (46%)
Unspecified	19 (38%)
Ability to Donate	
Yes	14 (28%)
No	36 (72%)

Discussion

With an increasing proportion of the population relying on social media for health information, it is necessary to understand how social networking websites are used for health information and communication. In this study, we found that there are over 600 pages and 500 groups on Facebook related to melanoma. There were a variety of different categories of Facebook pages, with community and nonprofit organizations being the most common, and these pages have an average of 5.6 posts per week. Since every like on a page suggests a visitor to that page, and since a user's Facebook friends will then see that the page was liked in their own feed, the 266,709 likes observed from the first 50 pages suggests that many people viewed these melanoma pages and that health care providers and organizations can potentially utilize Facebook pages to provide educational materials for a wider audience. The Center for Disease Control and Prevention estimates that comprehensive prevention programs could reduce the number of melanoma cases by nearly 230,000 and cut costs for melanoma treatment by US $ 2.7 billion over a 10-year period [13]. Facebook pages can also serve as a tool for patient empowerment and allow for communication with physicians and other patients. Given the high volume of posts, it is imperative that the information provided is accurate and aligns with the advice of medical professionals. One method to prevent false information could be to have page administrators consult dermatologists or have dermatology departments create Facebook pages to educate patients.

In addition to providing health information, Facebook is a source of support for patients. Online communities have been shown to provide patients with a safe space to discuss sensitive topics [14]. In our study, we found that 52% (26/50) of melanoma Facebook groups were formed primarily for support. Groups not only contribute to social support, but informational, emotional, and esteem support [3]. Melanoma patients can suffer from anxiety, social withdrawal, and denial [15] and online support groups could be therapeutic. Of the groups analyzed, 64% (32/50) were closed (private), allowing users to have a private space to communicate about their health. In addition to emotional support, Facebook groups are also used for awareness, fundraising, and personal blogs. Facebook groups are therefore s another avenue for unregulated health care information to be provided over the internet. The inclusion of dermatologists in Facebook groups may be beneficial to ensure there is no misleading or incorrect information provided within the group. One limitation of our study is the small sample size of groups and pages, selection bias, and lack of information regarding the nature of posts in each page.

Future studies should examine more closely how patients are able to interact in these platforms and their experience with Facebook groups and pages.

References

1. Cohen RA, Adams PF. Use of the internet for health information: United States, 2009. NCHS Data Brief 2011 Jul(66):1-8 [FREE Full text] [Medline: 22142942]
2. Cline RJ, Haynes KM. Consumer health information seeking on the Internet: the state of the art. Health Educ Res 2001 Dec;16(6):671-692 [FREE Full text] [Medline: 11780707]
3. Greene JA, Choudhry NK, Kilabuk E, Shrank WH. Online social networking by patients with diabetes: a qualitative evaluation of communication with Facebook. J Gen Intern Med 2011 Mar;26(3):287-292 [FREE Full text] [doi: 10.1007/s11606-010-1526-3] [Medline: 20945113]
4. Diaz JA, Griffith RA, Ng JJ, Reinert SE, Friedmann PD, Moulton AW. Patients' use of the Internet for medical information. J Gen Intern Med 2002 Mar;17(3):180-185 [FREE Full text] [Medline: 11929503]
5. Chou WS, Hunt YM, Beckjord EB, Moser RP, Hesse BW. Social media use in the United States: implications for health communication. J Med Internet Res 2009;11(4):e48 [FREE Full text] [doi: 10.2196/jmir.1249] [Medline: 19945947]
6. Moorhead SA, Hazlett DE, Harrison L, Carroll JK, Irwin A, Hoving C. A new dimension of health care: systematic review of the uses, benefits, and limitations of social media for health communication. J Med Internet Res 2013;15(4):e85 [FREE Full text] [doi: 10.2196/jmir.1933] [Medline: 23615206]
7. Amir M, Sampson BP, Endly D, Tamai JM, Henley J, Brewer AC, et al. Social networking sites: emerging and essential tools for communication in dermatology. JAMA Dermatol 2014 Jan;150(1):56-60. [doi: 10.1001/jamadermatol.2013.6340] [Medline: 24196212]
8. Elkarim GA, Alotaibi NM, Samuel N, Wang S, Ibrahim GM, Fallah A, et al. Social media networking in pediatric hydrocephalus: a point-prevalence analysis of utilization. J Neurosurg Pediatr 2017 May 26:1-6. [doi: 10.3171/2017.3.PEDS16552] [Medline: 28548615]
9. Abedin T, Al MM, Lasker MAA, Ahmed SW, Shommu N, Rumana N, et al. Social Media as a Platform for Information About Diabetes Foot Care: A Study of Facebook Groups. Can J Diabetes 2017 Feb;41(1):97-101. [doi: 10.1016/j.jcjd.2016.08.217] [Medline: 28126155]
10. Facebook. 2017. Pages URL: https://www.facebook.com/help/282489752085908/?helpref=hc_fnav[WebCite Cache ID 6zCT1EHK4]
11. Karimkhani C, Green AC, Nijsten T, Weinstock MA, Dellavalle RP, Naghavi M, et al. The global burden of melanoma: results from the Global Burden of Disease Study 2015. Br J Dermatol 2017 Mar 30. [doi: 10.1111/bjd.15510] [Medline: 28369739]
12. Leiter U, Garbe C. Epidemiology of melanoma and nonmelanoma skin cancer--the role of sunlight. Adv Exp Med Biol 2008;624:89-103. [doi: 10.1007/978-0-387-77574-6_8] [Medline: 18348450]
13. Guy GP, Thomas CC, Thompson T, Watson M, Massetti GM, Richardson LC, Centers for Disease ControlPrevention (CDC). Vital signs: melanoma incidence and mortality trends and projections - United States, 1982-2030. MMWR Morb Mortal Wkly Rep 2015 Jun 05;64(21):591-596 [FREE Full text] [Medline: 26042651]
14. Bender JL, Jimenez-Marroquin M, Jadad AR. Seeking support on facebook: a content analysis of breast cancer groups. J Med Internet Res 2011;13(1):e16 [FREE Full text] [doi: 10.2196/jmir.1560] [Medline: 21371990]
15. Söllner W, Gross R, Maislinger S. Psychotherapeutic interventions in melanoma patients. Recent Results Cancer Res 2002;160:362-369. [Medline: 12079235]

2

Facebook Intervention for Young-Onset Melanoma Patients and their Family Members

Elliot J Coups[1,2], PhD; Sharon L Manne[1,2], PhD; Sherry L Pagoto[3], PhD; Kevin R Criswell[1], PhD; James S Goydos[1,4], MD

[1]Rutgers Cancer Institute of New Jersey, Rutgers, The State University of New Jersey, New Brunswick, NJ, United States

[2]Department of Medicine, Rutgers Robert Wood Johnson Medical School, Rutgers, The State University of New Jersey, New Brunswick, NJ, United States

[3]Department of Allied Health Sciences, College of Agriculture, Health and Natural Resources, University of Connecticut, Storrs, CT, United States

[4]Department of Surgery, Rutgers Robert Wood Johnson Medical School, Rutgers, The State University of New Jersey, New Brunswick, NJ, United States

Corresponding Author:
Elliot J Coups, PhD
Rutgers Cancer Institute of New Jersey
Rutgers, The State University of New Jersey
195 Little Albany Street
New Brunswick, NJ, 08903
United States

Email: coupsej@cinj.rutgers.edu

Abstract

Background: Despite their elevated melanoma risk, young-onset melanoma patients and their families exhibit low rates of engagement in skin cancer surveillance and sun protection behaviors. Interventions that improve skin cancer surveillance (total cutaneous exam [TCE] and skin self-exam [SSE]) and prevention (sun protection) practices among young-onset patients and their family members would likely have an impact on skin cancer morbidity and mortality; however, such interventions are lacking.

Objective: The objective of our study was to examine the development, feasibility, and preliminary impact of a family-focused Facebook intervention to increase engagement in TCE, SSE, and sun protection among young-onset melanoma patients and their families.

Methods: In this study, 48 young-onset melanoma patients and their 40 family members completed measures of knowledge; beliefs; and TCE, SSE, and sun protection intentions before and 1 month after participating in 1 of 5 separate "secret" (ie, private) Facebook groups. The intervention content consisted of daily postings about skin cancer, skin cancer risk factors, TCE, SSE, and sun protection.

Results: Patient and family member participation rates differed by recruitment setting, with acceptance rates ranging from 24.6% to 39.0% among families recruited from a cancer center setting and from 12.7% to 61.5% among families recruited from a state registry. Among the 5 consecutive groups conducted, engagement, as measured by comments and likes in response to postings, increased across the groups. In addition, participants positively evaluated the intervention content and approach. Preliminary analyses indicated increases in TCE, SSE, and sun protection intentions.

Conclusions: Our family-focused Facebook intervention showed promise as a potentially feasible and efficacious method to increase sun protection and skin cancer surveillance among individuals at increased risk for melanoma.

KEYWORDS

young adults with melanoma; family interventions; sun protection; skin surveillance; skin examination; social media; Facebook

Introduction

The incidence of young-onset melanoma, defined as a diagnosis of melanoma before the age of 40, is increasing; the risk of developing melanoma is more than 6 times higher among young adults than it was 40 years ago [1]. Melanoma is the most common malignancy occurring among young adults aged 25-29 years and the second most common malignancy among persons aged 15-29 years [2]. Having a first-degree relative with melanoma more than doubles a person's melanoma risk, which can be attributed to genetics as well as shared environmental factors [3]. Furthermore, spouses or partners of melanoma patients are at increased risk for melanoma [4], which may be due to shared environmental or phenotypic risk factors. Thus, the population of family members at an elevated risk for melanoma is growing in tandem with the increase in the patient population.

Melanoma risk is known to be associated with the magnitude of ultraviolet radiation exposure [5-7]. The American Cancer Society and other agencies (eg, Skin Cancer Foundation) recommend prevention by avoiding exposure to ultraviolet light during peak exposure hours and recommend using sunscreen and sun-protective clothing. The American Cancer Society also recommends regular surveillance for adults, including total cutaneous exams (TCEs) by a health care provider and comprehensive skin self-exams (SSEs). TCE is a cost-effective and safe procedure that facilitates the identification of thinner lesions that can be treated more successfully than thicker ones [8,9]. Comprehensive SSE confers up to a 63% reduction in melanoma risk [10]. Reportedly, 40%-45% of diagnosed melanomas are initially detected by patients incidentally or while conducting a deliberate SSE [11]. Adherence to TCE and SSE is likely to reduce the cancer burden as well as the incidence of malignant melanomas diagnosed at advanced stages, particularly among populations at an elevated risk.

The US Preventive Services Task Force states that there is insufficient evidence to recommend regular TCE and SSE for the general population of average-risk adults. However, professional and preventive services groups recommend routine screening for higher-risk persons who have an first-degree relative with melanoma [2,12]. It is recommended that these at-risk family members should engage in regular sun protection and undergo routine TCEs and SSEs [2,12].

Despite their elevated melanoma risk, engagement in TCE, SSE, and sun protection is low among first-degree relatives of melanoma patients. Between 47% and 59% of first-degree relatives report ever having a TCE [13-15], and about one-third of first-degree relatives have not conducted an SSE in the past year [10,14-16]. Reportedly, engagement in regular sun protection ranges from 20% to 59% [13-15]. The limited work conducted to date has indicated that engagement in TCE, SSE, and sun protection is similarly low among first-degree relatives of young-onset melanoma patients (Manne, unpublished data).

Moreover, young-onset melanoma survivors are at a higher relative risk for a second malignancy than adults diagnosed with cancer who are over 39 years of age [17]. The cumulative incidence of secondary malignancies rises faster over time for young adult survivors than for childhood and older adult survivors [17]. Follow-up guidelines for melanoma patients recommend that they reduce their risk for secondary malignancies by receiving a periodic TCE, conducting a regular SSE, and engaging in regular sun avoidance and protection [18,19]. Although most melanoma patients receive a periodic TCE [20-22], only 14%-39% of patients conduct a thorough SSE on a regular basis [8,9,23,24]. Prior research has indicated that engagement in recommended TCE is very high among young-onset melanoma patients (Manne, unpublished). Only 59% of young-onset melanoma patients have reported engaging in SSE in the past year (Manne, unpublished). Even among those reporting a skin exam, comprehensiveness of self-exams is low (eg, 42% examine their feet, 29% examine their scalp; Manne, unpublished). Furthermore, engagement in regular sun protection is low (Manne, unpublished).

Young-onset melanoma patients and their family members are a growing and unique cancer population who are at elevated skin cancer risk. Effective interventions to improve their surveillance and prevention practices will likely have an impact on skin cancer morbidity and mortality. Prior behavioral interventions for melanoma patients and their family members have primarily been delivered in person or via individual print or telephone counseling [25,26]. Few of these interventions have targeted both patients and their family members. For example, Bowen et al [27] found that a Web-based family communication intervention improved skin surveillance and sun protection behaviors among melanoma patients and their family members compared with that among a wait-list control group. In another study, melanoma patients and their family members reported greater engagement in SSE behaviors after receiving a dyadic compared with a solo learning intervention [28].

An intervention that is delivered via a social media modality offers some advantages over other intervention modalities. One advantage is the high reach. Young adults are high users of Facebook [29]. Second, social media platforms allow users to interact with one another and create their own content. Closed social media platforms such as secret Facebook groups allow for the formation of a group environment where patients can engage with other patients who have undergone similar experiences, family members can interact with the families of other patients, and everyone can view all postings. This engagement may facilitate group support for behavior change and promote the setting of social norms and expectations for practices and attitudes. Normative influences drive attitudinal change and play a role in sun protection and SSE for individuals at increased risk for melanoma, including individuals with a personal or family history of melanoma [15,30]. Third, social media allows health care providers to interact with participants. For example, cutaneous oncologists can address questions about skin cancer that are viewed by all members of the group. Finally, social media modalities provide a less expensive way to disseminate information and skills [31]. Because of these advantages, social media modalities such as Facebook have been incorporated as a component of behavioral interventions to reduce tobacco use [32], improve physical activity [33,34], and enhance weight loss [35]. To date, there have been few stand-alone Facebook interventions [36].

This study reports on the development and acceptability of a family-focused Facebook intervention for young-onset melanoma patients and their family members. Young-onset survivors face unique challenges and have unique needs and preferences. They manage survivorship recommendations at a time when they manage other life tasks such as choosing life partners, starting or finishing new educational or occupational pursuits, and starting or caring for their own families [37,38]. In addition, their family members are likely younger than those of patients diagnosed at an older age and, therefore, may face similar challenges in engaging in skin cancer risk-reducing behaviors. This study had two aims. The first aim was to evaluate the feasibility of the intervention, which was measured by recruitment rates, participation in the Facebook groups, retention, and acceptability. The second aim was to provide a preliminary examination of the impact of the intervention on knowledge; beliefs (family perceptions and support, sun protection benefits and barriers, SSE benefits and barriers, and norms); and sun protection, SSE, and TCE intentions.

Methods

Procedure

Patients were recruited from the Rutgers Cancer Institute of New Jersey (CINJ) and via referral from the New Jersey State Cancer Registry (NJSCR). At CINJ, potentially eligible patients were identified by reviewing outpatient medical appointments and electronic medical records. Patients were either approached in the clinic area or sent a letter about the study, along with an informed consent form and postage-paid return envelope. The patients who were sent a letter were telephoned by a member of the research team. For the NJSCR, potentially eligible patients were identified through a case review of pathology reports and other surveillance records. Each patient's treating physician of record was contacted by a staff member from the NJSCR to ensure that the patient could be contacted. Physicians had 2 weeks to respond, after which an NJSCR staff member contacted patients via letters and telephone to obtain permission to share their contact information with the research team at CINJ. Patients who provided permission were mailed a letter about the study, along with the informed consent form and a postage-paid return envelope. They were then contacted via telephone to determine their eligibility and interest in the study. Eligible and interested patients were asked to provide the name and contact information of a spouse or partner and one or more first-degree relatives. These family members were recruited using the same procedures as outlined above for patients. All participants provided informed consent either by completing a hard-copy consent form or electronically using a secure Web-based form.

After providing informed consent, participants completed a Web-based or pencil and paper baseline survey that included questions on demographic factors; Facebook use; and skin cancer-related knowledge, beliefs, and behavioral intentions. Participants were then invited to join a study-specific "secret" Facebook group. A secret group on Facebook can only be viewed by invited individuals, and the name and existence of the group are not publicly disclosed on Facebook. Furthermore, posts to secret Facebook groups cannot be shared on Facebook outside of the group members.

Participants

Participants were melanoma patients and their family members (ie, spouses or partners, siblings, parents, and children). The eligibility criteria for patients were as follows: those diagnosed with melanoma within the past 5 years; diagnosed with stage 0-III melanoma between the ages of 18 and 45 years; not currently on active treatment for melanoma or any others cancer; able to speak and read English; with access to a computer with internet access and familiarity with social media platforms; with a spouse, partner, or first-degree relative(s) eligible and willing to participate in the study; and able to give meaningful informed consent. For family members, the eligibility criteria were as follows: those aged 18-89 years; able to speak and read English; with access to a computer with internet access and familiarity with social media platforms; and able to give meaningful informed consent.

Survey Measures

A copy of the survey is available in Multimedia Appendix 1.

Demographics and Facebook Use (Assessed at Baseline Only)

Participants reported their sex, age, and highest level of education. They also indicated the number of Facebook friends they have and the amount of time per day they spend on Facebook.

Knowledge and Beliefs (Assessed at Baseline and Follow-Up)

Knowledge about skin cancer risk factors was assessed using 13 true or false items drawn from prior research [15]. A total knowledge score was obtained by summing the number of correct responses for each participant. Family perceptions about skin cancer risk, sun protection, and SSE [15,39] is a 9-item measure assessing perceived benefits of sun protection and SSE to one's family as well as discussions with family about these topics (Cronbach alpha=.92 and .94 for the baseline and follow-up surveys, respectively). The family support measure was developed for this study; its 4 items measured the degree to which the participants supported their family members engaging in regular sun protection and regular SSE as well as how important it is that their family members engage in these behaviors (Cronbach alpha=.92 and .95, respectively). An 8-item measure assessed the benefits of sun protection (sunscreen, sun-protective clothing; Cronbach alpha=.84 and .82, respectively) [15]. A 15-item measure assessed perceived barriers to using sunscreen (Cronbach alpha=.87 and .83, respectively), and an 11-item measure assessed barriers to wearing sun-protective clothing (Cronbach alpha=.86 and .89, respectively) [40]. An 8-item measure assessed SSE benefits (Cronbach alpha=.79 and .87, respectively) [15], and an 11-item measure assessed barriers to SSE (Cronbach alpha=.76 and .80, respectively) [15]. Tanning norms (5 items) measured family and friends' sunbathing practices (Cronbach alpha=.74 and .72, respectively). Sun protection norms (7 items) measured family and friends' sun protection practices and attitudes (Cronbach alpha=.83 and .71, respectively). Furthermore, image norms for tanness (5 items) assessed participants' beliefs about societal beliefs regarding the importance of tanned appearance for celebrities and society (Cronbach alpha=.67 and .56, respectively) [41].

Behavioral Intentions (Assessed at Baseline and Follow-Up)

Sun protection intentions were assessed by averaging responses to 8 items (Cronbach alpha=.85 and .86 at baseline and follow-up, respectively) [42]. SSE intentions were assessed by averaging responses to 2 items (Cronbach alpha=.98 and .92, respectively) [42], and a single item was used to assess TCE intentions [42]. Furthermore, the measure of TCE intentions was only included in the final 2 Facebook groups.

Evaluations of the Facebook Groups (Assessed Immediately After Group Completion)

Drawing on prior research [42-44] and items developed for this project, 20 items assessed participants' evaluations in each Facebook group. Each item utilized a 7-point response scale. We created 3 subscales: evaluation of the content (7 items, Cronbach alpha=.92; eg, "The information I received was interesting"); helped prepare participants to discuss sun protection and exams with one's family (5 items, Cronbach alpha=.97; eg, "After participating in the group and viewing posts, I feel more prepared to talk to my family about engaging in regular sun protection, skin self-exams, and exams by a doctor"); and the overall Facebook experience (8 items, Cronbach alpha=.93; eg, "I felt comfortable participating in the discussions that we had on the Facebook group"). Correlations among the 3 subscales varied from r=.56 to r=.81. Additionally, we used open-ended questions to solicit additional feedback.

Overview of the Facebook Groups

We conducted 5 separate secret Facebook groups. After each group, the team met to decide upon changes to be made to content based on the information garnered from debriefing interviews with participants. An overview of the characteristics of the 5 groups is shown in Table 1. For each group, the research team posted approximately two times per day on average (typically morning and late afternoon), including weekends. The posts focused on the following broad topics: skin cancer risks, sun protection, SSE, and TCE. Additionally, the content of the posts was informed by the Preventive Health Model [45] and the Theory of Normative Social Behavior [46,47]. For example, posts focused on skin cancer knowledge, benefits and barriers to behavior change, goal setting, family support, and normative beliefs. As outlined later, some variation existed in the content and order of posts across the Facebook groups. In general, posts included a small amount of text content, typically accompanied by a photograph or graphic image. Some posts asked participants to respond to a poll, complete a quiz, or provide a viewpoint or answer to a question by commenting on the post. Example Facebook posts are shown in Figure 1 (a welcome message) and Figure 2 (a family support and engagement message).

For all Facebook groups, participants were asked to complete a Web-based, paper and pencil, or telephone Facebook evaluation survey immediately after the end of the group. The evaluation survey was completed by 76% (67/88) of the participants. In addition, participants were invited to complete a semistructured telephone interview at the end of the group that solicited feedback on study procedures and the content of the Facebook groups. For participants who had previously completed the Facebook evaluation survey, the interview provided them with an opportunity to expand on their survey responses. The number of individuals completing a semistructured interview for each group was as follows: group 1, n=4; group 2, n=8; group 3, n=5; group 4, n=19; group 5, n=17 (overall completion rate=53/88, 60%). Results of the Facebook evaluation surveys and semistructured interviews were reviewed by research team members and used to inform the content and approach of subsequent groups. Participants in groups 2-5 were asked to complete a follow-up Web-based or pencil and paper survey 1 month after the end of the group that included the questions on skin cancer-related knowledge, beliefs, and behavioral intentions from the baseline survey (overall completion rate=65/80, 81%). Furthermore, participants received a US $50 gift card for completing each of the baseline and follow-up surveys (but did not receive compensation for completing the Facebook evaluation survey or the telephone interview). This study was approved by the Rutgers Health Sciences Institutional Review Board.

Table 1. Characteristics of the Facebook groups.

Group number	Date of group	Length of group (days)	Posts (n)	Patients in the group (n)	Family members in the group (n)	Total group members (N)
1	May 2016	15	31	2	6	8
2	July-August 2016	28	53	7	4	11
3	November-December 2016	29	56	4	6	10
4	January-February 2016	28	54	14	10	24
5	June-July 2017	28	55	21	14	35

Figure 1. Example Facebook post 1. Photograph from Getty Images; credit: andres; creative #: 489039170; licensed under fair use.

Hi everyone! Welcome to the Young Melanoma Family Facebook Group. This group, which will last for one month, is made up of 21 young people who have been diagnosed with melanoma as well as 12 of their family members. In this Facebook group, we encourage participation in the form of comments and "likes" so that we can make this a great group experience for everyone! Even brief comments ("I agree!" or "I am not sure about that…") are encouraged!

Tell us a little about yourself or your family.

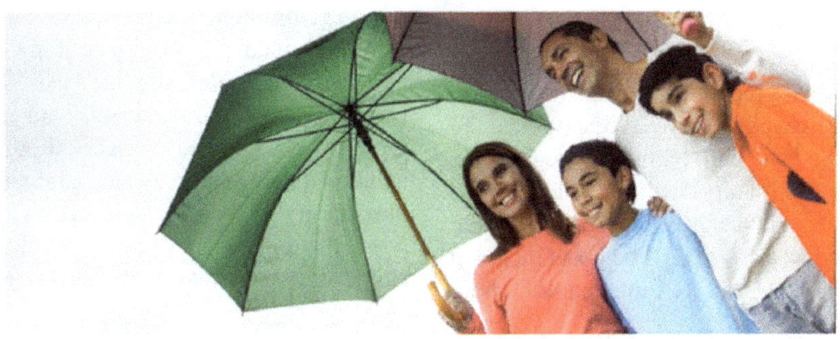

Figure 2. Example Facebook post 2.

We have brothers, sisters, and parents as well as people with skin cancer in this group. I know that families can really help one another with sun protection habits. For example, my mom has had skin cancer, and before we go to the car, I remind her to get her sunglasses.

What ways can you support your family members who are in this group with their sun protection goals?

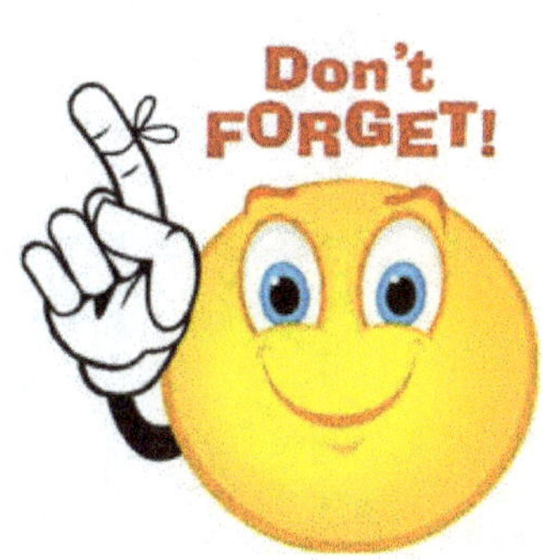

Facebook Group 1

For this group, participants received a 1-page handout in the mail after completing the baseline survey. As shown in Figure 3, the handout welcomed individuals to the program, described the goals of the program, and gave brief advice on how to reduce risk for skin cancer. There was no specific order to the Facebook posts, and the moderator only posted content but did not reply or engage in any conversation with participants in the group. The posts focused primarily on skin cancer risks and sun protection, with only 2 messages on SSE and 1 message on TCE. Several posts were memes or links to external sites. Changes suggested by one or more participants included the following: (1) organize messages by weekly topics; (2) increase the duration of the group to provide more content; (3) increase interactivity (eg, quizzes); (4) drop memes; and (5) use personal narratives.

Facebook Group 2

For this group, participants again received a 1-page handout in the mail after completing the baseline survey; we extended the length of the group to 28 days and included moderator's comments on most posts. Additionally, we grouped the posts into weekly topics: week 1, skin cancer risks; week 2, sun protection; week 3, SSE; and week 4, TCE. The posts included quizzes, personal narratives, polls, tailored information about the group's beliefs and behaviors (based on data from the baseline survey), and also addressed family influences. Several "ask the doctor" posts with prepared questions and answers were posted on behalf of a medical oncologist. Changes suggested by one or more participants included the following: (1) include information on planning behavior change; (2) provide alternate ways to consider barriers; (3) include more information on benefits; (4) include more pictures with posts; (5) reduce the length of posts; (6) add more discussion questions, and; (7) include more interaction with a medical oncologist.

Facebook Group 3

For this group and the subsequent groups, we removed the mailed 1-page handout. Posts for Facebook group 3 were revised to address the changes suggested by group 2 participants. For example, posts encouraged participants to develop behavior change goals and to identify potential barriers and solutions. In addition, a medical oncologist joined the group and answered questions on a more regular basis. Furthermore, more posts were made by moderators, and they encouraged group participation. Changes suggested by one or more participants included the following: (1) have larger groups to promote group interaction; (2) include more information about the dangers of indoor tanning; (3) increase the number of posts targeting young adults; and (4) include recent news or research about skin cancer.

Figure 3. Handout mailed to participants in Facebook groups 1 and 2.

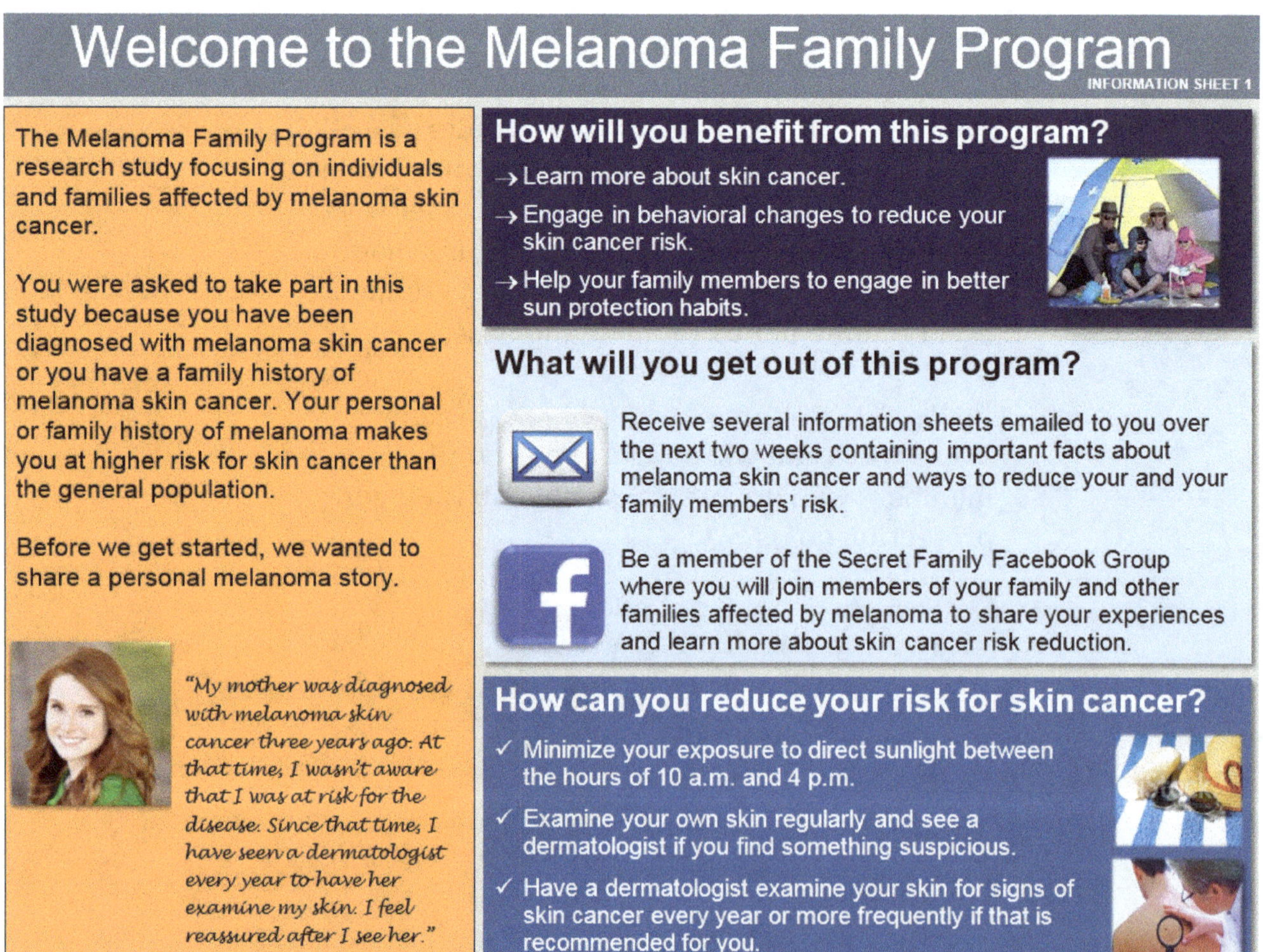

Facebook Group 4

The primary change for this group was to increase the number of group members to 24. Additionally, posts were revised to focus more on indoor tanning, young adults, and skin cancer-related news and research. Participants provided positive feedback about the group, with the primary suggestion being to have an even larger group.

Facebook Group 5

This group utilized the same posts and approach for group 4 but with a larger group of 35 individuals. Again, participants were enthusiastic about the group, suggested more encouragement of group support, and suggested a larger group size.

Results

Sample Characteristics

As detailed below, a total of 88 individuals (48 melanoma patients and 40 family members) participated across 5 separate Facebook groups. The demographic characteristics of the study sample are shown in Table 2. Among the 40 family members, 8 were the spouse or partner of the patient, 1 was the child, 19 were the sibling, and 12 were the parents. Among both patients and family members, the proportion of female participants was markedly higher than that of male participants. In part, this may be due to the higher rate of melanoma among young adult women than among men. The sample exhibited a relatively high level of education, with more than three-quarters of participants (71/88, 81%) reporting completing college or a graduate degree. Patients reported having a greater number of Facebook friends than their family members (P=.01), but the 2 groups did not differ with regard to the amount of time per week spent on Facebook (P=.81).

Acceptability

Enrollment

At CINJ, a total of 64 patients were approached for the study. Of them, 7 were ineligible and 40 declined to participate (either actively or passively); 17 patients consented and completed the baseline survey (consent rate=17/57, 30%) and 14 joined a Facebook group (overall Facebook joining rate=14/57, 25%). The 17 recruited patients provided contact information for a total of 44 spouses or partners and first-degree relatives. Of those 44 individuals, 3 were ineligible, 23 declined participation, 18 consented and completed the baseline survey (consent rate=18/41, 44%), and 16 joined a Facebook group (overall Facebook joining rate=16/41, 39%).

The staff of the NJSCR approached 292 patients regarding the study, 23 of whom were ineligible and 203 declined to provide permission to be contacted by the CINJ research team. Among 66 patients who gave permission to be contacted by the CINJ research team, 2 patients were ineligible, 27 declined to participate, 37 completed Web-based consent and the baseline survey (consent rate=37/267, 13.9%), and 34 joined a Facebook group (overall Facebook joining rate=34/267, 12.7%). The 37 recruited patients provided contact information for a total of 40 spouses or partners and first-degree relatives. Of those 40 individuals, 1 was ineligible, 11 declined participation, 28 completed Web-based consent and the baseline survey (consent rate=28/39, 72%), and 24 joined a Facebook group (overall Facebook joining rate=24/39, 62%).

Retention

Completion of the follow-up survey varied from 60% (6/10 for group 3) to 85% (50/59 for groups 4 and 5 combined).

Engagement

The engagement characteristics of the Facebook groups are shown in Multimedia Appendix 2. On average, participants viewed 66%-83% of posts. The average number of likes and comments per post was higher for groups 4 and 5, even after taking into account the higher number of participants in those groups and higher number of moderator posts in the latter groups. Furthermore, Multimedia Appendix 2 illustrates that the percentage of participants who liked and commented on 25% of the posts increased over the 5 subsequent groups. As outlined earlier, we increased the number of posts across each subsequent Facebook group.

Evaluation

The descriptive statistics for participants' evaluations of each Facebook group are shown in Table 3. Mean ratings of the intervention content in Facebook group 1 were relatively low compared with those in the subsequent groups. In groups 2-5, there were positive evaluations across the evaluation subscales, particularly with regard to the intervention content and feeling more prepared to discuss relevant issues with family members.

Comments made during the debriefing interview included input about the delivery method ("Facebook is a good medium for what you are doing"), content that was well liked ("I liked the Ask the Expert posts," "I liked the Mole Map," "I liked when we shared our personal stories"), impact on behavior ("I enjoyed information about sunscreen. I never used it before, and now I am more conscious," "I am going to see a dermatologist," "I need to ask my doctor to do a more thorough exam of my skin"), and how the material impacted discussions with family (eg, "I shared the posts with my children," "My mom talked to me about the posts"). Some participants commented that they wished there be more group discussion.

Changes in Outcomes From the Baseline to the Follow-Up

Changes in the outcomes from the baseline to the follow-up are shown in Table 4, which includes mean changes and their respective 95% CIs. Owing to the small sample sizes, we did not conduct formal inferential statistics. We provided CIs to provide a preliminary indication of potential effects. We conducted analyses separately for groups 2 and 3 due to the substantive differences between the messages and approach utilized in these groups. We analyzed results combined for groups 4 and 5 due to the strong similarity between their messages, approach, and sample sizes and to reduce the CI widths. There was some indication that knowledge scores improved across some groups, as did family perceptions and sun protection benefits. Counter to expectations, barriers to using sunscreen and sun-protective clothing were higher in several groups at follow-up compared with those at baseline. There was some indication that SSE benefits increased over time, but evidence was inconsistent with regard to changes in SSE barriers. Moreover, results were inconsistent with regard to changes in norms across the groups. Encouragingly, the most consistent beneficial effects were observed for behavioral intentions, particularly with regard to groups 4 and 5. For these groups, each of the CIs excluded zero and indicated increases in sun protection, SSE, and TCE intentions from baseline to follow-up.

Table 2. Demographic characteristics of the study sample (N=88).

Chacteristic	Patients (n=48)	Family members (n=40)
Recruitment site, n (%)		
Rutgers Cancer Institute of New Jersey	14 (29)	16 (40)
New Jersey State Cancer Registry	34 (71)	24 (60)
Relation to patient, n (%)		
Spouse or partner	—[a]	8 (20)
Daughter	—	1 (3)
Son	—	0 (0)
Sister	—	12 (30)
Brother	—	7 (18)
Mother	—	8 (20)
Father	—	4 (10)
Sex, n (%)		
Female	42 (88)	26 (65)
Male	6 (13)	14 (35)
Age (years), mean (SD)	34.5 (6.4)	39.5 (13.2)
18-25, n (%)	7 (15)	7 (18)
26-35, n (%)	17 (35)	10 (25)
36-45, n (%)	24 (50)	8 (20)
46-55, n (%)	0 (0)	8 (20)
≥56, n (%)	0 (0)	7 (18)
Education level, n (%)		
≤High school or General Educational Development	5 (10)	4 (10)
Some college	3 (6)	5 (13)
College graduate	27 (56)	19 (48)
Graduate degree	13 (27)	12 (30)
Number of Facebook friends, n (%)		
≤100	5 (11)	15 (40)
101-200	7 (15)	5 (13)
201-300	12 (26)	4 (11)
301-400	8 (17)	14 (37)
>400	15 (32)	0 (0)
Minutes per day of Facebook use, n (%)		
<10	8 (17)	5 (13)
10-60	18 (38)	18 (47)
61-120	10 (21)	6 (16)
>120	11 (23)	9 (24)

Table 3. Participants' evaluations of each Facebook group.

Variable[a]	Group 1 (n=6), mean (SD)	Group 2 (n=9), mean (SD)	Group 3 (n=7), mean (SD)	Group 4 (n=19), mean (SD)	Group 5 (n=26), mean (SD)	All groups, mean (SD)
Evaluation of content	4.86 (1.68)	6.19 (1.05)	6.31 (0.79)	5.66 (1.37)	6.21 (0.71)	5.94 (1.14)
Helped prepare me	3.56 (1.46)	6.37 (1.32)	6.16 (1.08)	5.05 (1.72)	6.14 (0.93)	5.63 (1.52)
Facebook experience	—[b]	—	5.25 (1.16)	5.45 (1.55)	5.87 (0.99)	5.63 (1.25)
Overall, mean (SD)	4.43 (1.53)	6.25 (1.13)	5.84 (0.93)	5.42 (1.38)	6.06 (0.79)	5.73 (1.19)

[a]All subscales were scored on a 1-7 scale, with higher numbers reflecting more positive evaluations.

[b]Subscale questions were not asked of participants in that Facebook group.

Table 4. Mean changes in outcomes from baseline (BL) to follow-up (FU) for the Facebook groups.

Outcomes	Group 2 (n=9)			Group 3 (n=6)			Groups 4 and 5 (n=50)		
	BL	FU	Change (95% CI)	BL	FU	Change (95% CI)	BL	FU	Change (95% CI)
Knowledge	11.67	11.89	0.22 (□0.42 to 0.86)	11.50	12.17	0.67 (0.12 to 1.21)	12.00	12.04	0.04 (□0.27 to 0.35)
Family perceptions	4.43	4.49	0.06 (□0.19 to 0.32)	4.39	4.69	0.30 (□0.28 to 0.88)	4.54	4.50	□0.04 (□0.25 to 0.17)
Family support	4.72	4.72	0.00 (□0.10 to 0.10)	4.88	4.83	□0.04 (□0.30 to 0.22)	4.79	4.74	□0.06 (□0.24 to 0.13)
Sun protection benefits	4.63	4.38	□0.25 (□1.03 to 0.53)	4.48	4.63	0.14 (□0.72 to 1.01)	4.62	4.67	0.05 (□0.04 to 0.14)
Sunscreen barriers	1.73	1.92	0.18 (□0.26 to 0.63)	2.43	2.53	0.11 (□0.48 to 0.69)	2.25	2.26	0.02 (□0.16 to 0.20)
Clothing barriers	2.47	2.92	0.45 (□0.83 to 1.74)	2.55	2.91	0.36 (□0.53 to 1.26)	3.01	2.97	□0.04 (□0.22 to 0.14)
Sun protection intentions	5.64	5.69	0.05 (□0.28 to 0.37)	5.15	5.30	0.15 (□1.98 to 2.28)	4.94	5.33	0.39 (0.17 to 0.61)
SSE[a] benefits	5.47	5.42	□0.05 (□0.58 to 0.49)	5.28	5.65	0.38 (□0.04 to 0.79)	5.16	5.28	0.12 (□0.11 to 0.35)
SSE barriers	3.05	3.18	0.14 (□0.82 to 1.10)	3.13	3.18	0.05 (□0.42 to 0.52)	2.98	2.93	□0.06 (□0.22 to 0.11)
SSE intentions	6.25	6.06	□0.19 (□1.23 to 0.86)	4.90	6.00	1.10 (□1.44 to 3.64)	5.29	6.13	0.84 (0.42 to 1.26)
TCE[b] intentions	—[c]	—	—	—	—	—	6.02	6.58	0.56 (0.18 to 0.94)
Tanning norms	3.95	3.48	□0.48 (□1.00 to 0.05)	4.52	4.28	□0.24 (□1.05 to 0.57)	3.73	3.76	0.02 (□0.22 to 0.27)
Sun protection norms	3.98	3.48	□0.50 (□0.94 to □0.06)	3.29	3.77	0.49 (□0.72 to 1.69)	3.79	3.70	□0.08 (□0.31 to 0.15)
Image norms	3.44	3.33	□0.12 (□0.81 to 0.57)	3.36	3.64	0.28 (□0.52 to 1.08)	3.66	3.53	□0.13 (□0.36 to 0.10)

[a]SSE: skin self-examination.

[b]TCE: total cutaneous examination.

[c]The measure was not included for that Facebook group.

Discussion

Principal Findings

To the best of our knowledge, this is one of the first studies to evaluate a family-based skin cancer risk reduction intervention for young adults with melanoma and their relatives and the first behavioral intervention for this population delivered entirely through Facebook. Interventions delivered through social media are innovative and a promising way to reach young adults and their family members. In addition, Facebook provides a novel way to engage family members with one another, encourage young survivors to interact with other young survivors and their relatives, and facilitate engagement between families in learning and discussion about skin cancer. During the year-long development of the Facebook group methodology and its content, our team learned several lessons.

First, group engagement, as defined by participation (ie, likes and comments to original posts), improved steadily over the groups (eg, 0% of group 1 members and 9% of group 2 members commented on at least 25% of posts compared with 40% of group 5 members). Several factors may have contributed to this increase. A higher number of group members were recruited into each group over time, which may have increased the likelihood that one or more participants would post comments, find commonalities, and promote discussion. Another factor that may have increased participation was the quality of the posts. Based on the postgroup debriefing with participants and team discussion, we created posts that were briefer and designed to elicit interaction (eg, posed a question). Posts such as personal stories, goal-setting exercises, quizzes, and the opportunity to have questions answered by a cutaneous oncologist were rated as particularly engaging by group members.

The second lesson learned was that recruitment was challenging. Patient provision of relatives' contact information, reaching out to and enrolling relatives, completion of surveys, and ultimate acceptance into the Facebook group represent different steps with the potential loss of participants associated with each step. The most common point for participant loss was at the initial patient contact. Acceptance rates among patients differed by recruitment source, with a lower acceptance rate from the cancer center recruitment (at CINJ) than from the NJSCR. Family members joined the Facebook groups at higher rates than did patients. It is possible that recruitment from the cancer center provides the advantage of patient trust on the oncologist and knowledge of the institution. However, registry recruitment has the advantage of provision of greater reach into the general patient population. Another challenge was the relatively small number of relatives provided by each patient. One possible explanation is that patients stated they did not have siblings, suggesting smaller family size to be a reason.

The third lesson learned was that despite the challenges of enrollment, once enrolled, engagement was high, particularly in the latter groups. In their comments, participants shared their personal experiences with melanoma, provided each other with encouragement to undergo SSE and TCE and to engage in sun protection, asked one another for advice about sun protection products and recommendations for dermatologists who could perform exams, discussed personal barriers to sun protection and skin exams, set skin exam and sun protection goals, and posed questions for the cutaneous oncologist about melanoma and skin exams. Negative, off-topic, or unhelpful comments were not observed, although some members stated in their debriefing interviews that they did not share as much as they might have to not upset the family member who was diagnosed with cancer.

The fourth lesson learned was that evaluations of the groups, other than group 1, were positive. Participants reported that the content was informative and valid, the group prepared them to discuss skin cancer prevention with their family, and they felt comfortable sharing their experiences and connected with other group members. Given one of the key goals of this intervention was to encourage family members to support one another's skin cancer risk reduction, the fact that participants reported that the posts prompted discussions with their family members and that the group facilitated interactions with family members who were not participating in the group was encouraging.

Owing to the small sample size and the fact that outcomes were reported separately by group, it is difficult to make firm conclusions about the efficacy of the intervention. Our preliminary data suggest that there were increases in sun protection, SSE, and TCE intentions for the final 2 groups. There were generally inconsistent results with regard to improvements in the knowledge and beliefs outcomes. Definitive conclusions with regard to the efficacy of the intervention will require larger randomized clinical trials.

Limitations

Limitations of this study include low recruitment rates for patients and the small sample size. Future research is warranted to examine patients' and their family members' preferences with regard to delivery platforms for skin cancer prevention and surveillance interventions. Additionally, efforts are needed to identify strategies for maximizing participant recruitment, engagement, and retention for interventions delivered via social media and other platforms. The fact that we conducted 5 separate Facebook groups allowed the team to develop and refine the intervention in a deliberate, iterative manner based on participant engagement and feedback, which was the primary purpose of this study. The sample size in this study meant that we were not able to conduct a factor analysis of the Facebook group evaluation survey items. This should be addressed in future studies with larger sample sizes.

Conclusions

This pilot and feasibility study demonstrated that a moderated family-focused Facebook intervention for young-onset melanoma survivors and their family members is feasible and acceptable. For future similar research, we recommend Facebook group durations of at least 1 month with ≥35 participants and regular posts by moderators. Because recruitment of patients was challenging, future studies may benefit from focusing on methods of enhancing patient recruitment. Additionally, although this study provided preliminary evidence of positive changes in outcomes, particularly with regard to behavioral intentions, further research is needed with larger sample sizes to determine the statistical and practical significance of such effects and to examine behavioral outcomes.

Acknowledgments

This research was supported by institutional funds to SLM, PhD. We thank Antoinette Stroup, PhD; Lisa Paddock, PhD; and other employees of the NJSCR for their valuable help in conducting this study and Evangelynn Murphy and Sara Frederick for assistance with data collection and management.

References

1. Reed KB, Brewer JD, Lohse CM, Bringe KE, Pruitt CN, Gibson LE. Increasing incidence of melanoma among young adults: an epidemiological study in Olmsted County, Minnesota. Mayo Clin Proc 2012 Apr;87(4):328-334 [FREE Full text] [doi: 10.1016/j.mayocp.2012.01.010] [Medline: 22469345]
2. Skin Cancer Foundation (SCF). Types of Melanoma URL: https://www.skincancer.org/skin-cancer-information/melanoma/types-of-melanoma [accessed 2018-04-24] [WebCite Cache ID 6yv5umVZn]
3. Olsen CM, Carroll HJ, Whiteman DC. Familial melanoma: a meta-analysis and estimates of attributable fraction. Cancer Epidemiol Biomarkers Prev 2010 Jan;19(1):65-73 [FREE Full text] [doi: 10.1158/1055-9965.EPI-09-0928] [Medline: 20056624]

4. Frank C, Fallah M, Ji J, Sundquist J, Hemminki K. The population impact of familial cancer, a major cause of cancer. Int J Cancer 2014 Apr 15;134(8):1899-1906 [FREE Full text] [doi: 10.1002/ijc.28510] [Medline: 24590453]
5. Fears TR, Bird CC, Guerry D, Sagebiel RW, Gail MH, Elder DE, et al. Average midrange ultraviolet radiation flux and time outdoors predict melanoma risk. Cancer Res 2002 Jul 15;62(14):3992-3996 [FREE Full text] [Medline: 12124332]
6. Swerdlow AJ, Weinstock MA. Do tanning lamps cause melanoma? An epidemiologic assessment. J Am Acad Dermatol 1998 Jan;38(1):89-98. [Medline: 9448211]
7. Evans RD, Kopf AW, Lew RA, Rigel DS, Bart RS, Friedman RJ, et al. Risk factors for the development of malignant melanoma--I: Review of case-control studies. J Dermatol Surg Oncol 1988 Apr;14(4):393-408. [Medline: 3280634]
8. Aitken JF, Elwood M, Baade PD, Youl P, English D. Clinical whole-body skin examination reduces the incidence of thick melanomas. Int J Cancer 2010 Jan 15;126(2):450-458 [FREE Full text] [doi: 10.1002/ijc.24747] [Medline: 19609948]
9. Margolis MJ, De Champlain AF, Klass DJ. Setting examination-level standards for a performance-based assessment of physicians' clinical skills. Acad Med 1998 Oct;73(10 Suppl):S114-S116. [Medline: 9795671]
10. Berwick M, Begg CB, Fine JA, Roush GC, Barnhill RL. Screening for cutaneous melanoma by skin self-examination. J Natl Cancer Inst 1996 Jan 3;88(1):17-23 [FREE Full text] [Medline: 8847720]
11. Hamidi R, Cockburn MG, Peng DH. Prevalence and predictors of skin self-examination: prospects for melanoma prevention and early detection. Int J Dermatol 2008 Oct;47(10):993-1003. [doi: 10.1111/j.1365-4632.2008.03780.x] [Medline: 18986343]
12. American Cancer Society (ACS). Cancer Prevention & Early Detection Facts & Figures 2015-2016 URL: https://www.cancer.org/content/dam/cancer-org/research/cancer-facts-and-statistics/cancer-prevention-and-early-detection-facts-and-figures/cancer-prevention-and-early-detection-facts-and-figures-2015-2016.pdf [accessed 2018-04-24] [WebCite Cache ID 6yv7NUqCJ]
13. Azzarello LM, Jacobsen PB. Factors influencing participation in cutaneous screening among individuals with a family history of melanoma. J Am Acad Dermatol 2007 Mar;56(3):398-406. [doi: 10.1016/j.jaad.2006.10.024] [Medline: 17184873]
14. Geller AC, Rutsch L, Kenausis K, Selzer P, Zhang Z. Can an hour or two of sun protection education keep the sunburn away? Evaluation of the Environmental Protection Agency's Sunwise School Program. Environ Health 2003 Nov 03;2(1):13 [FREE Full text] [doi: 10.1186/1476-069X-2-13] [Medline: 14613488]
15. Manne S, Fasanella N, Connors J, Floyd B, Wang H, Lessin S. Sun protection and skin surveillance practices among relatives of patients with malignant melanoma: prevalence and predictors. Prev Med 2004 Jul;39(1):36-47. [doi: 10.1016/j.ypmed.2004.02.028] [Medline: 15207984]
16. Friedman LC, Bruce S, Webb JA, Weinberg AD, Cooper HP. Skin self-examination in a population at increased risk for skin cancer. Am J Prev Med 1993;9(6):359-364. [Medline: 8311985]
17. Lee JS, DuBois SG, Coccia PF, Bleyer A, Olin RL, Goldsby RE. Increased risk of second malignant neoplasms in adolescents and young adults with cancer. Cancer 2016 Jan 01;122(1):116-123 [FREE Full text] [doi: 10.1002/cncr.29685] [Medline: 26441212]
18. Bichakjian CK, Halpern AC, Johnson TM, Foote HA, Grichnik JM, Swetter SM, American Academy of Dermatology. Guidelines of care for the management of primary cutaneous melanoma. American Academy of Dermatology. J Am Acad Dermatol 2011 Nov;65(5):1032-1047. [doi: 10.1016/j.jaad.2011.04.031] [Medline: 21868127]
19. National Comprehensive Cancer Network (NCCN). Guidelines for patients: Melanoma URL: https://www.nccn.org/patients/guidelines/melanoma/files/assets/common/downloads/files/melanoma.pdf[WebCite Cache ID 6yvO42lFQ]
20. Bowen DJ, Hay JL, Harris-Wai JN, Meischke H, Burke W. All in the family? Communication of cancer survivors with their families. Fam Cancer 2017 Oct;16(4):597-603. [doi: 10.1007/s10689-017-9987-8] [Medline: 28374161]
21. Rodríguez VM, Berwick M, Hay JL. Communication about melanoma and risk reduction after melanoma diagnosis. Psychooncology 2017 Dec;26(12):2142-2148. [doi: 10.1002/pon.4315] [Medline: 27862570]
22. Palesh O, Aldridge-Gerry A, Bugos K, Pickham D, Chen JJ, Greco R, et al. Health behaviors and needs of melanoma survivors. Support Care Cancer 2014 Nov;22(11):2973-2980. [doi: 10.1007/s00520-014-2286-0] [Medline: 24879390]
23. Coups EJ, Manne SL, Stapleton JL, Tatum KL, Goydos JS. Skin self-examination behaviors among individuals diagnosed with melanoma. Melanoma Res 2016 Feb;26(1):71-76. [doi: 10.1097/CMR.0000000000000204] [Medline: 26426762]
24. Manne S, Lessin S. Prevalence and correlates of sun protection and skin self-examination practices among cutaneous malignant melanoma survivors. J Behav Med 2006 Oct;29(5):419-434. [doi: 10.1007/s10865-006-9064-5] [Medline: 16855870]
25. Geller AC, Dickerman BA, Taber JM, Dwyer LA, Hartman AM, Perna FM. Skin cancer interventions across the cancer control continuum: A review of experimental evidence (1/1/2000-6/30/2015) and future research directions. Prev Med 2018 Jun;111:442-450. [doi: 10.1016/j.ypmed.2018.01.018] [Medline: 29425724]
26. Wu YP, Aspinwall LG, Conn BM, Stump T, Grahmann B, Leachman SA. A systematic review of interventions to improve adherence to melanoma preventive behaviors for individuals at elevated risk. Prev Med 2016 Dec;88:153-167 [FREE Full text] [doi: 10.1016/j.ypmed.2016.04.010] [Medline: 27090434]
27. Bowen DJ, Burke W, Hay JL, Meischke H, Harris JN. Effects of web-based intervention on risk reduction behaviors in melanoma survivors. J Cancer Surviv 2015 Jun;9(2):279-286 [FREE Full text] [doi: 10.1007/s11764-014-0412-0] [Medline: 25425205]
28. Robinson JK, Turrisi R, Stapleton J. Efficacy of a partner assistance intervention designed to increase skin self-examination performance. Arch Dermatol 2007 Jan;143(1):37-41. [doi: 10.1001/archderm.143.1.37] [Medline: 17224540]

29. Pew Research Center. Social Media Update 2016: Facebook usage and engagement is on the rise, while adoption of other platforms holds steady URL: http://assets.pewresearch.org/wp-content/uploads/sites/14/2016/11/10132827/PI_2016.11.11_Social-Media-Update_FINAL.pdf [accessed 2018-04-24] [WebCite Cache ID 6yvOUfUba]
30. Bruce A, Theeke L, Mallow J. A state of the science on influential factors related to sun protective behaviors to prevent skin cancer in adults. International Journal of Nursing Sciences 2017 Jul;4(3):225-235. [doi: 10.1016/j.ijnss.2017.05.005]
31. Pagoto SL, Baker K, Griffith J, Oleski JL, Palumbo A, Walkosz BJ, et al. Engaging Moms on Teen Indoor Tanning Through Social Media: Protocol of a Randomized Controlled Trial. JMIR Res Protoc 2016 Nov 29;5(4):e228 [FREE Full text] [doi: 10.2196/resprot.6624] [Medline: 27899339]
32. Naslund JA, Kim SJ, Aschbrenner KA, McCulloch LJ, Brunette MF, Dallery J, et al. Systematic review of social media interventions for smoking cessation. Addict Behav 2017 Oct;73:81-93. [doi: 10.1016/j.addbeh.2017.05.002] [Medline: 28499259]
33. Joseph RP, Keller C, Adams MA, Ainsworth BE. Print versus a culturally-relevant Facebook and text message delivered intervention to promote physical activity in African American women: a randomized pilot trial. BMC Womens Health 2015;15:30 [FREE Full text] [doi: 10.1186/s12905-015-0186-1] [Medline: 25886945]
34. Wójcicki TR, Grigsby-Toussaint D, Hillman CH, Huhman M, McAuley E. Promoting Physical Activity in Low-Active Adolescents via Facebook: A Pilot Randomized Controlled Trial to Test Feasibility. JMIR Res Protoc 2014;3(4):e56 [FREE Full text] [doi: 10.2196/resprot.3013] [Medline: 25357008]
35. Napolitano MA, Hayes S, Bennett GG, Ives AK, Foster GD. Using Facebook and text messaging to deliver a weight loss program to college students. Obesity (Silver Spring) 2013 Jan;21(1):25-31. [doi: 10.1002/oby.20232] [Medline: 23505165]
36. Cavallo DN, Tate DF, Ward DS, DeVellis RF, Thayer LM, Ammerman AS. Social support for physical activity-role of Facebook with and without structured intervention. Transl Behav Med 2014 Dec;4(4):346-354 [FREE Full text] [doi: 10.1007/s13142-014-0269-9] [Medline: 25584083]
37. Love C, Sabiston CM. Exploring the links between physical activity and posttraumatic growth in young adult cancer survivors. Psychooncology 2011 Mar;20(3):278-286. [doi: 10.1002/pon.1733] [Medline: 20238374]
38. Tai E, Buchanan N, Townsend J, Fairley T, Moore A, Richardson LC. Health status of adolescent and young adult cancer survivors. Cancer 2012 Oct 1;118(19):4884-4891 [FREE Full text] [doi: 10.1002/cncr.27445] [Medline: 22688896]
39. Manne SL, Coups EJ, Kashy DA. Relationship factors and couples' engagement in sun protection. Health Educ Res 2016 Aug;31(4):542-554. [doi: 10.1093/her/cyw027] [Medline: 27247330]
40. Glanz K, Lew RA, Song V, Murakami-Akatsuka L. Skin cancer prevention in outdoor recreation settings: effects of the Hawaii SunSmart Program. Eff Clin Pract 2000;3(2):53-61. [Medline: 10915324]
41. Jackson KM, Aiken LS. A psychosocial model of sun protection and sunbathing in young women: the impact of health beliefs, attitudes, norms, and self-efficacy for sun protection. Health Psychol 2000 Sep;19(5):469-478. [Medline: 11007155]
42. Manne SL, Meropol NJ, Weinberg DS, Vig H, Ali-Khan CZ, Manning C, et al. Facilitating informed decisions regarding microsatellite instability testing among high-risk individuals diagnosed with colorectal cancer. J Clin Oncol 2010 Mar 10;28(8):1366-1372 [FREE Full text] [doi: 10.1200/JCO.2009.25.0399] [Medline: 20142594]
43. Brug J, Conner M, Harré N, Kremers S, McKellar S, Whitelaw S. The Transtheoretical Model and stages of change: a critique: observations by five commentators on the paper by Adams, J. and White, M. (2004) why don't stage-based activity promotion interventions work? Health Educ Res 2005 Apr;20(2):244-258. [doi: 10.1093/her/cyh005] [Medline: 15618324]
44. Manne SL, Ostroff JS, Winkel G, Fox K, Grana G, Miller E, et al. Couple-focused group intervention for women with early stage breast cancer. J Consult Clin Psychol 2005 Aug;73(4):634-646. [doi: 10.1037/0022-006X.73.4.634] [Medline: 16173851]
45. Myers RE, Ross E, Jepson C, Wolf T, Balshem A, Millner L, et al. Modeling adherence to colorectal cancer screening. Prev Med 1994 Mar;23(2):142-151. [doi: 10.1006/pmed.1994.1020] [Medline: 8047519]
46. Real K, Rimal RN. Friends talk to friends about drinking: exploring the role of peer communication in the theory of normative social behavior. Health Commun 2007;22(2):169-180. [doi: 10.1080/10410230701454254] [Medline: 17668996]
47. Rimal RN, Lapinski MK, Cook RJ, Real K. Moving toward a theory of normative influences: how perceived benefits and similarity moderate the impact of descriptive norms on behaviors. J Health Commun 2005;10(5):433-450. [doi: 10.1080/10810730591009880] [Medline: 16199387]

Abbreviations

CINJ: Cancer Institute of New Jersey
NJSCR: New Jersey State Cancer Registry
SSE: skin self-exam
TCE: total cutaneous exam

3

Acceptability and Feasibility of a Trial Testing Allocation to Sunscreen and a Smartphone App for Sun Protection: Discontinued Randomized Controlled Trial

Angela M Rodrigues, MSc, PhD; Falko F Sniehotta, PhD; Mark A Birch-Machin, PhD; Patrick Olivier, PhD; Vera Araújo-Soares, PhD

Newcastle University, Newcastle, United Kingdom

Corresponding Author:
Angela M Rodrigues, MSc, PhD
Newcastle University
Baddiley-Clark Building
Richardson Road
Newcastle, NE2 4AX
United Kingdom

Email: angela.rodrigues@newcastle.ac.uk

Abstract

Background: Recreational sun exposure has been associated with melanoma prevalence, and tourism settings are of particular interest for skin cancer prevention. Effective, affordable, and geographically flexible interventions to promote sun protection are needed.

Objective: The aim of this study was to describe the protocol for a definitive randomized controlled trial (RCT) evaluating a smartphone mobile intervention (mISkin app) promoting sun protection in holidaymakers and to assess the acceptability and feasibility of the mISkin app and associated trial procedures in an internal pilot study.

Methods: Participants were recruited from the general community. Holidaymakers traveling abroad and owning a smartphone were enrolled in the internal pilot of a 2 (mISkin vs control) x 2 (sun protection factor [SPF] 15 vs SPF 30) RCT with a postholiday follow-up. The smartphone app is fully automated and entails a behavioral intervention to promote sun protection. It consisted of five components: skin assessment, educational videos, ultraviolet (UV) photos, gamification, and prompts for sun protection. Participants were also randomly allocated to receive sunscreen SPF 15 or SPF 30. Primary outcomes for the internal pilot study were acceptability and feasibility of trial procedures and intervention features. Secondary outcomes were collected at baseline and after holidays through face-to-face-assessments and included skin sun damage, sunscreen use (residual weight and application events), and sun protection practices (Web-based questionnaire).

Results: From 142 registers of interest, 42 participants were randomized (76% [32/42] female; mean age 35.5 years). Outcome assessments were completed by all participants. Random allocation to SPF 15 versus SPF 30 was found not to be feasible in a definitive trial protocol. Of the 21 people allocated to the mISkin intervention, 19 (91%) installed the mISkin on their phones, and 18 (86%) used it at least once. Participants were satisfied with the mISkin app and made suggestions for further improvements. Due to difficulties with the random allocation to SPF and slow uptake, the trial was discontinued.

Conclusions: The internal pilot study concluded that randomization to SPF was not feasible and that recruitment rate was slower than expected because of difficulties with gatekeeper engagement. Possible solutions to the problems identified are discussed. Further refinements to the mISkin app are needed before a definitive trial.

KEYWORDS

sunscreening agents; sun protection factor; smartphone; mobile applications; feasibility studies; randomized controlled trial; skin neoplasms; melanoma; skin aging; holidays; health promotion; health behavior

Introduction

Skin cancer is the most common form of all types of cancer diagnosed in the United Kingdom [1]. In 2014, about 15,400 new melanoma skin cancer and 132,000 new nonmelanoma cases were registered [2]. Melanoma incidence rates have increased by almost a half (45%) over the last decade in the United Kingdom [2]. Intermittent sun exposure, in particular, (eg, summer holidays in sunny destinations) has been shown to increase melanoma risk considerably [3]. Epidemiologic studies suggest that implementation of sun protection behaviors would decrease intermittent sun exposure and would reduce skin cancer incidence [4,5]. Although applying sunscreen has been widely promoted, there is some discrepancy regarding the recommended sunscreen protection factor. The National Institute for Health and Care Excellence (NICE) recommends using a sun protection factor (SPF) of 15, whereas the British Association of Dermatologists, Cancer Research UK, and the British Skin Foundation suggest the use of at least SPF 30 [6].

Tourism settings are of particular interest for skin cancer prevention [3]. Sunburn is a common experience [7,8], and sun-related behaviors such as intentional sun seeking associated with lifestyle changes (eg, holidays in sunny destinations and fashion trends) are increasingly high [9]. Holidaymakers are a volatile population present at different locations, which may make them difficult to reach. A scalable and geographically flexible mobile phone intervention might be an effective way of reaching this population. Mobile phone interventions have been shown to improve sun protection behaviors either by using SMS text messaging (short message service, SMS) interventions or mobile phone apps [10-12]. A novel mobile phone intervention (mISkin app) to promote sun protection among holidaymakers has recently been developed based on evidence [13,14], experts' knowledge and experience, and user involvement [15].

The starting point for this research was to address the main challenges identified by a recent systematic review of sun protection interventions, including (1) poor reporting of intervention development, design, and contents; (2) poor outcome measurement; and (3) poor study methodology [13]. In line with this, this study describes an internal pilot study evaluating an evidence-based behavior change intervention to promote sun protection among holidaymakers, using both objective and self-reported outcome measures. The study also provides evidence to inform guidelines regarding the recommended sunscreen SPF. The specific study objectives are to:

1. Test the acceptability of recruitment, allocation, measurement, and intervention procedures.
2. Assess the feasibility of a mobile phone intervention to promote sun protection (feasibility).
3. Collect feedback regarding satisfaction with the intervention (acceptability).
4. Explore users' engagement with the app and its active ingredients (fidelity).

Methods

Full details of the research protocol have been registered: ISRCTN3943558 [16]. Ethical approval was obtained from the Faculty of Medical Sciences at Newcastle University.

Trial Design

The study was initially designed as a single center assessor-blinded parallel group, individually randomized controlled trial (RCT), using a 2 (mISkin app intervention vs no intervention) x 2 (sunscreen provision: SPF 15 vs SPF 30) factorial design. This study sought to explore the independent main effects of both sunscreen SPF and mobile app that would result in consistent differences between the levels (SPF 15 vs SPF 30; app vs no app), rather than an interaction effect.

The intended number of participants to be recruited for the definitive trial was 200, with the first 30 comprising the internal pilot phase. The internal pilot was conducted from September 2012 to October 2013. A schedule of events is presented in Multimedia Appendix 1 (schedule of events for the trial, including enrollment, interventions, and outcome assessments).

Participants

Holidaymakers from the North East of England traveling abroad, older than 18 years, and owning an Android smartphone were recruited. The recruitment strategy involved placing posters in local urban community areas such as universities, travel agency; large companies; and using social media (ie, Twitter and Facebook). Interested individuals contacted the research team by email. Participants were assessed for inclusion criteria by a researcher (AR) and provided informed consent before participation.

Interventions

mISkin Intervention Group

Participants randomized to the intervention group engaged in a behavioral intervention (mISkin) delivered through a mobile phone (Android smartphone) during their holiday (see Template for Intervention Description and Replication checklist in Multimedia Appendix 2). The mISkin app (Figure 1) is fully automated and was designed to promote holidaymakers' sun protection behavior by providing information, addressing appearance-related concerns (eg, ultraviolet [UV] photo), and prompting sun protection based on location (ie, global positioning system, GPS) [15]. The content of the mISkin app was unchanged during the trial. The mISkin app had four main menus: (1) *My skin,* (2) *How to be sun smart,* (3) *Sun safety quiz,* and (4) *Sun alert service*. First, the *My skin* menu assessed skin sensitivity and provided advice depending on skin type. Second, the *How to sun smart* menu contained videos on sun protection recommendations, detailed information on how to apply sunscreen appropriately (quantity, frequency, SPF, when to apply, where to apply, and guidance on costs), and skin damage information depicted in UV photographs. Third, the *Sun safety quiz* component engaged participants by answering questions on general principles of sun protection practices, information on positive consequences of sun protection, tanning, vitamin D, and UV index.

Figure 1. Main screen of the mISkin app.

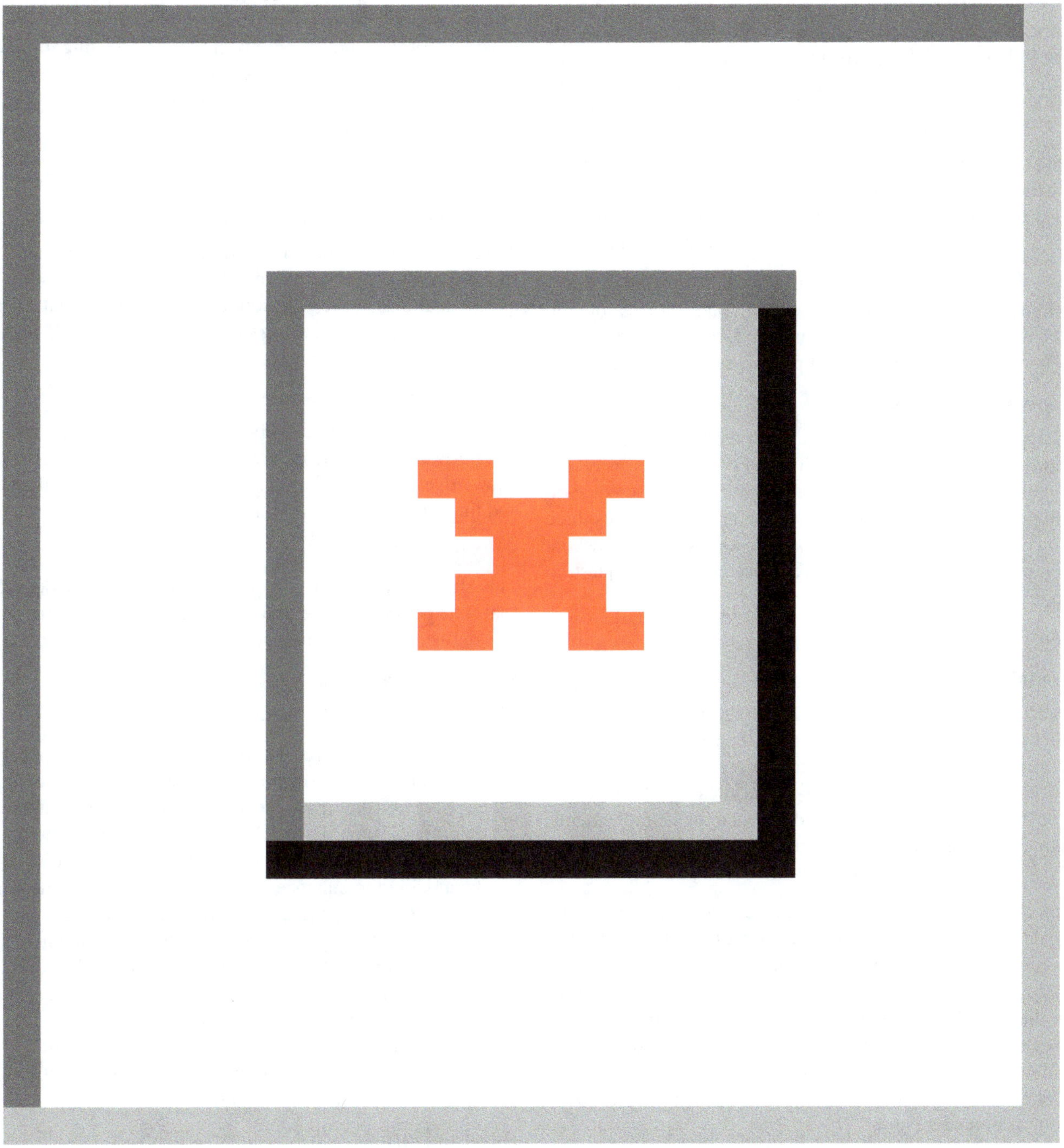

This involved a gamification component, by which participants received performance-based rewards (ie, positive feedback and a final score message), with immediate feedback on general recommendations for sun protection. Fourth, the *Sun alert service* menu allowed participants to receive sun protection reminders. The default setting for this feature comprised a minimum of two prompts, but participants could customize these to suit their preferences (eg, times and frequency). This menu also included a self-monitoring feature that recorded sun protection from 11 AM to 3 PM.

The development of the app was based on evidence [13,14], experts' knowledge and experience, and user involvement, and the systematic and iterative development process has been detailed elsewhere [15]. The process incorporated both theory and evidence-based approaches outlined by the Medical Research Council framework [17,18], engaging users' perspectives in the development process of the mISkin app [19,20].

No Mobile App Control Group

Participants allocated to the control condition did not receive the mISkin app on their phones.

Sunscreen Sun Protection Factor

All participants received two bottles of sunscreen (Ambre Solaire, 200 mL), and they were randomly allocated to receive either SPF 15 or SPF 30. To reflect the current guidelines for sunscreen use [21], the following instructions for sunscreen use were provided to all participants: (1) participant information sheet defined SPF 15 as medium SPF and SPF 30 as high SPF, stating that there is general agreement for the need of sunscreen use with an SPF of 15 or higher (SPF 15+); (2) the sunscreen bottles provided could not be shared with traveling partners; and (3) participants were asked to use the provided sunscreen.

The sunscreen bottles used in the study had a standard label, providing information on application, other forms of sun protection, dangers of overexposure, and long term prevention of UV-induced skin damage and premature skin ageing.

Protocol Deviations

Participant feedback over the course of the trial indicated that random allocation to the distinct SPF strengths was not acceptable. Although the random allocation to sunscreen SPF continued, the protocol was amended to give participants three options: (1) SPF 15, (2) SPF 30, or (3) both. Records were kept about participant allocation acceptance and any request to change allocation.

Primary Outcomes

Acceptability and Feasibility

The primary outcome of the internal pilot trial was to assess the quality and quantity of the delivery of the trial procedures and the mISkin intervention, including (1) acceptability and feasibility of trial procedures—procedures used to recruit holidaymakers, materials provided, meeting arrangements, outcomes assessment, and group allocation and (2) acceptability and fidelity of the intervention—satisfaction and app usage.

Postholiday, face-to-face interviews were conducted to obtain detailed information regarding acceptability and feasibility of recruitment, allocation, outcome measurement procedures, and intervention components. These interviews were conducted with the first 30 participants involved in the study providing consent to be recruited to the interviews and lasting 8 to 34 min for intervention participants and 3 to 8 min for control. The analyses focused on the general feedback and main issues arising from trial procedures.

Secondary Outcomes

This section describes the variables that would be the main outcomes for the definitive trial.

Mitochondrial Deoxyribonucleic Acid Damage

Skin damage caused by UV exposure was measured objectively using a reliable epithelial skin swab to test for mitochondrial deoxyribonucleic acid (mDNA) before and after holiday. These samples were taken at baseline and follow-up. Cotton swabs were collected from sterilized skin from the nose bridge and forearm and stored in a sterile collection tube until extraction following standard procedures [22].

Sunscreen Use

Participants were given sunscreen bottles with a built-in triaxial accelerometer (AX3; time- and date-stamped) recording sunscreen application. This method has shown to have a sensitivity of 91% and specificity of 98% in detecting sunscreen use events. Due to shortage, sensors were allocated to participants on the basis of availability at baseline (N=28). Sunscreen use (quantity) was also measured by weighing bottles at baseline and posttest. The same scale (Salter, model 1234SSDR) was used for all sunscreen assessments.

Self-Reported Sun Protection Behaviors

A web-based self-reported questionnaire with seven items on sun protection was also completed by all participants. This questionnaire assessed exposure times; sunscreen, hat, t-shirt, and sunglasses usage; seeking shade; and experience of sunburn [23].

Process Variables Assessment

Participants completed a Web-based questionnaire at baseline and posttest, adapted from previous studies [24-30], assessing knowledge, intentions, attitudes, self-efficacy, social influences, and time perspective (see Multimedia Appendix 3).

Sample Size

This study was originally intended to be a full-scale definitive trial. The period until the first 30 participants to enter the study was defined as the internal pilot study.

Stopping Guidelines

The following stop rules were defined:

- If more than 10 out of the first 30 participants do not accept the group allocation, measurement procedures, or other aspects of the trial procedures or if the postholiday interviews identify any significant problems with the acceptability of the trial protocol, the protocol will either be modified to enhance acceptability and feasibility based on the insights gained, or the trial will be discontinued.
- If during this period no significant problems with acceptability and feasibility are detected, the data from the internal pilot will become part of the main dataset and analyzed as part of the definitive trial.
- If any major modifications to the protocol needed to be implemented, the data from the internal pilot will not be analyzed alongside the definitive trial.

Randomization

A simple randomization was used with a 1:1:1:1 allocation ratio to assign participants to the experimental conditions. This was performed using a telephone-based randomization service provided by a staff member independent and blinded to the identity of individuals. An independent researcher generated and administered the randomization list. Only after baseline assessment were participants assigned to experimental groups.

Blinding

At baseline assessment, the outcome assessor was blinded to allocation. At follow-up, assessors were aware of the allocation, and it was hypothesized that outcome assessors could not influence outcome measurements as these were mainly objective. Researchers conducting the lab analyses for skin damage were blinded to allocation, and samples were given a code unrelated to the trial ID. This coding was performed by an independent lab researcher.

Analytical Methods

The analyses focused on descriptive data regarding recruitment rates and attrition, as well as acceptability and participants' satisfaction with the intervention. The main aim was to test whether the proposed protocol was viable for a definitive trial.

For the secondary outcomes, the focus of the analysis was on data yield and quality. Descriptive statistics are provided for participants' characteristics and trial outcomes at baseline and follow-up.

Results

Participants

A total of 42 participants were recruited from December 2012 to October 2013. Figure 2 shows the flow of participants through the feasibility study. As seen on the flow diagram, there were six protocol deviations.

Participants' characteristics and demographics can be found in Table 1. The mean age of the participants was 35.5 years (SD 9.7; N=42), with more women participating (76% [32/42]). The majority of participants reported that they usually burn and tan minimally (35% [15/42]). The most frequent holiday destination was Spain (N=12) and lasting more than 14 days (N=15).

Figure 2. Consolidated Standards of Reporting Trials (CONSORT) diagram for the trial.

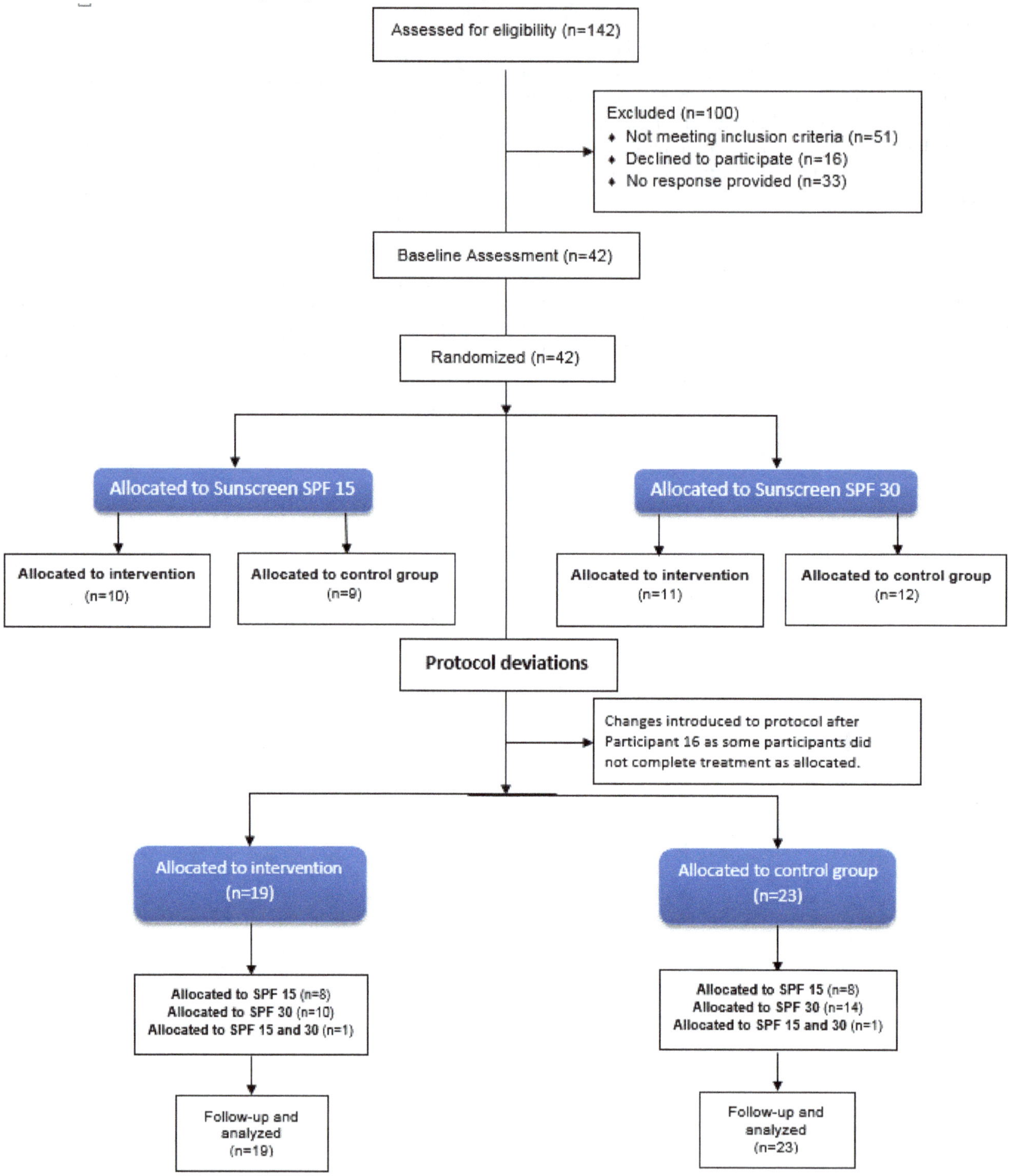

Table 1. Demographics of study participants by group (N=42).

Variables	SPF[a]15		SPF 30		Total
	mISkin app (N=10)	Control (N=9)	mISkin app (N=11)	Control (N=12)	
Age in years, mean (SD)	37.2 (11.2)	34.2 (9.1)	36.6 (9.3)	34.0 (10.1)	35.5 (9.7)
Gender (female), n (%)	5 (50)	7 (78)	9 (81)	11 (92)	32 (76)
Skin type, n (%)					
I—Burns easily, never tans	0 (0)	0 (0)	0 (0)	1 (8)	1 (3)
II—Burns easily, tans minimally	3 (30)	1 (14)	3 (33)	3 (25)	10 (26)
III—Burns and tans moderately	2 (20)	1 (14)	6 (67)	5 (42)	14 (37)
IV—Burns minimally, tans easily	4 (40)	4 (57)	0 (0)	2 (17)	10 (26)
V—Rarely burns, tans profusely	1 (10)	1 (14)	0 (0)	0 (0)	2 (5)
VI—Never burns, tans profusely	0 (0)	0 (0)	0 (0)	1 (8)	1 (3)

[a]SPF: sun protection factor.

Primary Outcomes for the Internal Pilot Study: Acceptability and Feasibility

Feasibility of Trial Procedures

Recruitment

Out of the 142 participants that registered interest, 42 (29.6%) met the inclusion criteria and provided consent to participate in this study. The main reasons for exclusion were as follows: (1) ineligible smartphone (eg, iPhone; 21.8% [31/142]) and (2) unwillingness to be randomized to SPF 15 or SPF 30 (3.5% [5/142]).

Randomization

Two breaches in the trial protocol occurred, as 2 participants were allocated to receive the mISkin app but were unable to install it because of smartphone technical issues.

Outcome Assessment

All participants consenting to participate in the study completed baseline and follow-up assessments.

Mitochondrial Deoxyribonucleic Acid Skin Damage

The skin swabs were obtained for all participants at both time points. Data on mDNA skin damage for the nose was retrieved from 34 (81% [34/42]) samples at baseline and 33 (79% [33/42]) at follow-up. Data were available for 31 (74% [31/42]) samples at baseline and 36 (86% [36/42]) at follow-up for the arm. Two reasons explain these missing data: (1) polymerase chain reaction analyses could not be computed (4.2% [7/168]; the total number of mDNA samples was 168, as a total of four samples were taken from each participant [nose and arm; before and after holiday]) and (2) samples were mislabeled during analyses and therefore lost when decoding (16.1% [27/168]).

Residual Sunscreen Weight

Sunscreen weight was available for 41 out of 42 participants at both baseline and follow-up. For one participant, a value could not be obtained because of a fault in the scale used.

Sunscreen Use Patterns (Accelerometry)

AX3 sensors measuring sunscreen-use events were allocated to only 28 participants out of 42 participants because of a lack of sensors at baseline. Reliable data detecting sunscreen use was extracted from 28 participants. Due to battery issues, data were missed at the end of the holiday period for 14 participants. Battery life lasts approximately 14 days, but sometimes the time between the initial assessment and the postholiday assessment was longer.

Self-Reported Sunburn and Sun Protection Practices

The survey was completed at baseline by 38 participants (90% [38/42]) and at follow-up by 41 participants (98% [41/42]).

Acceptability of Trial Procedures

A total of 30 interviews were conducted (mISkin app: N=13, no app: N=17), and data were collected about three main areas: consent, allocation to interventions, and assessment.

Consent

All participants stated that information received before or during enrollment was easy to understand and clear. All participants were also very positive about the arrangements made for the assessment meetings.

Allocation to Interventions

Participants were satisfied with being randomized to the mISkin app or control group. App installation was not possible because of technical difficulties in two cases. The randomized group allocation to SPF 15 versus SPF 30 was not acceptable to many participants. A total of 11 participants raised concerns about the random allocation to sunscreen SPF. From this, 10 were unwilling to be randomly allocated to SPF 15, as it was considered to be too low. Only one participant raised concerns about SPF 30 being too high. Overall, 7 people declined participation based on the random allocation to SPF.

Taking into account this information, after the initial 16 participants, the trial procedures were changed to give participants the option to choose from three options: (1) SPF 15, (2) SPF 30, or (3) both. With the introduction of this change, 6 participants chose a different SPF to what they had been allocated to: 3 participants asked to change allocation to SPF 30 instead of SPF 15, 1 participant asked to change allocation to SPF 15 instead of SPF 30, and 2 participants asked for one bottle of each.

Outcome Assessment

The main findings for secondary outcomes with descriptive data for the total sample at baseline and follow-up can be seen in Multimedia Appendix 4.

Mitochondrial Deoxyribonucleic Acid Skin Damage

The skin swabs procedure was described as painless and made easy by the provision of information detailing the procedure. Some participants reported that it might be helpful to mention that the swabs would remove makeup.

Sunscreen Use Patterns (Accelerometry)

Participants indicated that they did not experience problems carrying the AX3 sensors attached to the sunscreen bottle. A total of 5 participants (18% [5/28]) mentioned, though, that their silicone band snapped, which in some cases led to problems in calculating data events. To overcome this, when possible, participants were given an extra silicone band and were instructed on how to fit it.

Self-Reported Sun Protection Behaviors and Psychological Variables

Questionnaires were described as being straightforward, easy to understand, and the length was considered acceptable. One participant mentioned that some questions were difficult to understand, in particular questions about social norms and skin color.

Acceptability of the mISkin App Intervention

A total of 13 participants were interviewed to collect data on acceptability of the mISkin app. However, one interview was lost because of recording problems.

Data collected showed that 6 out of the 12 holidaymakers were very satisfied with the app, 4 were somehow satisfied, and 2 were dissatisfied. All participants commented and made suggestions to improve the app (Multimedia Appendix 5).

Participants were highly satisfied with the initial skin type identification, the videos, and the *Sun safety quiz*. Participants suggested that the *Sun alert service* could be improved by having a system that is able to learn from participants' sun protection habits, preferences, personal risk, and personalize prompts according to these (eg, time until sunburn risk). A few technical problems regarding the GPS functionality to detect indoor or outdoor location were also reported. Participants also recommended that the UV level forecast should be integrated with the *Sun alert service* to create a parsimonious system. Another reported issue was the disturbance created by keeping the phone on British time (Greenwich Mean Time) so that the sensor data could be synchronized with the app log usage data. This was described as disruptive, as time shown on the phones was incorrect and led to prompts not being received appropriately.

Acceptability of the Sunscreen Sun Protection Factor

One participant allocated to SPF 15 reported being slightly sunburnt at the beginning of the holiday. Some participants allocated to SPF 30 mentioned that using this SPF prevented them from being sunburnt. Others also reported the lack of a tan after their holidays as a consequence of using SPF 30. Participants felt that they used more sunscreen than they would normally (n=7). Two participants reported using sunscreens other than the ones provided.

Fidelity: mISkin App Usage

Data about the usage of the app can be seen in Table 2. A total of 19 participants (91% [19/21]) installed the mISkin on their phones, and 18 (86% [18/21]) used it at least once during holidays (ie, logging and utilized of the app features). Rates of usage were high, with a median of 60 log-in events. The median number of cues acknowledged by participants was 9 (range: 0-43). The *Sun safety quiz* was completed by 17 participants (81%). The median number of ecological momentary assessments completed was 2 (range: 0-11).

Optimization of the Trial Procedures

The problems identified and potential changes to the trial protocol are presented in Table 3. The main change introduced was the possibility of participants choosing their SPF: (1) SPF 15, (2) SPF 30, or (3) both.

Reasons for Stopped Trial

Modification and potential improvements have been recorded in Table 3, following guidelines to produce an informed decision on the internal pilot trial [31]. Evidence gathered during the internal pilot study identified significant problems influencing acceptability and feasibility of the internal pilot that led to stop the trial early, namely the SPF allocation and improvements to the app. The trial was stopped in October 2013, and a definitive trial on the mISkin app has not been conducted. The study was part of a PhD thesis [32], and funding ran out to relaunch the new protocol.

Table 2. Descriptive statistics about the mISkin app usage.

mISkin app features	Descriptive statistics				
	Frequencies	Median	Interquartile range	Maximum	Minimum
Log-in events	—	60	63	181	3
Ecological Momentary Assessments	—	2	4	11	0
Cues received	—	17	12	47	0
Cues acknowledged	—	9	7	43	0
Videos watched	—	0	5	7	0
Videos (any), n (%)	9 (47)	—	—	—	—
Video "Protecting sensitive skin," n (%)	6 (32)	—	—	—	—
Video "Sun protection tips," n (%)	5 (26)	—	—	—	—
Video "Choosing a good sunscreen," n (%)	7 (37)	—	—	—	—
Video "How to apply sunscreen," n (%)	8 (42)	—	—	—	—
Video "Preventing damage," n (%)	7 (37)	—	—	—	—
Video "Protecting children," n (%)	6 (32)	—	—	—	—
Video "Other's use of sun protection," n (%)	3 (16)	—	—	—	—
Sun safety quiz, n (%)	17 (81)	—	—	—	—

Table 3. Main problems and changes introduced to the trial protocol.

Trial procedures and problems	Changes introduced during pilot study	Suggestions for definitive trial
Recruitment		
Initial low recruitment rate	Recruitment was scaled up (eg, by involving local councils), and holiday duration was enlarged to 3 weeks.	Alternative pathways for recruitment, such as pharmacies where people buy their holiday medicines.
		mISkin app to be available in different platforms (ie, iPhone operating system)
mISkin app installation problems	Standard operating procedure (SOP) was changed to fully check participants' smartphone suitability for the mISkin app installation before the randomization procedure.	—
Measurement		
Samples lost during blinding procedure	Skin swabs blinding SOP was changed to ensure that trial number can be fully retrieved by keeping the original skin swab package where both trial number and new labeling is written.	—
Samples lost because of incorrect labeling during analyses	Skin swabs samples labeling SOP during lab analyses was changed to ensure samples have a more meaningful label (ie, date plus numbers from labeling procedure will not conducted more than 24 samples per day). SOP also now recommends that lab analyses are conducted in sets of 24 samples to prevent tiredness of the researcher and potential mistakes.	—
Loss of accelerometer data on final days of holiday	—	Important to keep the time between baseline and follow-up assessments constant as battery life of accelerometers only lasts up to 14 days.
Randomization		
Random allocation to SPF 15 or SPF 30 reported as problematic	SOP and materials were changed to give participants the possibility to choose form three options: (1) two bottles of SPF 15, (2) two bottles of SPF 30, or (3) one bottle of SPF 15 and one bottle of SPF 30.	A preference design trial might be appropriate. Alternatively participants could be given the possibility of buying their own sunscreen (eg, voucher for high-street retailer).
Intervention		
The need to keep phone time on British time (Greenwich Mean time) reported as problematic	SOP was changed to allow participants to keep their time preference on their smartphone. Data from sensors will be analyzed taking into account details provided by participants on the holiday location and local time.	—
Suggested changes to mISkin app (interviews)	—	Improve *Sun alert service* by having a system that is able to learn participants' sun protection habits and preferences.
		Ultraviolet levels forecast information should be integrated with the *Sun alert service*.

Discussion

Principal Findings

This study described an internal pilot study aimed at testing acceptability and feasibility of the trial procedures and the mISkin app. The internal pilot study revealed potential issues on participant recruitment, acceptability of the randomization to participants, and features of the intervention. A list of possible solutions to the problems identified within pilot and feasibility RCT was mapped (Table 3) following the algorithm for *decision making* after pilot and feasibility trials guidelines [33].

Despite most trial procedures being considered acceptable and feasible, the random allocation to SPF 15 versus SPF 30 was found not to be feasible in a definitive trial protocol. During the internal pilot, the SPF allocation procedures were modified to improve acceptability of participants' allocation. A preference design trial based on a participant's preference regarding sunscreen SPF could be a possible solution for a definitive trial.

Regarding the feasibility of recruitment, this was limited by the inclusion requirement to own an Android smartphone. Several participants were excluded because they owned other smartphones, showing the need to improve the interoperability of the mISkin app in a definitive trial. The relatively low rate of recruitment could also be improved by diversifying the pathways of recruitment (eg, pharmacies).

The key issue reported about the mISkin app was the *Sun alert service,* and future revisions of the app should consider improving this feature. The need for more intelligent and interactive systems has been reported previously [34]. The study by Buller and colleagues [35] also shows that participants were interested in a system that would (1) display how long they could be exposed to the sun without burning (including vitamin D synthesis), (2) show daily UV levels, (3) advice on recommended SPF, and (4) send prompts to reapply sunscreen. Nevertheless, such a system would need to tackle some of the uncertainties related to vitamin D synthesis and sunscreen use. The estimation of time needed to synthesize vitamin D is a complex and challenging calculation influenced by various factors, including skin type, age, body fat, genetic factors, lifestyle, sun protection, solar zenith angle, and atmospheric conditions [36,37]. For sunscreen, most calculations rely on the assumption that people apply the recommended amount (2 mg of sunscreen per $cm^2$of skin surface) to achieve the labeled protection [38,39]. However, evidence suggests that individuals tend to apply less than the recommended amount [14,40], dramatically reducing its protective features. In addition, NICE [41] does not recommend any specific amount of sunlight exposure to stimulate vitamin D production, only stating that longer periods of exposure may be needed for those with darker skin [21].

Comparison With Other Studies

Sun protection information delivered via a purpose-designed mobile phone app was feasible, attractive, and convenient, and usage was high with 86% using it at least once during holidays. Users were particularly interested in the *Sun alert service,* highlighting the value of receiving prompts and advice in convenient place (eg, holiday setting). These findings, although preliminary, are very promising and align with those found in other investigations of mobile apps to promote sun protection, in which usage and acceptability have been similarly demonstrated [11,12,35]. The systematic and iterative development of the app [15] and the theory-driven nature of the app [42], including active components shown to be key in interventions promoting sun protection [13], may have led to greater usage. Further research is required to assess whether the mISkin app can successfully change sun protection behaviors and to identify factors that can contribute to the uptake of the app. As it is easy and convenient to receive advice, delivering sun protection information via a mobile phone app is a promising alternative or addition to existing skin cancer prevention interventions.

Overall, sunscreen use was low in this study, with an average daily use of 14.46 g. This is a special concern if the average exposure time of 5.36 hours per day is taken into consideration. The guideline for sunscreen application thickness is 2 mg/cm^2 [43]. According to Diffey [44], a full body application will consist of 35 g of the sunscreen (ie, one-third of a bottle). In line with our findings, a study conducted by Nicol and colleagues [40], with 364 beachgoers, shows that the daily amount of sunscreen used was 7.67 g/day and 9.33 g/day for the intervention groups. Rodrigues and colleagues [14] also showed that participants used less than the recommended sunscreen amount (1.34 mg/cm^2) in an experimental setting. Future preventive strategies should provide more explicit instructions of sunscreen application thickness, possibly relating to practical examples (eg, "as much as a golf ball or a full shot glass" for whole body coverage).

Even though the use of gamification within the mISkin app is original, more efforts could be made to make this feature more engaging. Gamification can be defined as the use of gaming elements in a nongaming context to foster motivation [45]. Two core ingredients of gamification (linked to behavior change techniques) were used in the mISkin app: reinforcement and progress comparison. A key aspect of gamification is the concept of rewards that promote continuous participation, promoting not only engagement, but also behavior change [46]. Gamification applied to digital health has the potential to make the interventions more fun and engaging [45]. Recent findings have shown the potential of health apps to change behavior though gamification [47-49]. The current quiz has a set of questions that, despite allowing participants to go through it several times, does not change. A possible way to make this more attractive and further "gamify" would be to use gaming principles more systematically, such as allowing users to gain points every time they reapply sunscreen; or engage with app features; or by gradually increase the difficulty of the quiz (ie, different levels to increase challenge) [50].

Strengths and Limitations

This paper describes the efforts in addressing the main challenges identified in a previous systematic review on sun protection interventions: (1) poor reporting of intervention development, design, and contents; (2) poor outcome measurement; and (3) poor study methodology [13]. The tested intervention was developed based on the most recent evidence base available [13,14], and the development process followed a systematic approach, with a thorough report of the process and description of intervention [15]. In addition, the use of digital technologies followed the most recent advances in the area of behavioral science, with a close involvement of users in the design and development of the app [51]. The use of a combination of biologic, technological, and self-report outcome measures to understand and assess sun protection also provided a step forward in the field. Finally, the mISkin intervention was subject to intensive pilot testing, following the preregistered methods of a definitive trial. The methodology implemented aims to reduce the risk of bias by using robust procedures of blinding, allocation concealment, and intention to treat.

The process evaluation alongside the internal pilot trial is also a strength, as it provides relevant information on the mISkin intervention acceptability and how the trial procedures could be enhanced. However, the findings should be interpreted in the context of the study limitations given the nature of the study (ie, feasibility study), and some caution should be taken in generalizing these results.

The feedback on the app and trial procedures was collected through face-to-face interviews and could have introduced bias to the self-reported acceptability of the intervention and trial procedures. The possibility of measurement reactivity was also a concern, especially considering the comprehensive list of self-reported outcomes used. A recent systematic review on the topic [52] did not find any study assessing question-behavior effect on sun protection behavior and concluded that the "question-behavior effect" on health-related behavior is small and was therefore not considered when designing the protocol.

The amount of sunscreen provided might have not been enough, as it is possible that participants inferred (incorrectly) that by giving them 2 bottles (2 x 200 mL) this amount would be sufficient for their whole holiday, and therefore they tried to eke it out. The app highlighted that sunscreen should not be the first line of defense and targeted other forms of sun protection, such as wearing protective clothes and avoiding sun exposure at midday [4].

For practical reasons and resources available at the time of this study, the UV photos shown in the mISkin app were not personalized. Recent evidence suggests the importance of appearance-based beliefs and how interventions should aim at tackling those by showing personalized UV photos that depict damage [13,53,54]. Future studies should explore whether the effects of visualizing nonpersonalized UV photos are equivalent to personalized UV photos.

Unfortunately, this study faced considerable challenges in recruitment. Despite several attempts to involve high-street travel agencies and the local airport, the involvement of a gatekeeper to facilitate the access to holidaymakers was unsuccessful. It took several contacts to reach the relevant decision makers, and many highlighted that the aim of the study to promote sun protection would conflict with their products. This is consistent with other studies that have encountered similar difficulties when involving tourism industries [55,56].

Conclusions

This paper summarizes an internal pilot and feasibility RCT, testing the acceptability and feasibility of the trial procedures and the newly developed mISkin app. The evidence-based intervention was highly acceptable to participants, but the recruitment strategy and allocation to SPF 15 versus 30 were not feasible. This pilot study offers potential solutions to inform the trial procedures of a future trial and to improve the mISkin app, namely the possibility of participants choosing their sunscreen SPF, using alternative pathways to recruit holidaymakers (ie, pharmacies), and upgrading the interoperability of the mISkin app.

Acknowledgments

The work described in this paper was funded by a PhD fellowship from the Portuguese Science and Technology Foundation (FCT; Reference: SFRH/BD/60392/2009). AMR and FFS were funded by Fuse, the Centre for Translational Research in Public Health, a UK Clinical Research Collaboration Public Health Research Centre of Excellence based on funding from the British Heart Foundation, Cancer Research UK, the Economic and Social Research Council, Medical Research Council, and the National Institute for Health.

References

1. Cancer Research UK. Cancer Research UK. 2013. Skin cancer facts URL: http://www.cancerresearchuk.org/about-cancer/causes-of-cancer/sun-uv-and-cancer/skin-cancer-facts [accessed 2018-02-16] [WebCite Cache ID 6xHE6Duur]
2. Cancer Research UK. Cancer Research UK. 2016. Skin cancer statistics URL: http://www.cancerresearchuk.org/health-professional/cancer-statistics/statistics-by-cancer-type/skin-cancer [accessed 2018-02-16] [WebCite Cache ID 6xHDmmQXI]
3. Mitchell-Box K, Braun KL. Fathers' thoughts on breastfeeding and implications for a theory-based intervention. J Obstet Gynecol Neonatal Nurs 2012;41(6):E41-E50. [doi: 10.1111/j.1552-6909.2012.01399.x] [Medline: 22861175]
4. Armstrong BK, Kricker A. The epidemiology of UV induced skin cancer. J Photochem Photobiol B 2001 Oct;63(1-3):8-18. [Medline: 11684447]
5. English DR, Armstrong BK. Identifying people at high risk of cutaneous malignant melanoma: results from a case-control study in Western Australia. Br Med J (Clin Res Ed) 1988 May 07;296(6632):1285-1288 [FREE Full text] [Medline: 3133052]
6. The British Skin Foundation. The British Skin Foundation. 2011. Responde to NICE about skin cancer Guidance URL: http://www.bad.org.uk//site/734/default.aspx [accessed 2018-02-16] [WebCite Cache ID 6xHDg4znD]
7. Cancer Research UK. Cancer Research UK. 2013. Advice for tour operators URL: http://www.sunsmart.org.uk/advice-and-prevention/touroperators/ [accessed 2018-02-16] [WebCite Cache ID 6xHDYTO4S]
8. World Health Organisation. WHO. 2002. Sun protection: an essential element of health-promoting schools URL: http://www.who.int/hpr/gshi/ [accessed 2018-02-16] [WebCite Cache ID 6xHDS1wGs]
9. de Vries E, Coebergh JW. Cutaneous malignant melanoma in Europe. Eur J Cancer 2004 Nov;40(16):2355-2366. [doi: 10.1016/j.ejca.2004.06.003] [Medline: 15519506]
10. Finch L, Janda M, Loescher LJ, Hacker E. Can skin cancer prevention be improved through mobile technology interventions? a systematic review. Prev Med 2016 Sep;90:121-132. [doi: 10.1016/j.ypmed.2016.06.037] [Medline: 27374946]
11. Buller DB, Berwick M, Lantz K, Buller MK, Shane J, Kane I, et al. Smartphone mobile application delivering personalized, real-time sun protection advice: a randomized clinical trial. JAMA Dermatol 2015 May;151(5):497-504 [FREE Full text] [doi: 10.1001/jamadermatol.2014.3889] [Medline: 25629710]

12. Buller DB, Berwick M, Lantz K, Buller MK, Shane J, Kane I, et al. Evaluation of immediate and 12-week effects of a smartphone sun-safety mobile application: a randomized clinical trial. JAMA Dermatol 2015 May;151(5):505-512 [FREE Full text] [doi: 10.1001/jamadermatol.2014.3894] [Medline: 25629819]
13. Rodrigues A, Sniehotta FF, Araujo-Soares V. Are interventions to promote sun-protective behaviors in recreational and tourist settings effective? a systematic review with meta-analysis and moderator analysis. Ann Behav Med 2013 Apr;45(2):224-238. [doi: 10.1007/s12160-012-9444-8] [Medline: 23229160]
14. Rodrigues AM, Sniehotta FF, Birch-Machin MA, Araujo-Soares V. Aware, motivated and striving for a 'safe tan': an exploratory mixed-method study of sun-protection during holidays. Health Psychol Behav Med 2017 Jun;5(1):276-298 [FREE Full text] [doi: 10.1080/21642850.2017.1335205] [Medline: 28670503]
15. Rodrigues AM, Sniehotta FF, Birch-Machin MA, Olivier P, Araújo-Soares V. Systematic and iterative development of a smartphone app to promote sun-protection among holidaymakers: design of a prototype and results of usability and acceptability testing. JMIR Res Protoc 2017 Jun 12;6(6):e112 [FREE Full text] [doi: 10.2196/resprot.7172] [Medline: 28606892]
16. Controlled-trials.: Current Controlled Trials, c/o BioMed Central; 2013. A factorial randomised controlled trial of the mISkin smartphone intervention and sunscreen with SPF 15 vs. SPF 30 to prevent epidermal DNA skin damage amongst holidaymakers URL: http://www.controlled-trials.com/isrctn/pf/63943558 [accessed 2018-02-16] [WebCite Cache ID 6xHDJY5DV]
17. Craig P, Dieppe P, Macintyre S, Michie S, Nazareth I, Petticrew M. Developing and evaluating complex interventions: the new medical research council guidance. BMJ 2008 Sep 29;337(sep29 1):a1655. [doi: 10.1136/bmj.a1655]
18. Peter C, Paul D, Sally M, Susan M, Irwin N, Mark P. Developing and evaluating complex interventions: an introduction to the new Medical Research Council guidance. In: Killoran A, Kelly M, editors. Evidence-based Public Health: Effectiveness and efficiency. Oxford: Oxford Scholarship Online; 2010.
19. Eun-Ok B, Kursat C, Elizabeth B, Theodore F. User-centered design and development. In: Spector MJ, Merrill DM, Elen J, Bishop MJ, editors. Handbook of research on educational communications and technology. New York: Lawrence Erlbaum Associates; 2008:659-670.
20. Yardley L, Morrison L, Bradbury K, Muller I. The person-based approach to intervention development: application to digital health-related behavior change interventions. J Med Internet Res 2015 Jan;17(1):e30 [FREE Full text] [doi: 10.2196/jmir.4055] [Medline: 25639757]
21. NICE. NICE. 2016. Sunlight exposure: risks and benefits URL: https://www.nice.org.uk/guidance/ng34/ [accessed 2018-02-16] [WebCite Cache ID 6xHD8UjzX]
22. Harbottle A, Maki J, Reguly B, Wittock R, Robinson K, Parr R, et al. Real-time polymerase chain reaction analysis of a 3895-bp mitochondrial DNA deletion in epithelial swabs and its use as a quantitative marker for sunlight exposure in human skin. Br J Dermatol 2010 Dec;163(6):1291-1295. [doi: 10.1111/j.1365-2133.2010.10001.x] [Medline: 20731654]
23. Glanz K, Yaroch AL, Dancel M, Saraiya M, Crane LA, Buller DB, et al. Measures of sun exposure and sun protection practices for behavioral and epidemiologic research. Arch Dermatol 2008 Feb;144(2):217-222. [doi: 10.1001/archdermatol.2007.46] [Medline: 18283179]
24. Mitchell-Box K, Braun KL. Fathers' thoughts on breastfeeding and implications for a theory-based intervention. J Obstet Gynecol Neonatal Nurs 2012;41(6):E41-E50. [doi: 10.1111/j.1552-6909.2012.01399.x] [Medline: 22861175]
25. Bandura A. Social cognitive theory: an agentic perspective. Annu Rev Psychol 2001;52(1):1-26. [doi: 10.1146/annurev.psych.52.1.1] [Medline: 11148297]
26. Mahler HI, Kulik JA, Gibbons FX, Gerrard M, Harrell J. Effects of appearance-based interventions on sun protection intentions and self-reported behaviors. Health Psychol 2003 Mar;22(2):199-209. [Medline: 12683740]
27. Jackson KM, Aiken LS. A psychosocial model of sun protection and sunbathing in young women: the impact of health beliefs, attitudes, norms, and self-efficacy for sun protection. Health Psychol 2000 Sep;19(5):469-478. [Medline: 11007155]
28. Adams J. Consideration of immediate and future consequences, smoking status, and body mass index. Health Psychol 2012 Mar;31(2):260-263. [doi: 10.1037/a0025790] [Medline: 22103393]
29. Orbell S, Kyriakaki M. Temporal framing and persuasion to adopt preventive health behavior: moderating effects of individual differences in consideration of future consequences on sunscreen use. Health Psychol 2008 Nov;27(6):770-779. [doi: 10.1037/0278-6133.27.6.770] [Medline: 19025273]
30. Schüz N, Schüz B, Eid M. Adding perspective: predicting adolescent sunscreen use with an extended health action process approach. Appl Psychol Health Well Being 2016 Jul;8(2):155-171. [doi: 10.1111/aphw.12066] [Medline: 27040606]
31. Charlesworth G, Burnell K, Hoe J, Orrell M, Russell I. Acceptance checklist for clinical effectiveness pilot trials: a systematic approach. BMC Med Res Methodol 2013 Jun 13;13:78 [FREE Full text] [doi: 10.1186/1471-2288-13-78] [Medline: 23758922]
32. Rodrigues AM. NCL. 2014. Systematic development of a behavioural intervention to promote sun-protection behaviours amongst holidaymakers URL: https://theses.ncl.ac.uk/dspace/bitstream/10443/2569/1/Rodrigues%2C%20A.%202014.pdf [accessed 2018-02-20] [WebCite Cache ID 6xMiJcaYo]
33. Bugge C, Williams B, Hagen S, Logan J, Glazener C, Pringle S, et al. A process for decision-making after pilot and feasibility trials (ADePT): development following a feasibility study of a complex intervention for pelvic organ prolapse. Trials 2013

Oct 25;14:353 [FREE Full text] [doi: 10.1186/1745-6215-14-353] [Medline: 24160371]

34. Dennison L, Morrison L, Conway G, Yardley L. Opportunities and challenges for smartphone applications in supporting health behavior change: qualitative study. J Med Internet Res 2013 Apr;15(4):e86 [FREE Full text] [doi: 10.2196/jmir.2583] [Medline: 23598614]
35. Buller DB, Berwick M, Shane J, Kane I, Lantz K, Buller MK. User-centered development of a smart phone mobile application delivering personalized real-time advice on sun protection. Transl Behav Med 2013 Sep;3(3):326-334 [FREE Full text] [doi: 10.1007/s13142-013-0208-1] [Medline: 24058385]
36. Faurschou A, Beyer DM, Schmedes A, Bogh MK, Philipsen PA, Wulf HC. The relation between sunscreen layer thickness and vitamin D production after ultraviolet B exposure: a randomized clinical trial. Br J Dermatol 2012 Aug;167(2):391-395. [doi: 10.1111/j.1365-2133.2012.11004.x] [Medline: 22512875]
37. Rhodes L. NICE. 2015. Sunlight-induced vitamin D synthesis URL: https://www.nice.org.uk/guidance/ng34/evidence/expert-paper-5-sunlightinduced-vitamin-d-synthesis-pdf-2311152881 [accessed 2018-02-16] [WebCite Cache ID 6xHCaCA6X]
38. Faurschou A, Wulf HC. Ecological analysis of the relation between sunbeds and skin cancer. Photodermatol Photoimmunol Photomed 2007 Aug;23(4):120-125. [doi: 10.1111/j.1600-0781.2007.00289.x] [Medline: 17598864]
39. Schalka S, Dos Reis VM, Cucé LC. The influence of the amount of sunscreen applied and its sun protection factor (SPF): evaluation of two sunscreens including the same ingredients at different concentrations. Photodermatol Photoimmunol Photomed 2009 Aug;25(4):175-180. [doi: 10.1111/j.1600-0781.2009.00408.x] [Medline: 19614894]
40. Nicol I, Gaudy C, Gouvernet J, Richard MA, Grob JJ. Skin protection by sunscreens is improved by explicit labeling and providing free sunscreen. J Invest Dermatol 2007 Jan;127(1):41-48 [FREE Full text] [doi: 10.1038/sj.jid.5700509] [Medline: 17068486]
41. National Institute for Health and Care Excellence. 2016. Vitamin D deficiency in adults - treatment and prevention URL: https://cks.nice.org.uk/vitamin-d-deficiency-in-adults-treatment-and-prevention#!topicsummary[WebCite Cache ID 6xHD2FfWo]
42. Michie S, Ashford S, Sniehotta FF, Dombrowski SU, Bishop A, French DP. A refined taxonomy of behaviour change techniques to help people change their physical activity and healthy eating behaviours: the CALO-RE taxonomy. Psychol Health 2011 Nov;26(11):1479-1498. [doi: 10.1080/08870446.2010.540664] [Medline: 21678185]
43. British Association of Dermatologists. British Association of Dermatologists. 2013. Sunscreen factsheet URL: http://www.bad.org.uk/desktopDefault.aspx?TabId=734 [accessed 2018-02-16] [WebCite Cache ID 6xHCkydd7]
44. Diffey BL. People do not apply enough sunscreen for protection. BMJ 1996 Oct 12;313(7062):942. [doi: 10.1136/bmj.313.7062.942]
45. Cugelman B. Gamification: what it is and why it matters to digital health behavior change developers. JMIR Serious Games 2013 Dec;1(1):e3 [FREE Full text] [doi: 10.2196/games.3139] [Medline: 25658754]
46. Nour M, Yeung SH, Partridge S, Allman-Farinelli M. A narrative review of social media and game-based nutrition interventions targeted at young adults. J Acad Nutr Diet 2017 May;117(5):735-52.e10 [FREE Full text] [doi: 10.1016/j.jand.2016.12.014] [Medline: 28238894]
47. Miller AS, Cafazzo JA, Seto E. A game plan: gamification design principles in mHealth applications for chronic disease management. Health Informatics J 2016 Jun;22(2):184-193. [doi: 10.1177/1460458214537511] [Medline: 24986104]
48. King D, Greaves F, Exeter C, Darzi A. 'Gamification': influencing health behaviours with games. J R Soc Med 2013 Mar;106(3):76-78. [doi: 10.1177/0141076813480996] [Medline: 23481424]
49. Lister C, West JH, Cannon B, Sax T, Brodegard D. Just a fad? gamification in health and fitness apps. JMIR Serious Games 2014 Aug;2(2):e9 [FREE Full text] [doi: 10.2196/games.3413] [Medline: 25654660]
50. Hale AR, Young VL, Grand A, McNulty CA. Can gaming increase antibiotic awareness in children? a mixed-methods approach. JMIR Serious Games 2017 Mar 24;5(1):e5 [FREE Full text] [doi: 10.2196/games.6420] [Medline: 28341618]
51. Pagoto S, Bennett GG. How behavioral science can advance digital health. Transl Behav Med 2013 Sep;3(3):271-276 [FREE Full text] [doi: 10.1007/s13142-013-0234-z] [Medline: 24073178]
52. Rodrigues AM, O'Brien N, French DP, Glidewell L, Sniehotta FF. The question-behavior effect: genuine effect or spurious phenomenon? a systematic review of randomized controlled trials with meta-analyses. Health Psychol 2015 Jan;34(1):61-78. [doi: 10.1037/hea0000104] [Medline: 25133835]
53. Dodd LJ, Forshaw MJ. Assessing the efficacy of appearance-focused interventions to prevent skin cancer: a systematic review of the literature. Health Psychol Rev 2010 Sep;4(2):93-111. [doi: 10.1080/17437199.2010.485393]
54. Williams AL, Grogan S, Clark-Carter D, Buckley E. Appearance-based interventions to reduce ultraviolet exposure and/or increase sun protection intentions and behaviours: a systematic review and meta-analyses. Br J Health Psychol 2013 Feb;18(1):182-217. [doi: 10.1111/j.2044-8287.2012.02089.x] [Medline: 22989352]
55. Buller DB, Andersen PA, Walkosz BJ, Scott MD, Beck L, Cutter GR. Rationale, design, samples, and baseline sun protection in a randomized trial on a skin cancer prevention intervention in resort environments. Contemp Clin Trials 2016 Jan;46:67-76 [FREE Full text] [doi: 10.1016/j.cct.2015.11.015] [Medline: 26593781]
56. Buller DB, Andersen PA, Walkosz BJ, Scott MD, Beck L, Cutter GR. Effect of an intervention on observed sun protection by vacationers in a randomized controlled trial at North American resorts. Prev Med 2017 Jun;99:29-36 [FREE Full text]

[doi: 10.1016/j.ypmed.2017.01.014] [Medline: 28189810]

Abbreviations

AX3: triaxial accelerometer
GPS: global positioning system
mDNA: mitochondrial deoxyribonucleic acid
NICE: National Institute for Health and Care Excellence
RCT: randomized controlled trial
SMS: short message service
SPF: sun protection factor
UV: ultraviolet

4

Development of Smartphone Apps for Skin Cancer Risk Assessment: Progress and Promise

Tiago M de Carvalho[1], PhD; Eline Noels[1], MD; Marlies Wakkee[1], MD, PhD; Andreea Udrea[2], PhD; Tamar Nijsten[1], MD, PhD

[1]Department of Dermatology, Erasmus Medical Center, Rotterdam, Netherlands

[2]Department of Automatic Control and System Engineering, Polytechnic University of Bucharest, Bucharest, Romania

Corresponding Author:
Tiago M de Carvalho, PhD
Department of Dermatology
Erasmus Medical Center
Doctor Molewaterplein 40
Rotterdam, 3015 GD
Netherlands

Email: t.decarvalho@erasmusmc.nl

Abstract

Skin cancer is a growing public health problem. Early and accurate detection is important, since prognosis and cost of treatment are highly dependent on cancer stage at detection. However, access to specialized health care professionals is not always straightforward, and population screening programs are unlikely to become implemented. Furthermore, there is a wide margin for improving the efficiency of skin cancer diagnostics. Specifically, the diagnostic accuracy of general practitioners and family physicians in differentiating benign and malignant skin tumors is relatively low. Both access to care and diagnostic accuracy fuel interest in developing smartphone apps equipped with algorithms for image analyses of suspicious lesions to detect skin cancer. Based on a recent review, seven smartphone apps claim to perform image analysis for skin cancer detection, but as of October 2018, only three seemed to be active. These apps have been criticized in the past due to their lack of diagnostic accuracy. Here, we review the development of the SkinVision smartphone app, which has more than 900,000 users worldwide. The latest version of the SkinVision app (October 2018) has a 95% sensitivity (78% specificity) for detection of skin cancer. The current accuracy of the algorithm may warrant the use of this app as an aid by lay users or general practitioners. Nonetheless, for mobile health apps to become broadly accepted, further research is needed on their health impact on the health system and the user population. Ultimately, mobile health apps could become a powerful tool to reduce health care costs related to skin cancer management and minimize the morbidity of skin cancer in the population.

KEYWORDS

skin cancer; early detection; mhealth; smartphone app; mobile phone

Rationale for Using Mobile Health Apps for Early Detection of Skin Cancer

There are three main types of skin cancers—malignant melanoma (MM), squamous cell carcinoma (SCC), and basal cell carcinoma (BCC)—with the latter two also known as keratinocyte carcinoma (KC). In the United States, it was estimated that about 91,000 people will be diagnosed with melanoma and 9300 will die due to MM in 2018 [1]; in addition, in 2012, more than 5 million people were diagnosed and 3 million received treatment for KC, which is more than the values for all other cancers combined [2]. Globally, in 2015, there were about 351,000 new incident melanoma cases and 60,000 melanoma-related deaths [3], with the highest burden of disease in Australasia, North America, and Europe. In the last 30 years, the incidence of MM, adjusted for changes in the age distribution of the population, more than doubled in the United States (among Caucasians) and the United Kingdom; nearly doubled in Norway, Sweden, and New Zealand; and increased by approximately 75% in Australia [4]. This is mostly due to changes in risk factors such as increased exposure to ultraviolet light and indoor tanning [4-6]. Since these risk factors are mostly preventable, comprehensive prevention programs aimed at better sun protection behavior have been implemented in several countries, such as SunSmart in Australia [7].

Although several organizations have issued recommendations on how often to check skin lesions for individuals at higher risk (eg, Fitzpatrick scale I-III, a family history of melanoma, a history of sun-damaged skin, and multiple atypical nevi), ranging from every 3 months to every year [8], most countries do not have an organized early detection program for skin cancer. The US Preventive Services Task Force has issued an I-recommendation for skin cancer screening [9], indicating that there is insufficient evidence to evaluate the harms and benefits of skin cancer screening. Currently, there are only two major skin screening programs: (1) In the United States, the American Academy of Dermatology, which started in 1985, includes screening and skin cancer awareness education [10] and (2) in Germany, a national screening program was started in 2008 [11]; the program in Germany does not seem to be effective in reducing skin cancer–related mortality and morbidity [12].

In practice, it is difficult to provide a high-quality skin checks, even for high-risk individuals. Waiting times and, in some areas, dermatologist shortages, out-of-pocket costs, and distance to the nearest dermatologist [13] may discourage people at risk from receiving dermatological care. For example, in the United States, a study found that availability of a dermatologist within the county is associated with a 35% decrease in melanoma mortality [14]. Another US estimate found that only a quarter of individuals at higher risk of skin cancer have ever received a total skin body examination [8].

In several countries, namely, in the United Kingdom and the Netherlands, skin checks are first carried out by a general practitioner (GP, also sometimes referred to as primary care provider), who may then choose to refer a patient to a dermatologist if there is a suspicion of skin cancer. However, several studies suggest that the accuracy of GPs to detect skin cancer is relatively low [15-20]. The sensitivity of GPs without specific training to detect skin cancer was estimated to be below 60% in British and Dutch studies [15,16]. One US study found that only 35% of patients had a correct diagnosis [17]. Altogether, this may result in a delay in diagnosis or missing the cancer in its earlier stages when patient survival is more favorable and treatment is less costly. Furthermore, many GP consultations and subsequent referrals to a specialist to examine the skin for cancer result in a benign diagnosis. A Dutch study found that 69% of GP consultations related to suspicious skin lesions result in a benign diagnosis [19], and two separate studies in the Netherlands estimated that a large proportion (40%) of referral cases to the dermatologist due to suspicion of skin cancer turned out to be benign cases [19,20]. Two studies (in the United States and Germany) including more than 70 dermatologists found that dermatologists' disease classification decisions have a specificity of 60%-80% [21,22], which may result in unnecessary biopsies/excisions.

Early detection and surveillance of skin cancer could be more efficient with mobile health (mHealth) apps, which are easily accessible due to the ubiquity of smartphone usage. One example of a smartphone app for self-assessment of skin lesions for skin cancer is the SkinVision app (SVA), developed by SkinVision, BV, The Netherlands). In the next section, we review the development of SkinVision app over time.

Development of a Smartphone App for Skin Cancer Detection

SkinVision is a smartphone app built as a digital dermatology service for self-monitoring skin lesions. It was launched in 2011 and as of October 2018, it was on its fifth major version. The workflow of the app is given in Figure 1.

Figure 1. Workflow of the SkinVision app service. SVA: SkinVision app.

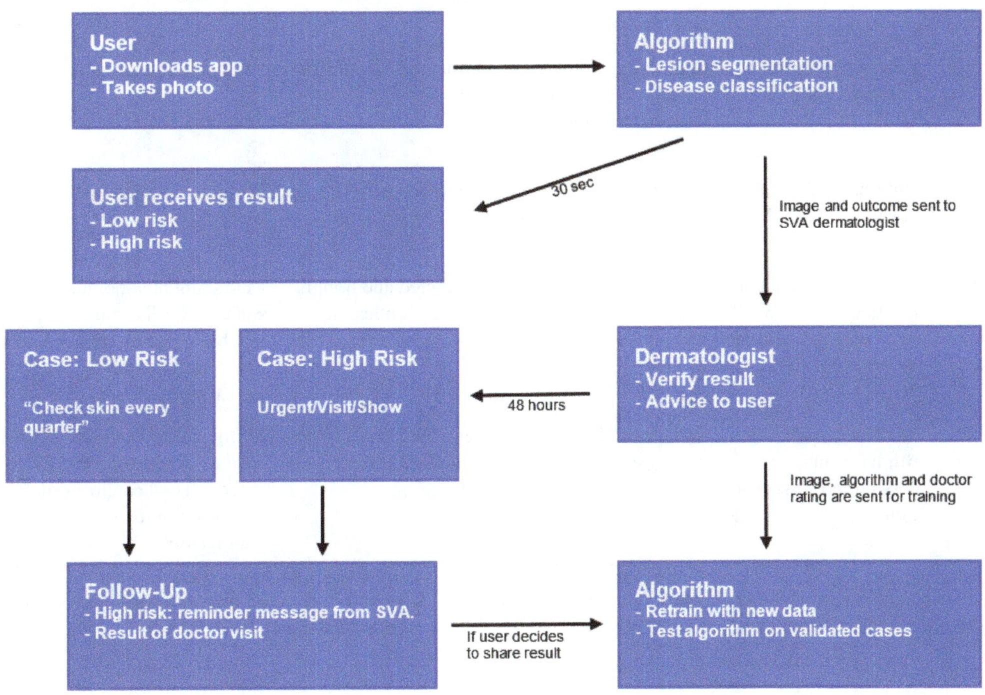

A user can self-assess the risk of a skin lesion for skin cancer by taking a photo with his/her smartphone, which is processed by an algorithm. The outcome of the procedure is a binary risk rating, which can be low or high. This smartphone app does not provide a diagnosis (eg, "you have melanoma"). For high-risk cases, the user receives advice from the costumer care team based on the image assessment of an in-house dermatologist.

Development of the SkinVision App Service

The history of the SkinVision app service is shown in Table 1. It went through several upgrades throughout its history, modifying the camera, the algorithm and its evaluation, type of lesions analyzed, and communication of the algorithm result to its user. One of the major initial challenges was related to image acquisition. In the beginning, there was no filter on the images sent for analyses, which meant that a significant proportion of the pictures taken by users was of insufficient quality to be analyzed by the disease classification algorithm or did not even contain a lesion to be analyzed. Since version 3 of the SkinVision app (2014), a special camera module [23] has been embedded, which only lets the camera take a photo after certain minimal quality conditions are met. Compared to unfiltered images taken with a standard smartphone camera, the camera module reduces the number of blurry photos by about 52% on an average (determined using 2018 data). Altogether, improvements in the camera module (namely, image quality checks) and the algorithm pipeline led to a reduction in the number of assessments that failed to produce a risk rating, from 26% in 2016 to 2% in 2018 on an average.

An overview of studies on the diagnostic accuracy of the SkinVision app is shown in Table 2. Diagnostic accuracy is evaluated based on two measures: sensitivity (proportion of lesions correctly classified as high risk) and specificity (the proportion of lesions correctly rated as benign). The first algorithm for skin lesion assessment was a rule-based fractal algorithm [24]. Initially, it was focused on pigmented skin lesions and only able to analyze whether MM was present in the lesion, and it was tested based on clinical review of images. The Munich University Hospital study was the first peer-reviewed publication where the SkinVision app algorithm was evaluated against histopathology [24], and thereafter, the algorithm achieved 73% sensitivity (83% specificity). During the Catharina Hospital Eindhoven study [25], the algorithm was recalibrated to analyze pigmented and nonpigmented lesions. Currently, it can detect several types of skin cancer (MM, SCC, and BCC) and skin conditions that can lead to skin cancer, namely, actinic keratosis and Bowen disease. It achieved 80% sensitivity (78% specificity) after inclusion of user clinical information. Although in the Eindhoven study, only 233 lesions were used for calibration, in 2018, the SkinVision app assembled a training dataset of more than 130,000 images that were risk classified by a dermatologist from the app's user database. This led to replacement of the rule-based classification algorithm by a machine learning approach (A Udrea et al, PhD, unpublished material, 2019).

Table 1. Development of the SkinVision smartphone app.

Version	Launch date	Algorithm	Camera	Type of skin lesion	Type of skin cancer detected	Testing
1	May 2011	Rule-based fractal algorithm version 1	Standard smartphone camera	Pigmented skin lesion only	Malignant melanoma	Preclinical testing using 600 images against the opinion of two dermatologists
2	December 2012	Rule-based fractal algorithm version 2	Standard smartphone camera, exclusion criteria introduced	Pigmented skin lesion only	Malignant melanoma	Preclinical testing using 600 images against the opinion of two dermatologists
3	September 2014	Rule-based fractal algorithm version 2	Camera module: exclusion criteria automated	Pigmented skin lesion only	Malignant melanoma	Clinical study, Munich University Hospital
4	July 2016	Rule-based fractal algorithm version 3, all outcomes checked by dermatologists (Sept 2016)	Camera module version 1	Pigmented and nonpigmented skin lesions	Malignant melanoma, squamous cell carcinoma, basal cell carcinoma, some premalignant lesions	Clinical study, Catharina Hospital Eindhoven (more types of skin cancer)
5	January 2018	Machine learning algorithm for image processing and classification	Camera module major version 2[a]	Pigmented and nonpigmented skin lesions	Malignant melanoma, squamous cell carcinoma, basal cell carcinoma, some premalignant lesions	Data from previous clinical studies and user database with new algorithm

[a]New features include a dynamic grey threshold to differentiate between normal skin and lesion and a feature that prevents taking pictures without uniform luminosity.

Table 2. Studies on the accuracy of the SkinVision app's risk assessment. All studies presented here were sponsored by the SkinVision app.

Study	Data	Algorithm	Test set	Sensitivity (%)	Specificity (%)	Remarks
Maier et al, 2014 [24]	University Hospital Munich	Rule-based fractal algorithm version 2	26 lesions with melanoma	73	83	Algorithm tested only on malignant melanoma
Thissen et al, 2017 [25]	Catharina Hospital Eindhoven	Rule-based fractal algorithm version 3	108 lesions including several types of skin cancer	80[a]	78[a]	Algorithm tested mostly on keratinocyte carcinoma (Munich data also used for testing)
Udrea et al, 2019[b]	Clinical studies and SkinVision app user database	Machine learning–based algorithm	285 lesions with skin cancer, from clinical studies and a user database with histopathology information	95	78	All types of skin cancer

[a]After incorporating answers into a questionnaire about the skin lesion.

[b]Manuscript under peer review (June 2019). For more details on these results, see Multimedia Appendix 1.

SkinVision App Service in 2018

Camera

Before downloading the app, the smartphone should be equipped with a camera capable of producing a video stream with sufficiently high resolution. Although the app uses a regular smartphone camera, the camera module embedded in the app automatically places some restrictions to ensure minimal quality requirements of the images are met: The image needs to be focused, the lesion should be present and contained in the image, and there should be no hair or shadows covering the lesion. The module also prevents the camera from taking images that cannot be assessed by the algorithm (eg, lesions under a nail or near clothing in a skin fold).

Algorithm for Lesion Assessment

There are several steps to analyze the lesion. The first task of the algorithm is to identify and separate the lesion from normal skin. This is done using a machine learning technique called conditional Generative Adversarial Neural Network [26] (A Udrea et al, PhD, unpublished material, 2019). After the lesion is segmented, all "noise" (eg, hair surrounding the lesion) is removed in the image by applying an inpainting procedure [27]. The third step is to extract the features from the lesion that are used in the disease classification algorithm. These features include 24 shape, color, and texture attributes that characterize the lesion. A Support Vector Machines (SVM) classifier is used to provide a risk rating, which can be high or low. The SVM model is obtained by maximizing sensitivity to detect cancer subject to a constraint of a minimal specificity value (eg, 80%). The optimization is performed using a Particle Swarm Optimization algorithm [28]. The classification algorithm is regularly updated and retrained with new data. This is necessary to maintain robustness to variation due to imaging, newer devices, and the user population adopting the app.

Training and Testing

For training of the algorithm, we used images obtained from the user database (more than 130,000 pictures from 30,000 users), which received either a low- or high-risk tag during quality control of the algorithm by a dermatologist affiliated with SkinVision. A selection of cases clinically validated as low risk were randomly selected from the user database, while all cases rated as high risk or with a histopathological report were used, since there were considerably fewer of them. For testing the sensitivity, we used 285 skin lesions derived from both previous clinical studies (Munich and Catharina Hospital, 195 skin lesions, containing most common forms of skin cancer) and the user database (90 cases of melanoma that received histopathological confirmation from users). Furthermore, to test the specificity, we used 6000 randomly selected cases from the user database (June to August 2018), which were tagged as benign by SkinVision-affiliated dermatologists and were not used in training. An overview of these datasets together with the participant flowcharts are shown in Multimedia Appendix 1.

Performance Evaluation

The gold standard (main comparator) to evaluate algorithm sensitivity is comparison against histopathologically validated cancers. The second comparator is the performance of the algorithm against the image assessment of the dermatologist (which is comparable to a teledermatology consult). In order to calculate the specificity, we use images of lesions that were classified by dermatologists as benign cases, since these are not usually biopsied, and therefore, there is no histopathology report. Sensitivity has improved from 73% in the first peer-reviewed study, where only MM was detectable, to 95% in the current version of the algorithm (78% specificity), where the SkinVision app can detect all forms of skin cancer (Table 2 and Multimedia Appendix 1).

Postassessment Follow-Up

Since 2016, images processed by the algorithm are reviewed by at least one affiliated dermatologist. To help users with the interpretation of high-risk cases, a senior dermatologist adds advice depending on the probable severity of the disease. The advice can contain the labels "Show," "Visit," or "Urgent." "Show" indicates that the lesion should be shown at the next planned doctor appointment, "Visit" indicates that the appointment should be made soon, and "Urgent" advises the user to show the lesion to a doctor as soon as possible. Users with a low-risk rating only receive a reminder to check their skin regularly.

Assessments with a high-risk rating given by the dermatologist are followed up by the customer support department of the SkinVision app. If the user does not respond, he/she may receive additional messages encouraging a visit to the doctor, depending on the perceived severity of the disease. Some users share their diagnosis of skin cancer with the SkinVision app (n=3806, Multimedia Appendix 1). Of these, a small proportion (338/3806, 8.8%) share the histopathology report. At the end of September 2018, about 338 users had shared histopathological reports, of which 58% (178/338) were of MM diagnosis. The histopathologically validated cases are used for training and testing the algorithm.

Smartphone App Users

In Table 3, we show self-reported demographic data on SkinVision app users. As of September 2018, the SkinVision app has performed more than 1.8 million assessments. Some of these users shared their demographic data with the SkinVision app: 56% (355,491/635,807) shared their age group and 28.5% (181,706/635,807) shared their gender. Although skin cancer is more prevalent in older age groups, only 7% of the people were older than 60 years of age (19,358/355,491) in the user database and about 31% (110,529/355,491) were younger than 30 years of age. More than 60% of the users were female (118,182/181,706). A majority of the users come from the following countries: The Netherlands (n=111,063, 17.4%), United Kingdom (n=109,178, 17.2%), Australia (n=109,126, 17.2%), New Zealand (n=70,244, 11%), and Belgium (n=21,328, 3.3%).

Table 3. Self-reported demographic characteristics of the SkinVision app users. The data are from the SkinVision app proprietary user database, accessed in September 2018. Numbers are based on users, who made a picture that was evaluated by the algorithm, and filled the online questionnaire.

Characteristic	Users
Number of registered users	931,789
Total number of users with an assessment	635,807[a]
Gender[b], n (%)	
Male	62,914 (9.9)
Female	118,182 (18.6)
Missing	454,731 (71.5)
Age group[b] (years), n (%)	
<30	110,529 (17.4)
30-39	98,327 (15.5)
40-49	74,928 (11.8)
50-59	46,840 (7.4)
60-69	19,358 (3.0)
>70	5509 (0.9)
Missing	280,316 (44.0)
Country, n (%)	
The Netherlands	111,063 (17.4)
Australia	109,178 (17.2)
United Kingdom	109,126 (17.2)
New Zealand	70,244 (11.0)
Belgium	21,128 (3.3)
Others	215,355 (33.9)

[a]Some users may be health care providers taking pictures of multiple patients, so this is likely an underestimate.

[b]For the gender and age categories, about 75% and 44%, respectively, did not fill any data.

State of the Field

Available Mobile Health Apps for Skin Cancer Detection

A recent review [29] found that there are 43 smartphone apps developed for skin cancer detection, monitoring, and education. Of these, nine smartphone apps use an algorithm for image analysis [29]. We verified the current status of these smartphone apps in December 2018 with Google search and PubMed and in app stores. The results are presented in Table 4. We confirm that seven apps claim to use an algorithm for image analysis. Of these, four do not seem to be active as of October 2018. Compared to a previous review conducted in July 2014 [30], there are now less apps available for risk assessment of skin lesions through image analysis (three instead of four).

Table 4. List of smartphone apps that claim to perform skin lesion image analyses to detect skin cancer, based on a systematic review [29].[a]

Commercial name	Algorithm[b]	Evidence on PubMed	Status	Source[c]
DermaCompare	Machine learning	Not found	Removed from app store, last update on January 2017	[31]
Lubax	Content-based image retrieval, k-nearest neighbor	Yes, one supported peer-reviewed publication[d]	Removed from app store, last update on February 2015	[32,33]
MSkinDoctor[e]	Grab cut algorithm (segmentation) and SVM[f] (classification)	Not found; there is a conference abstract only	Removed from app store, update on February 2016	[34]
MySkinMap	Machine learning	Not found	Removed from app store, last update on September 2016	[35]
SkinScan	Image processing techniques, ABCDE rule	Unclear[g]	Available	[36]
SkinVision	Conditional generative adversarial neural network (segmentation) and SVM (classification)	Yes, two supported peer-reviewed publications, evaluated in independent publications	Available	[23-25,37], A Udrea et al, PhD, unpublished material, 2019
SpotMole	Image processing techniques, ABCDE rule	Yes, evaluated in independent publications	Available[h]	[38]

[a]After verifying the websites of every app (if available), it seems that two of the apps mentioned in the Ngoo et al study [29] with commercial names—Myskinpal and Skin Prevention - Photo Body—do not claim to perform automated image analysis for risk assessment. They only store images of moles to track changes.

[b]If available, the information is retrieved from scientific publications; otherwise, it is collected from the company's own website or app store description.

[c]Accessed on Dec 12, 2018.

[d]Results obtained in this publication [32] only for melanomas and large lesions.

[e]There is another app available with the same name; however, that one does not perform image analyses.

[f]SVM: support vector machines.

[g]There is an associated reference to an app of the same name from 2011; however, this does not appear to be the same app.

[h]This smartphone app has a website (spotmole.com); however, it was offline at the last time of access (Dec 12, 2018). It is unclear if this project is still alive, given the fact that the last update was in March 2016 and that it seems this app is being developed by a single individual.

Comparison of the SkinVision App With Other Apps

Currently, there seem to be three apps available for detection of skin cancer, including SkinVision app, SpotMole, and skinScan. All three allow the user to take a picture with the smartphone camera. The SkinVision app algorithm is based on machine learning techniques, while SpotMole and skinScan use algorithms inspired by the ABCDE rule [39]. The SkinVision app involves quality control by a dermatologist; however, the other apps do not seem to offer any further follow-up or advice to users.

Tables 2 and 5 show the diagnostic accuracy results from recent publications. We found five peer-reviewed studies and one submitted study about two available mHealth apps and two mHealth apps that do not exist anymore. Of the three currently available apps, no diagnostic accuracy or other studies were found for skinScan. The other two smartphone apps were evaluated in at least one study [40], and only one app (ie, SkinVision app) [24,25] has published evidence to show whether their proprietary algorithm is accurate.

mHealth apps for skin cancer assessment (including SkinVision app) have been criticized in past studies [40,41], because their accuracy was found to be significantly lower than that of a dermatologist. In Tables 2 and 5, only three studies showed a diagnostic accuracy close to that of a dermatologist, and one of these studies [32] only showed a high accuracy for large melanoma lesions. Although some of these studies are recent, these findings are possibly already outdated, as this is a rapidly evolving field. These results could also be explained by the limited sample size, including too few skin cancer cases and selected samples, which may be inadequate to calculate sensitivity or specificity or, in the case of SkinVision app, nonutilization of the full service with the dermatologists' advice.

Overall, the amount of evidence on the diagnostic accuracy of smartphone apps is still scarce, as there are few mHealth apps providing this service. It is also difficult to make an accurate comparison between different apps, since the rate of service or algorithm change is faster than the process of peer-review publication. It could also be the case that some developers may choose to publish their results in sources that are not referenced in PubMed, namely, ArXiv. An illustrative example of these difficulties is a Cochrane review [42] published in December 2018 on the diagnostic accuracy of smartphone apps, which only found two studies but only included articles published before August 2016, making it possibly obsolete at the time of publication. For these reasons, one should be cautious when interpreting the available literature.

Table 5. Recent studies on the diagnostic accuracy of smartphone apps for risk assessment of skin lesions.

App, study, year	Location for data collection	Algorithm	Test Set	Sensitivity (95% CI)	Specificity (95% CI)	Remarks
SkinVision app, Ngoo et al, 2018 [40]	Princess Alexandra Hospital, Brisbane	Rule-based fractal algorithm version 2	1 malignant melanoma, 41 clinically suspicious lesions[a]	iOS: 57% (41-73), Android: 72% (58-87)[b]	iOS: 50% (22-78), Android: 27% (1-56)[b]	Only 1 malignant melanoma was found
SpotMole, Ngoo et al, 2018 [40]	Princess Alexandra Hospital, Brisbane	Algorithm based on the ABCDE rule	1 malignant melanoma, 41 clinically suspicious lesions[a]	43% (28-58)	80% (60-100)	Only 1 malignant melanoma was found
Dr Mole, Ngoo et al, 2018 [40]	Princess Alexandra Hospital, Brisbane	Algorithm based on the ABCDE rule	1 malignant melanoma, 41 clinically suspicious lesions[a]	21% (9-34)	100% (100-100)	Only 1 malignant melanoma was found
Lubax, Cheng et al, 2015 [32]	DermNetNZ, New Zealand, and Los Angeles[c]	Content-based image retrieval	208 lesions with melanoma[d]	90% (86-94)	92% (85-95)	Algorithm tested only on malignant melanoma (large lesions only)
Not reported, Dorairaj et al, 2017 [41][e]	Galway University Hospital	Not reported	9 malignant melanomas	80% (52-96)	9% (0-41)	Algorithm tested only on malignant melanoma

[a]All lesions had a benign final histopathology diagnosis with the exception of one melanoma in situ.

[b]Ngoo et al 2017 [40] reported the results per type of operating system: iOS/Android.

[c]DermNetZN is a publicly accessible skin lesion image database from New Zealand containing about 20,000 images. Images collected within the Los Angeles county were collected by the app company. No reference to a clinical site of the data collection was given in the publication.

[d]Algorithm was only tested on "large lesions" defined as melanomas with a diameter ≥10 mm.

[e]Despite the study being published in 2017, the study took place in 2012.

Improving the Diagnostic Accuracy of Mobile Health Apps

A promising avenue to improve the diagnostic accuracy of mHealth apps is to train machine learning algorithms on large databases of skin cancer images. Several algorithms for skin cancer classification were recently developed based on clinical or dermoscopic images, with algorithm accuracy routinely on par with a dermatologist [21,22,43]. For mHealth apps, the task of skin lesion classification is more difficult, as the images are taken by the users themselves, with variability in angle, luminosity, and smartphone model. The SkinVision app showed that skin lesion classification based on smartphone images can also achieve high accuracy (Table 2; A Udrea et al, PhD, unpublished material, 2019).

Alternatives to Mobile Health Apps

Early detection of skin cancer could be significantly improved by launching a population screening program, but this is unlikely to become common due to the high costs and lack of evidence on harms and benefits [9,44]. As the main risk factors for skin cancer like indoor tanning or ultraviolet exposure are, in large part, preventable [45], primary prevention and awareness campaigns (eg, Melanoma Monday and SunSmart in Australia) could have a better cost-benefit ratio than early detection [46]. These campaigns are a way for the general public to proactively adopt preventive behaviors and possibly learn how to recognize suspicious skin lesions [7]; they seemed to have resulted in better sun protection behavior [47]. On the other hand, this success can be reversed if these awareness efforts are not continuous [47] and they do not solve the shortages or difficulties in access to high-quality skin checks.

Training GPs or nurses with a special interest in recognizing skin cancer increases the capacity for early and accurate detection. However, compared to mHealth apps, it still requires face-to-face contact, and it is likely not enough to address all needs [13,48]. Store-and-forward teledermatology [49] allows users to take a photo and have it analyzed remotely by a dermatologist. This may solve some of the problems with access to care, but is solely based on a clinical assessment of a health care professional and is thus not automated. Smartphone apps with good performance are likely to be more efficient and could lead to larger cost savings for the health system compared to the above mentioned alternatives.

Usability Risks of Smartphone Apps

Smartphone apps pose some risks for the user, specifically, if the algorithm returns a negative result while the user has cancer, and detection and treatment of skin cancer are delayed. It is very challenging to study the rate of false-negatives due to a lack of histological verification. The user may also fail to assess all relevant skin lesions, in particular, if they are located in places that are hard to reach or that the user cannot see. Given that the specificity of SkinVision app is about 80%, there will be a few false-positive cases. This may cause unnecessary stress on users or unnecessary visits to the GP/dermatologist. Finally, the user may not follow the advice given in the smartphone app due to a lack of trust or unawareness.

Evaluating the Health Impact of Mobile Health Apps

Impact of Mobile Health Apps on Health Care Costs

A Dutch study based on national claims data observed an increase of about 67% in skin cancer–related costs between 2007 and 2017 (E. Noels, MD, unpublished data, 2019). This is due to higher costs of skin cancer treatments, for example, newly available expensive targeted immunotherapies for late-stage melanomas and, to a lesser extent, due to an increase in the skin cancer incidence. mHealth apps for self-assessment of skin lesions could limit this cost increase by (1) by detecting cancers early, which will reduce the average cost of treatment (ie, less advanced disease) and recovery and (2) reducing the need for doctor visits, since many primary care (GP)–related consultations either result in a benign diagnosis or in referrals to a specialist of cases that are later diagnosed as benign [19].

Impact of Mobile Health Apps on Public Health

Easy access to a high-quality assessment of skin lesions may lead to detection of skin cancers at an earlier stage, when their prognosis and treatment are more favorable. On the other hand, this could also cause overdiagnosis and overtreatment. Currently, evidence on the benefits and harms of skin cancer screening is insufficient [9,44]. To date, there are no randomized skin cancer screening trials, and it is unlikely that there will be new trials launched in the near future, since they would require a substantial number of patients and a long follow-up and it would be difficult and possibly unethical to guarantee that people in the control group would not access skin cancer detection methods. Consequently, it is difficult to determine whether early detection of skin cancer reduces skin cancer specific mortality. Another important target outcome could be the incidence of advanced melanoma. Therefore, indirect evidence on harms and benefits could be obtained by comparing the stage distribution of cancers detected early with a smartphone app from national registries.

Implementation of Mobile Health Apps in the Health System

The health impact of mHealth apps also depends on where it is implemented, that is, whether it is restricted to health care professionals such as GPs or dermatologists or accessible to the lay population. Offering apps directly to lay users could result in significantly greater efficiency gains for the health system; however, some regulatory bodies may prefer to restrict the usage to health care professionals to minimize usability risks. The regulatory framework is evolving quickly, with the National Institute for Health and Care Excellence in the United Kingdom suggesting a comprehensive approach to regulate mHealth technologies, taking into account not only the safety and efficacy of the app, which can be shown by carrying out a diagnostic accuracy study, but also whether it can plausibly improve current health care pathways, acceptability with users, and cost-effectiveness compared to usual care [50].

Barriers to Access of Mobile Health Apps

After implementation, the health impact of mHealth apps will also depend on the persistence of barriers to adoption among users (either lay persons or care providers). Zhao et al [51] described a technology acceptance model for mobile health [51]. For lay users, age can play a role in the rate of adoption [51]. Middle-aged and older users (the ones who are at a higher risk of skin cancer) may give more importance to the perceived amount of effort needed to learn how to use the smartphone app and the perceived personal risk for skin cancer. For clinicians, we believe the perceived ease of use also plays an important role, since clinicians have a limited amount of time. Other important factors may include perceived usefulness and efficacy of the smartphone apps, namely, whether clinicians believe in the quality of the app and whether they believe it provides the necessary information to make a clinical decision.

Postmarket Surveillance of Mobile Health Apps

A key point for mHealth apps for skin cancer detection consists of performing appropriate market surveillance activities in order to minimize usability risks, since data based on clinical studies in a controlled setting are likely not sufficient to control for differences in image-taking behavior or characteristics of the smartphone model. Algorithms used in mHealth apps should then be updated periodically, given the feedback from its users, whether they are lay users or clinicians. It is not easy to have complete follow-up from users, since due to privacy reasons, it is not straightforward for the smartphone apps to obtain access to the final clinical or histopathological diagnosis after the lesion is assessed by the algorithm.

Future Research

Research is still needed to establish the societal value of mHealth apps. First, there remains a need for more high-quality studies on their diagnostic accuracy in different populations. Second, given that these smartphone apps are accurate enough to be used by laypersons and GPs, its health and cost effects are yet to be evaluated.

The impact on the health system in terms of cost reduction due to less skin lesion–related visits still needs to be tested, ideally with a randomized control trial (RCT) accompanied by a cost-effectiveness analysis. However, performing an RCT may prove difficult. To design a trial capable of detecting a difference in the number of doctor visits, the sample size needed to carry out such a study is in the thousands, as shown by the Dutch data from 2010 [52] suggesting that about 93 consultations for every 1000 patients are related to skin cancer. The main problem is that this type of RCT has a high risk of contamination in the control group (no smartphone app), since access to smartphone apps and their usage is relatively simple. An alternative solution could be to follow a quasi-experimental approach for the design of the study [53].

In the absence of large RCTs and long-term follow-up data, modelling could be used to estimate the harms and benefits of early detection of skin cancer. There are a few studies in the literature that modelled the incidence and mortality of skin cancer [54-56]. The main drawback of these modelling studies is the difficulty in estimating tumor onset and progression. This could be addressed by forming a coalition of multiple modelling groups for skin cancer, like the Cancer Intervention and Surveillance Modelling Network (CISNET) group has done for other cancer sites [57].

Summary and Conclusions

Given the difficulties in access to high-quality care for early detection of skin cancer, there is considerable interest in developing algorithms and apps for skin cancer lesion assessment. Although mHealth apps have been criticized in the past due to their poor accuracy, the SkinVision app has a high accuracy to evaluate the risk of skin lesions for skin cancer. This was achieved due to improvements in the processing of images taken with the smartphone camera and a large risk-labeled image database from users, which was used to train a machine learning algorithm.

However, there are still many open questions regarding the usage of mHealth apps. National health authorities need to decide where to position these apps in the health care system (lay population, GPs, or dermatologists). Health effects of early and more accurate detection are difficult to estimate. There is currently no high-quality evidence on the health and cost benefits and harms of early detection of skin cancer, namely, on the trade-off between doctor visits and lives saved/advanced cases avoided. The reduction of the skin cancer burden on the health system and in the population could be substantial, as earlier detection of skin cancer could result in a lower average cost of treatment and a reduction in the number of doctor visits. However, further studies are needed to confirm this.

References

1. Siegel R, Miller KD, Jemal A. Cancer statistics, 2018. CA Cancer J Clin 2018 Dec;68(1):7-30 [FREE Full text] [doi: 10.3322/caac.21442] [Medline: 29313949]
2. Rogers HW, Weinstock MA, Feldman SR, Coldiron BM. Incidence Estimate of Nonmelanoma Skin Cancer (Keratinocyte Carcinomas) in the U.S. Population, 2012. JAMA Dermatol 2015 Oct;151(10):1081-1086. [doi: 10.1001/jamadermatol.2015.1187] [Medline: 25928283]
3. Karimkhani C, Green AC, Nijsten T, Weinstock MA, Dellavalle RP, Naghavi M, et al. The global burden of melanoma: results from the Global Burden of Disease Study 2015. Br J Dermatol 2017 Jul 30;177(1):134-140 [FREE Full text] [doi: 10.1111/bjd.15510] [Medline: 28369739]
4. Whiteman DC, Green AC, Olsen CM. The Growing Burden of Invasive Melanoma: Projections of Incidence Rates and Numbers of New Cases in Six Susceptible Populations through 2031. J Invest Dermatol 2016 Jun;136(6):1161-1171 [FREE Full text] [doi: 10.1016/j.jid.2016.01.035] [Medline: 26902923]
5. Erdmann F, Lortet-Tieulent J, Schüz J, Zeeb H, Greinert R, Breitbart EW, et al. International trends in the incidence of malignant melanoma 1953-2008--are recent generations at higher or lower risk? Int J Cancer 2013 Jan 15;132(2):385-400 [FREE Full text] [doi: 10.1002/ijc.27616] [Medline: 22532371]
6. Apalla Z, Nashan D, Weller RB, Castellsagué X. Skin Cancer: Epidemiology, Disease Burden, Pathophysiology, Diagnosis, and Therapeutic Approaches. Dermatol Ther (Heidelb) 2017 Jan;7(Suppl 1):5-19 [FREE Full text] [doi: 10.1007/s13555-016-0165-y] [Medline: 28150105]
7. Iannacone MR, Green AC. Towards skin cancer prevention and early detection: evolution of skin cancer awareness campaigns in Australia. Melanoma Manag 2014 Aug;1(1):75-84 [FREE Full text] [doi: 10.2217/mmt.14.6] [Medline: 30190812]
8. Johnson MM, Leachman SA, Aspinwall LG, Cranmer LD, Curiel-Lewandrowski C, Sondak VK, et al. Skin cancer screening: recommendations for data-driven screening guidelines and a review of the US Preventive Services Task Force controversy. Melanoma Manag 2017 Mar;4(1):13-37 [FREE Full text] [doi: 10.2217/mmt-2016-0022] [Medline: 28758010]
9. US Preventive Services Task Force, Bibbins-Domingo K, Grossman DC, Curry SJ, Davidson KW, Ebell M, et al. Screening for Skin Cancer: US Preventive Services Task Force Recommendation Statement. JAMA 2016 Jul 26;316(4):429-435. [doi: 10.1001/jama.2016.8465] [Medline: 27458948]
10. Okhovat J, Beaulieu D, Tsao H, Halpern AC, Michaud DS, Shaykevich S, et al. The first 30 years of the American Academy of Dermatology skin cancer screening program: 1985-2014. J Am Acad Dermatol 2018 Nov;79(5):884-891.e3 [FREE Full text] [doi: 10.1016/j.jaad.2018.05.1242] [Medline: 30057360]
11. Geller AC, Greinert R, Sinclair C, Weinstock MA, Aitken J, Boniol M, et al. A nationwide population-based skin cancer screening in Germany: proceedings of the first meeting of the International Task Force on Skin Cancer Screening and

Prevention (September 24 and 25, 2009). Cancer Epidemiol 2010 Jun;34(3):355-358. [doi: 10.1016/j.canep.2010.03.006] [Medline: 20381443]
12. Trautmann F, Meier F, Seidler A, Schmitt J. Effects of the German skin cancer screening programme on melanoma incidence and indicators of disease severity. Br J Dermatol 2016 Nov;175(5):912-919. [doi: 10.1111/bjd.14758] [Medline: 27203791]
13. Kimball AB, Resneck JS. The US dermatology workforce: a specialty remains in shortage. J Am Acad Dermatol 2008 Nov;59(5):741-745. [doi: 10.1016/j.jaad.2008.06.037] [Medline: 18723242]
14. Aneja S, Aneja S, Bordeaux JS. Association of increased dermatologist density with lower melanoma mortality. Arch Dermatol 2012 Feb;148(2):174-178. [doi: 10.1001/archdermatol.2011.345] [Medline: 22351816]
15. Goulding JMR, Levine S, Blizard RA, Deroide F, Swale VJ. Dermatological surgery: a comparison of activity and outcomes in primary and secondary care. Br J Dermatol 2009 Jul;161(1):110-114. [doi: 10.1111/j.1365-2133.2009.09228.x] [Medline: 19438854]
16. Koelink CJL, Vermeulen KM, Kollen BJ, de Bock GH, Dekker JH, Jonkman MF, et al. Diagnostic accuracy and cost-effectiveness of dermoscopy in primary care: a cluster randomized clinical trial. J Eur Acad Dermatol Venereol 2014 Nov;28(11):1442-1449. [Medline: 25493316]
17. Swetter SM, Chang J, Shaub AR, Weinstock MA, Lewis ET, Asch SM. Primary Care-Based Skin Cancer Screening in a Veterans Affairs Health Care System. JAMA Dermatol 2017 Dec 01;153(8):797-801 [FREE Full text] [doi: 10.1001/jamadermatol.2017.1324] [Medline: 28593242]
18. Beecher SM, Keogh C, Healy C. Dedicated general practitioner education sessions can improve diagnostic capabilities and may have a positive effect on referral patterns for common skin lesions. Ir J Med Sci 2018 Nov;187(4):959-963. [doi: 10.1007/s11845-018-1788-z] [Medline: 29541934]
19. Ahmadi K, Prickaerts E, Smeets JGE, Joosten VHMJ, Kelleners-Smeets NWJ, Dinant GJ. Current approach of skin lesions suspected of malignancy in general practice in the Netherlands: a quantitative overview. J Eur Acad Dermatol Venereol 2018 Feb;32(2):236-241. [doi: 10.1111/jdv.14484] [Medline: 28750138]
20. van Rijsingen MCJ, Hanssen SCA, Groenewoud JMM, van der Wilt GJ, Gerritsen MP. Referrals by general practitioners for suspicious skin lesions: the urgency of training. Acta Derm Venereol 2014 Mar;94(2):138-141 [FREE Full text] [doi: 10.2340/00015555-1752] [Medline: 24352366]
21. Esteva A, Kuprel B, Novoa RA, Ko J, Swetter SM, Blau HM, et al. Dermatologist-level classification of skin cancer with deep neural networks. Nature 2017 Dec 02;542(7639):115-118. [doi: 10.1038/nature21056] [Medline: 28117445]
22. Haenssle HA, Fink C, Schneiderbauer R, Toberer F, Buhl T, Blum A, Reader study level-Ilevel-II Groups. Man against machine: diagnostic performance of a deep learning convolutional neural network for dermoscopic melanoma recognition in comparison to 58 dermatologists. Ann Oncol 2018 Aug 01;29(8):1836-1842. [doi: 10.1093/annonc/mdy166] [Medline: 29846502]
23. Udrea A, Lupu C. Real-time acquisition of quality verified non-standardized color images for skin lesions risk assessment? A preliminary study, 18th International Conference on System Theory, Control and Computing (ICSTCC), 2014. 2014 Presented at: 18th International Conference on System Theory; 2014; Sinaia, Romania. [doi: 10.1109/ICSTCC.2014.6982415]
24. Maier T, Kulichova D, Schotten K, Astrid R, Ruzicka T, Berking C, et al. Accuracy of a smartphone application using fractal image analysis of pigmented moles compared to clinical diagnosis and histological result. J Eur Acad Dermatol Venereol 2015 Apr;29(4):663-667. [doi: 10.1111/jdv.12648] [Medline: 25087492]
25. Thissen M, Udrea A, Hacking M, von Braunmuehl T, Ruzicka T. mHealth App for Risk Assessment of Pigmented and Nonpigmented Skin Lesions-A Study on Sensitivity and Specificity in Detecting Malignancy. Telemed J E Health 2017 May 31. [doi: 10.1089/tmj.2016.0259] [Medline: 28562195]
26. Isola P, Zhou JY, Zhou T, Efros A. Image-to-Image Translation with Conditional Adversarial Networks. 2017 Presented at: IEEE Conference on Computer Vision and Pattern Recognition; 2017; Honolulu, Hawai, United States p. 3.
27. Telea A. An Image Inpainting Technique Based on the Fast Marching Method. Journal of Graphics Tools 2004;9(1):25-36. [doi: 10.1080/10867651.2004]
28. Li J, Li B. Parameters Selection for Support Vector Machine Based on Particle Swarm Optimization. Intelligent Computing Theory 2014;8588:41-47. [doi: 10.1007/978-3-319-09333-8_5]
29. Ngoo A, Finnane A, McMeniman E, Soyer H, Janda M. Fighting Melanoma with Smartphones: A Snapshot of Where We are a Decade after App Stores Opened Their Doors. Int J Med Inform 2018;118:99-112. [Medline: 30153928]
30. Kassianos AP, Emery JD, Murchie P, Walter FM. Smartphone applications for melanoma detection by community, patient and generalist clinician users: a review. Br J Dermatol 2015 Jun;172(6):1507-1518. [doi: 10.1111/bjd.13665] [Medline: 25600815]
31. AppAdvice. Derma Compare by Emerald Medical Applications URL: https://appadvice.com/app/derma-compare/982517772 [accessed 2019-07-02]
32. Chen R, Snorrason M, Enger S, Mostafa E, Ko J, Aoki V, et al. Validation of a Skin-Lesion Image-Matching Algorithm Based on Computer Vision Technology. Telemed J E Health 2016 Jan;22(1):45-50. [doi: 10.1089/tmj.2014.0249] [Medline: 26218353]
33. AppAdvice. Lubax - Skin lesion ID using image recognition by Lubax, Inc URL: https://appadvice.com/app/lubax-skin-lesion-id-using-image-recognition/956423382 [accessed 2019-07-02]
34. AppBrain. mSkin Doctor Mobile Application for Skin Cancer Detection by Aleem Technologies URL: https://www.

appbrain.com/app/mskin-doctor/com.maleemtaufiq.mSkinDoctor [accessed 2019-07-02]

35. AppAdvice. MySkinMap by Xyrupt Technologies, LLC URL: https://appadvice.com/app/myskinmap/1151655127 [accessed 2019-07-02]
36. AppAdvice. SkinScan by TeleSkin ApS URL: https://appadvice.com/app/skinscan/1025190936 [accessed 2019-07-02]
37. SkinVision. URL: https://www.skinvision.com/ [accessed 2019-07-02]
38. Google Play. SpotMole URL: https://play.google.com/store/apps/details?id=com.spotmole&hl=nl [accessed 2019-07-02]
39. American Cancer Society. Signs and Symptoms of Melanoma Skin Cancer URL: https://www.cancer.org/cancer/melanoma-skin-cancer/detection-diagnosis-staging/signs-and-symptoms.html [accessed 2019-07-02]
40. Ngoo A, Finnane A, McMeniman E, Tan J, Janda M, Soyer HP. Efficacy of smartphone applications in high-risk pigmented lesions. Australas J Dermatol 2017 Feb 27. [doi: 10.1111/ajd.12599] [Medline: 28240347]
41. Dorairaj JJ, Healy GM, McInerney A, Hussey AJ. Validation of a Melanoma Risk Assessment Smartphone Application. Dermatol Surg 2017 Feb;43(2):299-302. [doi: 10.1097/DSS.0000000000000916] [Medline: 28165352]
42. Chuchu N, Takwoingi Y, Dinnes J, Matin R, Bassett O, Moreau J, Cochrane Skin Cancer Diagnostic Test Accuracy Group. Smartphone applications for triaging adults with skin lesions that are suspicious for melanoma. Cochrane Database Syst Rev 2018 Dec 04;12:CD013192. [doi: 10.1002/14651858.CD013192] [Medline: 30521685]
43. Brinker TJ, Hekler A, Utikal JS, Grabe N, Schadendorf D, Klode J, et al. Skin Cancer Classification Using Convolutional Neural Networks: Systematic Review. J Med Internet Res 2018 Dec 17;20(10):e11936 [FREE Full text] [doi: 10.2196/11936] [Medline: 30333097]
44. Brunssen A, Waldmann A, Eisemann N, Katalinic A. Impact of skin cancer screening and secondary prevention campaigns on skin cancer incidence and mortality: A systematic review. J Am Acad Dermatol 2017;76(1):e10. [Medline: 27707591]
45. Linos E, Katz KA, Colditz G. Skin Cancer-The Importance of Prevention. JAMA Intern Med 2016;176(10):1435-1436. [Medline: 27459394]
46. Gordon L, Rowell D. Health system costs of skin cancer and cost-effectiveness of skin cancer prevention and screening: a systematic review. Eur J Cancer Prev 2015;24(2). [Medline: 25089375]
47. Makin JK, Warne CD, Dobbinson SJ, Wakefield MA, Hill DJ. Population and age-group trends in weekend sun protection and sunburn over two decades of the SunSmart programme in Melbourne, Australia. Br J Dermatol 2013 Jan;168(1):154-161. [doi: 10.1111/bjd.12082] [Medline: 23039760]
48. Porter M, Kimball A. Predictions, Surprises, and the Future of the Dermatology Workforce. JAMA Dermatol 2018;154(11):1253-1255. [Medline: 30193360]
49. Bashshur R, Shannon G, Tejasvi T, Kvedar J, Gates M. The Empirical Foundations of Teledermatology: A Review of the Research Evidence. Telemed J E Health 2015;21(12). [Medline: 26394022]
50. National Institute for Health and Care Excellence. 2019. Evidence Standards Framework for Digital Health Technologies, March 2019 URL: https://www.nice.org.uk/Media/Default/About/what-we-do/our-programmes/evidence-standards-framework/digital-evidence-standards-framework.pdf [accessed 2019-07-02]
51. Zhao Y, Ni Q, Zhou R. What factors influence the mobile health service adoption? A meta-analysis and the moderating role of age. International Journal of Information Management 2018 Dec;43:342-350. [doi: 10.1016/j.ijinfomgt.2017.08.006]
52. Koelink C, Kollen B, Groenhof F, van der Meer K, van der Heide W. Skin lesions suspected of malignancy: an increasing burden on general practice. BMC Fam Pract 2014;15. [Medline: 24517098]
53. Geldsetzer P, Fawzi W. Quasi-experimental study designs series-paper 2: complementary approaches to advancing global health knowledge. J Clin Epidemiol 2017;89:12-16. [Medline: 28365307]
54. Eisemann N, Waldmann A, Garbe C, Katalinic A. Development of a microsimulation of melanoma mortality for evaluating the effectiveness of population-based skin cancer screening. Med Decis Making 2015;35(2):243-254. [Medline: 25145574]
55. Pil L, Hoorens I, Vossaert K, Kruse V, Tromme I, Speybroeck N, et al. Cost-effectiveness and Budget Effect Analysis of a Population-Based Skin Cancer Screening. JAMA Dermatol 2017 Feb 01;153(2):147-153. [doi: 10.1001/jamadermatol.2016.4518] [Medline: 28002834]
56. Losina E, Walensky R, Geller A, Beddingfield F, Wolf L, Gilchrest B, et al. Visual screening for malignant melanoma: a cost-effectiveness analysis. Arch Dermatol 2007 Jan;143(1):21-28 [FREE Full text] [doi: 10.1001/archderm.143.1.21] [Medline: 17224538]
57. Lansdorp-Vogelaar I, Gulati R, Mariotto A, Schechter C, de Carvalho T, Knudsen A, et al. Personalizing age of cancer screening cessation based on comorbid conditions: model estimates of harms and benefits. Ann Intern Med 2014 Jul 15;161(2):104-112 [FREE Full text] [doi: 10.7326/M13-2867] [Medline: 25023249]

Abbreviations

BCC: basal cell carcinoma
CISNET: Cancer Intervention and Surveillance Modelling Network
GP: general practitioner
mHealth: mobile health
MM: malignant melanoma
RCT: randomized control trial
SCC: squamous cell carcinoma
SVM: support vector machine

5

Information About Sunscreen on YouTube and Considerations for Sun Safety Promotion: Content Analysis

Anne K Julian[1], MA, PhD; Jessica Welch[1], BS; Maddison M Bean[2], MS; Sarah Shahid[1], BS; Frank M Perna[1], EdD, PhD

[1]Behavioral Research Program, Division of Cancer Control and Population Sciences, National Cancer Institute, Rockville, MD, United States
[2]College of Public Health and Human Sciences, Oregon State University, Corvallis, OR, United States

Corresponding Author:
Anne K Julian, MA, PhD
Behavioral Research Program
Division of Cancer Control and Population Sciences
National Cancer Institute
9609 Medical Center Dr
Rockville, MD, 20877
United States

Email: anne.julian@nih.gov

Abstract

Background: Sunscreen use is a popular sun protection method; however, application of sunscreen rarely meets the standards recommended for effectiveness. Access to information about how to effectively use sunscreen may play a role in proper sunscreen application. The internet is a common health information source; however, the quality of sunscreen-related content varies.

Objective: The objective of this study was to examine information about sunscreen in YouTube videos by video source.

Methods: In November 2017, the authors identified the 20 most popular YouTube videos (sorted by view count and relevance) for each of these 5 search terms: sunscreen cancer, sunscreen health, sunscreen information, sunscreen ingredients, and sunscreen natural. The inclusion criteria were English language and view count >1000 (N=111 unique videos). We double-coded videos for standard recommendations for sunscreen use (eg, apply 20 minutes before sun exposure), use of outdated terminology, and recommendation of complementary sun safety strategies.

Results: The view counts ranged from 1100 to 671,142 (median 17,774, SD 109,651) and the average daily views ranged from 1 to 1448 (median 23, SD 234). End users (46/111, 41.4%) and health care providers (24/111, 21.6%) were the most common sources, and none of the most popular videos were produced by federal agencies or cancer-related nongovernmental organizations. Health care provider videos included marginally more recommendations than end user videos (mean 1.46, SD 1.96 vs mean 1.05, SD 1.20), but few (19/111, 17.1%) mentioned reapplication. The videos were generally positive toward sunscreen (82/111, 73.9%); however, some videos were negative (29/111, 26.1%), with warnings about the health risks of chemical sunscreens and their ingredients. Do-it-yourself sunscreen tutorials represented 19/111 (17.1%) of the sample.

Conclusions: YouTube is a potential source for disseminating sun safety messages; however, the quality of its sunscreen content varies. Most of the videos in our study failed to include important sunscreen use recommendations. Clinicians should be prepared to address the information needs of patients by discussing effective, evidence-based sunscreen application and recommending a combined sun safety approach.

KEYWORDS

sunscreen; social media; sun safety; cancer prevention

Introduction

Skin cancer affects an estimated 5 million people annually in the United States, with a treatment cost of over $8.1 billion [1]. Ultraviolet (UV) radiation is a known carcinogen that causes direct and indirect DNA damage; intentional or unintentional UV exposure is responsible for the majority of skin cancer incidence [2]. Sunscreen is a primary sun protection strategy that is used by approximately one third of US adults [3]; however, sunscreen application rarely reflects the standards necessary to meet the advertised protection levels [4,5]. Furthermore, sunscreen is intended for use in combination with other sun protection strategies [6]. In 2012, the US Food and Drug Administration (FDA) issued new regulations for sunscreen labeling [7]; however, research has demonstrated that sunscreen application rarely reflects the thickness, evenness, and timing (of both initial application and reapplication) necessary to meet the advertised protection level of the sunscreen [8]. In 2014, the Surgeon General's Call to Action to Prevent Skin Cancer included a renewed call to promote a combination sun protection strategy (eg, wearing sunscreen, a hat, and protective clothing) [5].

The Centers for Disease Control and Prevention (CDC) and the American Academy of Dermatology support the daily use of sunscreen with a sun protection factor (SPF) of at least 15 and 30, respectively, for UV protection, and dermatologists report recommending the use of sunscreen to their patients [9]. Although health care providers are trusted sources of health information, individuals increasingly supplement these sources with information garnered from the internet and social media [10]. In 2012, 72% of US adults had sought health information on the internet within the past 12 months [10]. The growing influence of social media in health decision making is not equally distributed across demographic and age groups; young age is a consistent predictor of social media use [11]; however, social media usage among adults is steadily increasing [12,13]. YouTube, the most prominent user-generated video-sharing website, allows any person to upload content on any topic [10]; based on traffic, it was the top-ranked website on the internet as of 2019 [14]. Furthermore, YouTube is increasingly being used as a platform to disseminate health information [15]. The American Cancer Society, National Institutes of Health, and National Cancer Institute have adopted this outlet to communicate health messages to broad audiences.

Despite these efforts, misleading or incorrect health information is common on YouTube [15]. For example, over one half of videos on the topic of immunization feature negative views or contradict the reference standard, which may lead viewers to make unsafe health decisions [16]. With respect to skin cancer, Basch et al [17] found YouTube content promoting untested home remedies for skin cancer, such as black salve; this finding highlights the challenge of health communication on social media. Moreover, a study of sun safety topics on YouTube [18] found that 17% of videos retrieved using the search term "sunscreen" included false or misleading information; however, less than a quarter of the videos in their sample were English language videos. Sunscreen use in practice is less thorough than recommended, and the question remains whether this is due in part to incomplete or misleading information available on social media platforms such as YouTube; this is especially likely to be the case if the content is not derived from governmental or professional medical organizations who create sun safety recommendations. Here, we analyzed a large sample of English language YouTube videos about sunscreen to address the following research questions: What primary sources, content types, positive/negative product attributions (valence), and adherence to standard recommendations [7] are included in YouTube videos about sunscreen? Do these videos contain the terms "sunblock" and "waterproof," which the FDA prohibits on sunscreen packaging? What complementary sun protection strategies do these videos include?

These data may inform public health video messaging to improve sun safety practices for effective sunburn prevention.

Methods

We conducted direct YouTube searches between November 13 and November 15, 2017 (search terms: sunscreen cancer, sunscreen health, sunscreen information, sunscreen ingredients, and sunscreen natural), deleting cookies after each search to avoid influencing subsequent results [19]. The YouTube region was set to United States. We identified the 20 most frequently appearing videos for each search term and removed duplicates to obtain the analytic sample of videos (see Figure 1).

We developed an early draft codebook in consultation with sun safety and communication experts to reflect common metrics in YouTube-based health information studies and sunscreen recommendation reference standards. This draft was then expanded and refined to include the recommendation of nonsunscreen sun safety methods, use of the outdated terms "sunblock" and "waterproof," and possible themes related to sunscreen safety. The codebook was pilot-tested using a test set of 5 videos by a team that included 3 experts in sun safety and 1 postbaccalaureate fellow. These videos were chosen using an extreme cases approach and reflected a diverse range of content and positions toward sunscreen. The codebook development team met to discuss and resolve coding discrepancies, generate additional constructs and codes, and refine coding response options.

After the initial codebook refinement, the coding team (MG, SS, JW, and AJ) double-coded all videos for the presence of 6 standard recommendations for effective sunscreen use based on FDA and CDC recommendations: SPF level, broad spectrum classification, application timing (20 minutes before exposure), liberal/generous application, and reapplication (every 2 hours and separately after toweling). We coded the overall valence toward sunscreen as negative or positive. We coded the use of the terms "sunblock" and "waterproof"; since 2011, the FDA has prohibited these terms on sunscreen labels, as they may be misleading [7]. We further coded the video source based on the posting source of the video and the posting channel's thumbnail and description. Lastly, we coded recommendation of the following complementary sun protection strategies (operationalized as instruction to adopt): seeking shade, wearing a hat, wearing protective clothing, wearing sunglasses, and staying indoors during peak UV hours (Cohen kappa range 0.80-0.96). Viewer attention to social media content is short [20]; therefore, we stopped coding each video after 5 minutes. Any final disagreement was resolved through discussion. We used Stata/SE 14 [21] to calculate descriptive statistics (means, medians and standard deviations, ranges and percentages) overall and stratified by video source.

Figure 1. YouTube video search flow chart depicting the number of unique videos retrieved from YouTube in November 2017 using the search terms sunscreen information, sunscreen health, sunscreen natural, sunscreen ingredients, and sunscreen cancer and the final number of videos meeting the English language requirement. Relevance is a proprietary search algorithm owned by YouTube.

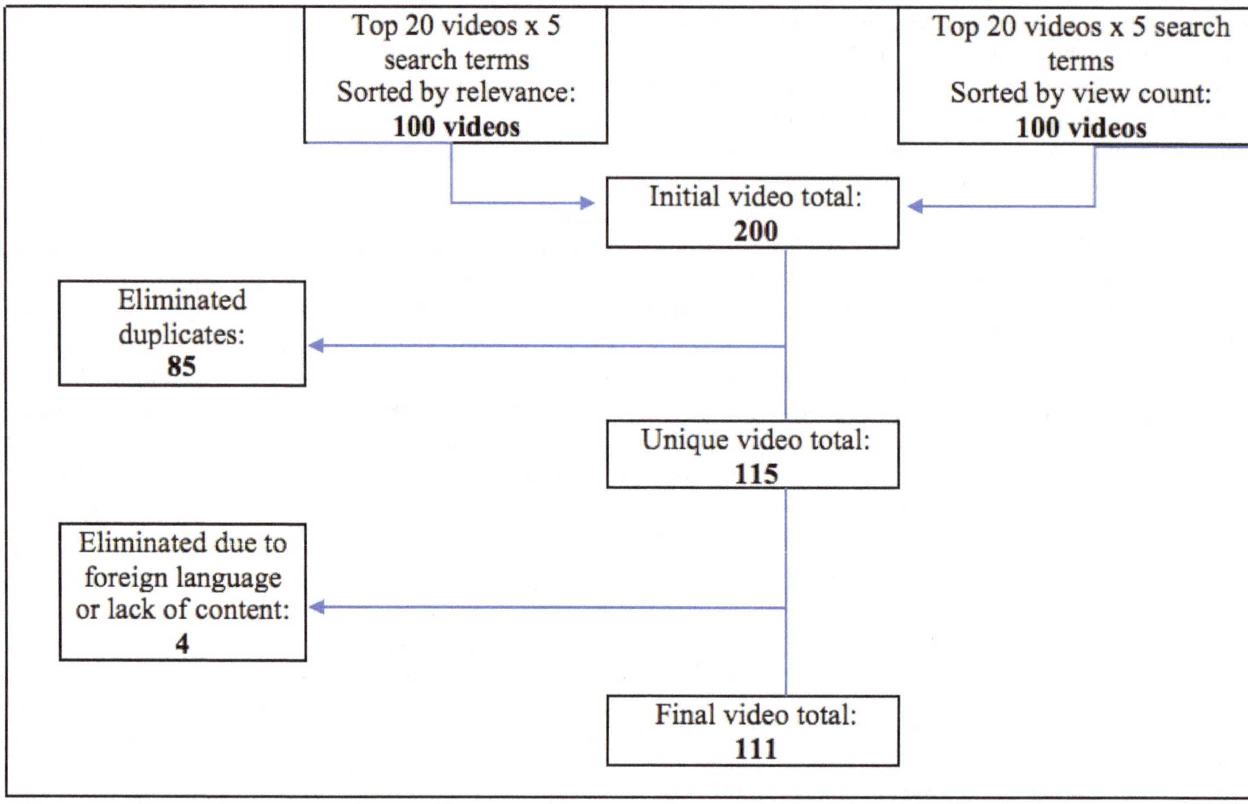

Results

The videos had view counts of 1100 to 671,142 (mean 58,642, median 17,774, SD 109,651), were between 40 seconds and 41 minutes long (mean 5:54 minutes, median 4:19 minutes), and were uploaded between 2009 and 2017 (average post duration 1127 days, median 1101, range 64-3135, SD 784). Average daily views ranged from 1 to 1448 (mean 96.8, median 23, SD 234). Primary video sources were health care providers or their associations (24/111, 21.6%), end users (51/111, 45.9%), and corporate entities (15/111, 13.5%) (see Table 1 for the descriptive characteristics of the videos). No government health agencies were among the sources of videos retrieved. Valence toward sunscreen use was generally positive (82/111, 73.9%); however, positive content included promotion of mineral sunscreens that warned about health risks of chemical sunscreens. Videos that discouraged sunscreen use (29/111, 26.2%) included misleading content, such as overstatement of the benefits of vitamin D, and outright falsehoods, such as the claim that sunscreen causes cancer.

Of the 6 recommendations for effective sunscreen use, the most frequently mentioned were SPF (35/111, 31.5%) and broad-spectrum classification (30/111, 27.0%); meanwhile, application timing, generous application, reapplication every 2 hours, and reapplication after toweling were each mentioned in fewer than 20% of videos (see Table 2). Most videos included 0, 1, or 2 recommendations. SPF was mentioned in 5/9 (55%) of news and television coverage videos. Corporate entities, such as sunscreen or skin care companies, most frequently recommended generous application (4/14 videos, 29%); however, 6/14 (43%) of these videos paired this message with a poor demonstration of sunscreen application.

Few videos advocated the use of complementary sun protection strategies in conjunction with sunscreen (19/111, 17.1%). Of videos with positive valence toward sunscreen, 15/82 (18.3%) suggested complementary sun protection strategies, compared to 3/29 (10.3%) of videos with negative valence (see Table 2).

Few videos cited scientific sources for the presented information (30/111, 27.0%). Sources of scientific information were the Environmental Working Group (EWG), an environmental advocacy group (13/111, 11.7%), the FDA (7/111, 6.3%), and peer-reviewed articles (5/111 videos, 4.5%). Lastly, an unexpected finding was that 19/111 (17.1%) of videos demonstrated do-it-yourself recipes for how to make sunscreen at home.

Table 1. Video content types, sources, and characteristics (N=111).

Video characteristic	Frequency, n (%)
Content type	
Public service announcement	4 (3.6)
Medical advice	24 (21.5)
Scientific explanation	12 (10.8)
Product demonstration/promotion	14 (12.6)
Do-it-yourself sunscreen tutorial	19 (17.1)
Opinion/commentary	23 (20.7)
Televised news clip	15 (13.5)
Source	
Nongovernmental organization	5 (4.5)
News organization	9 (8.1)
Health care provider[a]	24 (21.6)
End user	51 (45.9)
Corporation	15 (13.5)
Topic-based group channel	7 (6.3)
Use of outdated terms[b]	
Sunblock	13 (11.7)
Waterproof	5 (4.5)
Valence[c]	
Positive	82 (73.9)
Negative	29 (26.1)
Total number of recommendations	
0	54 (48.6)
1	20 (18.0)
2	19 (17.1)
3	9 (8.1)
4	3 (2.7)
5	4 (3.6)
6	2 (1.8)

[a]"Health care provider" was broadly defined to include physicians, nurses, and their organizations as well as people who self-identified as doctors but whose credentials did not include a medical degree. Videos featuring a doctor as the primary messenger were coded for the credentials of the provider; these included allopathic doctors (MD, DO), nonmedical doctors (PhD), and complementary or alternative medicine practitioners (DC, ND, MD(H)).

[b]In videos using the terms "sunblock" and "waterproof," 5 and 2 respectively used it in the context of an explanation that the term is considered misleading and should no longer be used.

[c]Videos coded as positive toward sunscreen include those that promoted the use or home manufacture of mineral or "natural" sunscreens but that also included warnings about potential negative effects of chemical or commercial sunscreens on humans or the environment.

Table 2. Standard recommendations for sunscreen use, overall and by video source[a].

Recommendation	Overall (N=111)	Health care provider (n=24)	Corporation (n=14)	News (n=9)	End user (n=47)
Sunscreen application, n (%)					
Choose a broad spectrum	30 (27)	5 (22)	2 (14)	4 (44)	14 (30)
SPF level 15+	35 (32)	8 (36)	3 (21)	5 (55)	16 (37)
Apply 20 minutes before exposure	14 (13)	6 (26)	2 (14)	1 (11)	2 (3)
Reapply every 2 hours	16 (14)	5 (22)	2 (14)	1 (11)	2 (3)
Apply a generous amount	19 (17)	5 (22)	4 (29)	1 (11)	5 (10)
Reapply after toweling	12 (11)	4 (17)	2 (14)	1 (11)	2 (3)
Complementary sun protection, n (%)					
Wear a wide-brimmed hat	1 (4)	1 (4)	1 (0)	2 (22)	2 (4)
Wear protective clothing	12 (11)	1 (4)	0 (0)	3 (33)	3 (6)
Wear sunglasses	8 (7)	1 (4)	0 (0)	2 (22)	1 (2)
Seek shade/use an umbrella	11 (10)	0 (0)	0 (0)	3 (33)	3 (6)
Stay indoors during peak UV periods	6 (5)	0 (0)	0 (0)	1 (11)	1 (2)

[a]Due to small cell sizes, videos from nongovernmental organizations and sources coded as "Other," which included topic-based group channels and sources that were not classifiable, were omitted from these group analyses. Therefore, the rows do not total 100%.

Discussion

Principal Findings

Incomplete or misleading information about sunscreen is common on YouTube and may play a role in sunscreen misuse, as reported in the literature [4,5]. In light of research on the quality of videos covering other areas of health information, the variable accuracy we found with respect to sunscreen use is not surprising [9]. Consistent with previous literature, no videos produced by government health agencies or cancer-related NGOs were among the most popular or relevant [13]. The EWG was the most-cited source of scientific information, but these video references were typically decontextualized statements about possible harms of common sunscreen chemicals (eg, oxybenzone and octinoxate) used in pitches to promote and sometimes sell other products. The outdated terms "sunblock" and "waterproof" were rarely used, but the videos generally failed to include all standard recommendations for effective sunscreen use or to recommend a combined sun protection approach. In the absence of instruction on application thickness, reapplication, and complementary sun protection measures, the emphasis we observed on SPF and broad-spectrum classification may perpetuate ineffective sunscreen use.

Unexpected Findings

Some videos contradicted sun safety recommendations, warned about health risks or dangerous ingredients of sunscreen, or included do-it-yourself recipes. Although these videos were not the majority, this finding is surprising and somewhat alarming in that some of these videos featured health care–affiliated spokespersons. These providers represented a subset of health care providers on YouTube and were primarily promoters of alternative or naturopathic medicine. The do-it-yourself sunscreen tutorial was a concerning and unexpected content category, as our search strategy did not target this content. Do-it-yourself sunscreen recipes have not undergone the testing that is required by the FDA and cannot be assumed to be effective. Some "recipes" included no approved sunscreen ingredients and instead promoted ingredients such as green tea and coconut oil. Clinicians should be aware of such videos and should be prepared to address the topic with patients who are considering making their own sunscreen. While recent research on sunscreen absorption [22] may raise public concern, especially about the use of sunscreen by children, the extant recommendations are unchanged; we can conclude from available evidence that sunscreen is safe and that its use is superior to unprotected exposure for children and adults (for infants under 6 months of age, sunscreen is not recommended; rather, sun exposure should be avoided completely) [23]. Guidance such as use of a mineral sunscreen, sun avoidance strategies, and use of protective clothing and hats [23] may be particularly useful to parents who are concerned about using sunscreen products on children.

Limitations

The YouTube videos analyzed here represent one point in time. Videos that are highly popular at one point may fade in popularity over time and may therefore not be prominent in subsequent searches. In our approach, we intentionally used neutral search terms associated with sunscreen and then gauged the valence of the most popular and relevant videos. Positive or negative search terms may yield different types of content; also, the search algorithms such as "relevance" used by YouTube are proprietary and may change over time, thus yielding different search results. Sunscreen videos are a narrow topic, and the most popular videos still do not qualify as generally popular, as viral videos have millions of views. Furthermore, not all adults use sunscreen, and individuals seeking information about sunscreen specifically from government health agencies may not use the YouTube application programming interface and may instead use Google or search the agency's website. The number of videos contradicting standard recommendations for sun safety or demonstrating do-it-yourself sunscreen was unanticipated; however, the behavioral significance of this finding is unclear.

Conclusion

Sunscreen use is a common and important form of sun protection, and YouTube is a common source of health information; it is especially popular among teens and young adults, which are the developmental groups with the highest rates of sunburn [3]. This study fills an important gap in the literature by offering a comprehensive examination of sunscreen information on YouTube, a common source of information for young people. The public currently bears the burden of judging the credibility of sunscreen messages; however, a challenge inherent in our findings is that health care providers depicted in videos (who are generally trusted sources of information) were not, as a rule, arbiters of high-quality sunscreen information. While the popular videos sampled were generally positive toward sunscreen use, the information content appears to be problematic in 2 ways. First, sunscreen-related content on YouTube infrequently recommends complementary sun safety strategies. This is particularly problematic when videos explicitly discourage sunscreen use [24]. Second, a small but not unimportant percentage of popular videos contained misleading information.

YouTube is a promising tool to share information on effective sunscreen use; however, incomplete or negative content about sunscreen is common, and in some cases, this content is communicated by health care–affiliated messengers. Further, health agencies that produce YouTube videos related to sun protection were not among the more popular or relevant video sources. These data highlight a challenge of using YouTube for public health communication: how to create eye-catching content that will reliably be identified by social media search algorithms. To better harness YouTube for disseminating sun safety messages, health agencies may look to increase their content visibility by better incorporating features such as memorable titles and keyword tags to increase their popularity. Considering the increasing popularity of YouTube as a source of health information, further research is warranted to examine viewer response to these videos and to determine whether exposure to the videos impacts subsequent sun safety behavior.

Acknowledgments

The authors would like to acknowledge the contributions of Anne Hartman, who assisted in codebook development.

References

1. Guy GP, Machlin SR, Ekwueme DU, Yabroff KR. Prevalence and costs of skin cancer treatment in the U.S., 2002-2006 and 2007-2011. Am J Prev Med 2015 Feb;48(2):183-187 [FREE Full text] [doi: 10.1016/j.amepre.2014.08.036] [Medline: 25442229]
2. Armstrong BK, Kricker A. The epidemiology of UV induced skin cancer. J Photoch Photobio B 2001 Oct;63(1-3):8-18. [doi: 10.1016/s1011-1344(01)00198-1]
3. Holman DM, Ding H, Guy GP, Watson M, Hartman AM, Perna FM. Prevalence of Sun Protection Use and Sunburn and Association of Demographic and Behaviorial Characteristics With Sunburn Among US Adults. JAMA Dermatol 2018 May 01;154(5):561-568 [FREE Full text] [doi: 10.1001/jamadermatol.2018.0028] [Medline: 29541756]
4. Pratt H, Hassanin K, Troughton LD, Czanner G, Zheng Y, McCormick AG, et al. UV imaging reveals facial areas that are prone to skin cancer are disproportionately missed during sunscreen application. PLoS One 2017;12(10):e0185297 [FREE Full text] [doi: 10.1371/journal.pone.0185297] [Medline: 28968413]
5. US Dept of Health and Human Services, Office of the Surgeon General. 2014. The Surgeon General's Call to Action to Prevent Skin Cancer URL: https://www.hhs.gov/sites/default/files/call-to-action-prevent-skin-cancer.pdf [accessed 2020-04-16]
6. Morris KL, Perna FM. Decision Tree Model vs Traditional Measures to Identify Patterns of Sun-Protective Behaviors and Sun Sensitivity Associated With Sunburn. JAMA Dermatol 2018 Aug 01;154(8):897. [doi: 10.1001/jamadermatol.2018.1646]
7. 21CFR201.: U.S. Food and Drug Administration Code of Federal Regulations Title 21 URL: https://www.accessdata.fda.gov/scripts/cdrh/cfdocs/cfCFR/CFRSearch.cfm?fr=201.327 [accessed 2019-10-25]
8. Petersen B, Wulf HC. Application of sunscreen--theory and reality. Photodermatol Photoimmunol Photomed 2014;30(2-3):96-101. [doi: 10.1111/phpp.12099] [Medline: 24313722]
9. Farberg AS, Glazer AM, Rigel AC, White R, Rigel DS. Dermatologists' Perceptions, Recommendations, and Use of Sunscreen. JAMA Dermatol 2017 Jan 01;153(1):99. [doi: 10.1001/jamadermatol.2016.3698]
10. Koch-Weser S, Bradshaw YS, Gualtieri L, Gallagher SS. The Internet as a health information source: findings from the 2007 Health Information National Trends Survey and implications for health communication. J Health Commun 2010 Dec;15 Suppl 3:279-293. [doi: 10.1080/10810730.2010.522700] [Medline: 21154099]
11. Chou WS, Hunt YM, Beckjord EB, Moser RP, Hesse BW. Social media use in the United States: implications for health communication. J Med Internet Res 2009 Nov;11(4):e48 [FREE Full text] [doi: 10.2196/jmir.1249] [Medline: 19945947]

12. Perrin A. Social Media Usage: 2005-2015. 2005. Pew Research Center 2015 Oct 8 URL: https://www.pewinternet.org/2015/10/08/social-networking-usage-2005-2015/ [accessed 2019-10-25]
13. Mitchell SJ, Godoy L, Shabazz K, Horn IB. Internet and Mobile Technology Use Among Urban African American Parents: Survey Study of a Clinical Population. J Med Internet Res 2014 Jan 13;16(1):e9. [doi: 10.2196/jmir.2673]
14. Alexa. The top 500 sites on the web URL: https://www.alexa.com/topsites [accessed 2019-10-25]
15. Madathil KC, Rivera-Rodriguez AJ, Greenstein JS, Gramopadhye AK. Healthcare information on YouTube: A systematic review. Health Informatics J 2015 Sep;21(3):173-194. [doi: 10.1177/1460458213512220] [Medline: 24670899]
16. Keelan J, Pavri-Garcia V, Tomlinson G, Wilson K. YouTube as a source of information on immunization: a content analysis. JAMA 2007 Dec 5;298(21):2482-2484. [doi: 10.1001/jama.298.21.2482] [Medline: 18056901]
17. Basch CH, Basch CE, Hillyer GC, Reeves R. YouTube Videos Related to Skin Cancer: A Missed Opportunity for Cancer Prevention and Control. JMIR Cancer 2015 Mar 02;1(1):e1. [doi: 10.2196/cancer.4204]
18. Ruppert L, Køster B, Siegert A, Cop C, Boyers L, Karimkhani C, et al. YouTube as a source of health information: Analysis of sun protection and skin cancer prevention related issues. Dermatol Online J 2017 Jan 15;23(1) [FREE Full text] [Medline: 28329465]
19. Sampson M, Cumber J, Li C, Pound CM, Fuller A, Harrison D. A systematic review of methods for studying consumer health YouTube videos, with implications for systematic reviews. PeerJ 2013 Sep;1:e147 [FREE Full text] [doi: 10.7717/peerj.147] [Medline: 24058879]
20. Does Video Length Matter?. URL: https://wistia.com/learn/marketing/does-length-matter-it-does-for-video-2k12-edition [accessed 2020-04-16]
21. StataCorp. Stata Statistical Software: Release 14. College Station, TX: Statacorp LP; 2015. URL: https://www.stata.com/stata14/ [accessed 2020-04-16]
22. Matta MK, Zusterzeel R, Pilli NR, Patel V, Volpe DA, Florian J, et al. Effect of Sunscreen Application Under Maximal Use Conditions on Plasma Concentration of Sunscreen Active Ingredients. JAMA 2019 Jun 04;321(21):2082. [doi: 10.1001/jama.2019.5586]
23. Holman DM, Qin J, Gottschlich EA, Balk SJ. Clinical counseling on sun protection and indoor tanning avoidance: A survey of current practices among U.S. health care providers. Prev Med 2019 Sep;126:105783. [doi: 10.1016/j.ypmed.2019.105783]
24. Bleakley A, Lazovich D, B Jordan A, Glanz K. Compensation Behaviors and Skin Cancer Prevention. Am J Prev Med 2018 Dec;55(6):848-855. [doi: 10.1016/j.amepre.2018.06.019] [Medline: 30344038]

Abbreviations

CDC: Centers for Disease Control and Prevention
EWG: Environmental Working Group
FDA: Food and Drug Administration
SPF: sun protection factor
UV: ultraviolet

6

Understanding Social Media Use and Engagement Among Dermatology Patients to Inform Dermatological Prevention and Care in Vietnam

Sau Huu Nguyen[1,2], MD; Giang Thu Vu[3], MSc; Long Hoang Nguyen[4], MPH; Cuong Tat Nguyen[5,6], MPH; Thu Hoai Thi Le[1,2], MD; Tung Hoang Tran[7], MD; Bach Xuan Tran[8,9], PhD; Carl A Latkin[9], PhD; Wilson W S Tam[3,10], PhD; Cyrus S H Ho[11], MBBS; Roger C M Ho[4,12,13], MBBS

[1]National Hospital of Dermatology and Venereology, Hanoi, Vietnam
[2]Department of Dermatology and Venereology, Hanoi Medical University, Hanoi, Vietnam
[3]Center of Excellence in Evidence-based Medicine, Nguyen Tat Thanh University, Ho Chi Minh City, Vietnam
[4]Center of Excellence in Behavioral Medicine, Nguyen Tat Thanh University, Ho Chi Minh City, Vietnam
[5]Institute for Global Health Innovations, Duy Tan University, Da Nang, Vietnam
[6]Faculty of Medicine, Duy Tan University, Da Nang, Vietnam
[7]Institute of Orthopaedic and Trauma Surgery, Vietnam-Germany Hospital, Hanoi, Vietnam
[8]Institute for Preventive Medicine and Public Health, Hanoi Medical University, Hanoi, Vietnam
[9]Bloomberg School of Public Health, Johns Hopkins University, Baltimore, MD, United States
[10]Alice Lee Centre for Nursing Studies, Yong Loo Lin School of Medicine, National University of Singapore, Singapore, Singapore
[11]Department of Psychological Medicine, National University Hospital, Singapore, Singapore
[12]Department of Psychological Medicine, Yong Loo Lin School of Medicine, National University of Singapore, Singapore, Singapore
[13]Institute for Health Innovation and Technology (iHealthtech), National University of Singapore, Singapore, Singapore

Corresponding Author:
Bach Xuan Tran, PhD
Institute for Preventive Medicine and Public Health
Hanoi Medical University
No 1 Ton That Tung Street
Dong Da District
Hanoi, 100000
Vietnam

Email: bach.ipmph@gmail.com

Abstract

Background: Social media has emerged as a common source of dermatological information. Monitoring the patterns of social media use and engagement is important to counteract the limitations of social media. However, evidence in Vietnamese dermatology patients is lacking.

Objective: This study aimed to explore social media use and engagement by dermatology patients and to identify factors associated with social media use and engagement.

Methods: A cross-sectional study was conducted with 519 participants at the Vietnam National Hospital of Dermatology and Venereology during September to November 2018. Data about sociodemographic characteristics, social media use, and social media engagement were collected. Multivariate logistic and tobit regression models were used to identify factors associated with social media use and engagement.

Results: Interest in information about "cosmetic, beauty, and skincare techniques" was the greatest (184/519, 46.2%). The mean engagement score was 8.4 points (SD 2.4 points). Female patients were more likely to use social media (odds ratio [OR] 2.23, 95% CI 1.23-4.06) and be interested dermatological information on social media (OR 3.09, 95% CI 1.35-7.09). Women also had higher social media engagement scores (coefficient=0.68, 95% CI 0.17-1.18). Higher social media engagement scores were related with Instagram use (coefficient=0.58, 95% CI 0.00-1.15) and higher credibility scores for "family members" (coefficient=0.15, 95% CI 0.03-0.26) and "dermatology companies" (coefficient=0.22, 95% CI 0.04-0.39).

Conclusions: This study discovered high social media usage among dermatology patients. However, only moderate utilization and credibility levels were reported regarding the use of social media as a source of dermatological information. More efforts should focus on involving dermatologists in the development of individualized information on social media targeting specific groups of dermatology patients.

KEYWORDS

dermatology; social media; engagement; prevention; Vietnam

Introduction

Dermatological diseases are popular health issues and the leading causes of disability and mortality worldwide. Skin diseases contributed to 1.79% of the global burden of diseases in 2017; of the skin diseases, dermatitis, acne vulgaris, psoriasis, and urticaria represented the greatest burden [1]. Dermatological diseases are also the most common reasons for health care service utilization [2,3], accounting for 8.4% of primary care visits [4]. People with dermatological diseases often have low quality of life [5] and self-esteem as well as feelings of stigmatization [6]. However, lack of access to dermatology services, particularly in low and middle-income countries [1], still challenges the provision of appropriate care for dermatology patients. As a result, patients seek other ways for self-treatment, including finding information on the internet and social media platforms.

Internet has played a key role in health care by reducing the cost of health service delivery [7], providing health information for specific disorders [8,9], delivering behavioral interventions [10], reducing harm for adverse health habits [11,12], facilitating physical rehabilitation [13], providing access to potential patients during health care crises [14], and supporting caregivers [15,16]. Social media is a popular method of communication [17] that enables internet users to generate information and share their opinions or media (eg, photos, clips) [18,19]. The term social media encompasses a diversity of platforms such as social networking sites (eg, Facebook, Instagram), blogs (eg, Twitter, Tumblr), or media sharing (eg, YouTube) [20-22]. It is estimated that more than 3.1 billion people worldwide were active social media users in 2018 [23]. The use of social media by patients to access medical information has accelerated with overall internet use [24].

Social media is well-recognized as a useful aid for health care providers to communicate and support patients [25-27]. Moreover, it empowers patients by encouraging active information seeking about disease prevention and treatment [28,29], providing support among peers [29,30], improving self-efficacy and self-management [27], supplementing information provided by health professionals [28], and facilitating the patient-health care professional relationship [31]. Social media is a dynamic teaching tool for health professionals [32,33] and has modernized dermatology training [34]. Although social media is a convenient source for health information, there is a paucity of literature that has evaluated the quality [35] and credibility [27] of the information on social media. Therefore, patient misinformation through social media use is a major concern among health professionals [25].

Social media is frequently used by patients to solicit advice related to dermatological concerns, has the potential to advance professional training in dermatology, and can facilitate new research methods [36]. Additionally, for dermatology, social media has the advantages of enabling the sharing of visual components such as images and videos that are important for diagnosis and consultancy. Nonetheless, little is known about the impact of social media on dermatology patients in developing countries.

Vietnam is among the countries with a high burden of dermatological diseases. A recent estimate indicates that skin disorders accounted for 2.3% of the disease burden in Vietnam in 2017 [1]. In addition, the growth in internet and social media use in Vietnam is substantial. In 2015, Vietnam had 44.4 million internet users, and this number grew to 55.8 million in 2018 [37,38]. Social media has been used widely in Vietnam, with about 46 million active users of some of the dominant social media platforms including Facebook, YouTube, Zalo, and Instagram [23]. Despite a call to understand social media use and engagement for seeking health information among dermatology patients or people interested in dermatological issues [39-43], no studies have determined social media use in this population in Vietnam. Hence, this study aimed to explore social media use and engagement by dermatology patients and to identify factors associated with social media use and engagement.

Methods

Study Design and Sampling Method

A cross-sectional study was performed at the Vietnam National Hospital of Dermatology and Venereology (NHDV) from September to November 2018. The NHDV was chosen due to the diversity of dermatology illnesses and the background of treated patients. As a leading hospital for dermatology and venereology diagnosis and treatment in Vietnam, the NHDV receives patient referrals from health facilities at various levels. A convenient sampling technique was adopted to recruit participants for this study. Sample size calculation was conducted using inputs determined based on a study of a similar topic in 13 European countries [44]: an expected mean social engagement score of 0.70, expected standard deviation of 0.20, and a confidence level of 95%. The calculation resulted in a minimum sample size of 385 participants. We selected from the pool of patients attending the outpatient department at the NHDV using the pre-determined eligibility criteria of age ≥18 years, a diagnosis of any dermatology disease, receiving services in the outpatient clinic, ability to provide coherent answers to the interview questions, and agreeing to participate by providing written consent. A total of 519 participants was successfully recruited for the study. The response rate was 100%.

Measurements and Instruments

We built a structured questionnaire to collect data concerning the sociodemographic status of participants and their social media use and engagement regarding dermatological issues and information. The questionnaire also assessed various aspects of health status and service utilization, based on data from other studies exploring these topics [45]. The questionnaire was first piloted in 10 patients to validate the language and logic of each item. After revising the questionnaire based on the patient feedback, face-to-face interviews were conducted by undergraduate medical students from the Hanoi Medical University, who were well-trained in conducting community interviews. A private room at the hospital was used to hold the interviews to ensure the confidentiality and comfort of the participants.

Sociodemographic Characteristics

Data about age, gender, education, marital status, occupation, and living location were collected.

Social Media Use

In this study, we collected information about the type of social network sites the participants visited and used frequently for dermatology care (eg, What are the social media sites that you use frequently for dermatology care?) and the types of dermatological information in which they were interested to find online. In addition, we asked the participants to rate the credibility of the dermatological information sources on social media including family members, friends/relatives, celebrities (including medical professionals/clinics), television programs/magazines, dermatological product retailers (people who sell dermatology-related products), and dermatology companies (companies manufacturing and selling dermatology-related products). To obtain the credibility score, each source was rated on a scale from 0 points (Totally not credible) to 10 points (Totally credible).

Engagement With Social Media

Data on social media engagement were collected using three questionnaire items: searching for dermatological information on social media, sharing dermatological information on social media, and applying dermatological information obtained from social media. Each item used a Likert scale with five response levels: "always" (5 points) to "never" (1 point). Then, we calculated the engagement score by summing the scores of the three items. The highest possible score was 15 points, and the lowest possible score was 3 points. This approach was adapted from the Social Media Engagement theory [46].

Statistical Analysis

We analyzed the data using Stata version 15.0 (Stata Corp. LP, College Station, TX). Multivariable logistic regression analysis was used to determine the factors correlated with social media use and interest in any dermatological information on social media. Multivariable tobit regression analysis was used to identify the factors associated with the engagement score. Potential explanatory variables included sociodemographic characteristics (age, gender, education, marital status, and occupation), social network platforms, and the credibility score. Stepwise forward selection strategies were combined with the multivariable regressions to reduce the models. A value of 0.2 of the log-likelihood's *P* value was considered the threshold of variable selection. The results of a previous study indicated that engagement depended heavily on specific contexts, ie, specific social network platforms as well as the credibility of the information from each platform [47]. $P<.05$ was considered statistically significant.

Ethical Approval

The Institutional Review Board of the NHDV approved the study protocol (document number 855/HDDDBVDLTU dated September 7, 2018).

Results

Of the 519 dermatology patients participating in the study, 62.8% (326/519) resided in urban areas. The mean age was 35.7 years (SD 13.7 years), and the greatest proportion of participants was 18-30 years old. Participants were mostly women (282/506, 55.7%), had completed at least a vocational education (341/517, 66.0%), and were married or had a partner (323/518, 62.4%). The most commonly reported occupation was freelancing (176/518, 34.0%), followed by white-collar job (145/518, 28.0%). Atopic dermatitis accounted for the greatest proportion of dermatology diseases (127/519, 24.4%), followed by contact dermatitis (75/519, 14.5%) and skin fungal infections (57/519, 11.0%; Table 1).

Facebook (359/392, 91.6%) and Zalo (247/392, 63.2%) were the most commonly used social media platforms. Information about "cosmetic, beauty, and skin care techniques" was sought by the most participants (184/397, 46.3%), followed by "general information about dermatology diseases" (168/397, 42.5%) and "medical institutions for dermatology disease treatment" (132/397, 32.6%). Regarding the credibility score of information sources on social media, "family members" and "television programs/magazines" scored the highest (mean 6.9 points, SD 2.3 points; mean 6.9 points, SD 2.2 points, respectively). Information from dermatological product retailers scored the lowest (mean 4.8 points, SD 2.3 points). No differences were found between men and women regarding the credibility of information sources or the social network platforms used (Table 2).

Table 1. Sociodemographic and clinical characteristics of the participants, N=519.

Characteristics	n (%)
Living location	
Urban	326 (62.8)
Rural	193 (37.2)
Age group (n=507)	
18-30 years	239 (47.1)
31-40 years	114 (22.5)
41-50 years	72 (14.2)
51-60 years	46 (9.1)
>60 years	36 (7.1)
Gender (n=506)	
Male	224 (44.3)
Female	282 (55.7)
Education (n=517)	
Up to secondary school	73 (14.1)
Upper secondary school	103 (19.9)
Vocational education and higher	341 (66.0)
Marital status (n=518)	
Single	195 (37.6)
Having a partner/married	323 (62.4)
Occupation (n=518)	
Unemployed	13 (2.5)
Freelancer	176 (34.0)
White-collar worker	145 (28.0)
Blue-collar worker	70 (13.5)
Student	62 (12.0)
Other	52 (10.0)
Dermatology diseases (n=519)	
Atopic dermatitis	127 (24.4)
Contact dermatitis	75 (14.5)
Psoriasis	29 (5.6)
Skin infections	13 (2.5)
Skin fungal infections	57 (11.0)
Urticaria	44 (8.5)
Warts	16 (3.1)
Zona	31 (6.0)
Age (n=507), years	35.7 (13.7)[a]

[a]Mean (SD).

Table 2. Social media use among dermatology patients, with comparisons between genders.

Characteristics	Total sample	Men	Women	*P* value
Uses a social network, n (%) (n=493)				
Yes	393 (79.7)	156 (71.9)	237 (85.9)	.00[a]
No	100 (20.3)	61 (28.1)	39 (14.1)	
Social network platform, n (%)				
Facebook (n=392)	359 (91.6)	144 (92.3)	215 (91.1)	.67[a]
Instagram (n=391)	103 (26.3)	35 (22.4)	68 (28.8)	.16[a]
Zalo (n=392)	247 (63.2)	89 (57.4)	158 (66.9)	.06[a]
Other (n=392)	18 (4.6)	5 (3.2)	13 (5.5)	.29[a]
Type of dermatological information sought on social network sites, n (%)				
Cosmetic, beauty, and skin care techniques (n=397)	184 (46.3)	30 (19.1)	154 (64.2)	<.001[a]
Medical institution for cosmetic surgery or beauty salons (n=397)	95 (23.9)	18 (11.5)	77 (32.1)	<.001[a]
Beauty or cosmetic surgery experts (n=397)	60 (15.1)	10 (6.4)	50 (20.8)	.10[a]
General information about dermatology diseases (n=397)	168 (42.3)	68 (43.3)	100 (41.7)	.75[a]
Preventive methods for dermatology disease (n=397)	90 (22.7)	41 (26.1)	49 (20.4)	.19[a]
Treatment methods for dermatology diseases (n=397)	95 (23.9)	41 (26.1)	54 (22.5)	.41[a]
Medical institutions for dermatology disease treatment (n=397)	132 (33.2)	51 (32.5)	81 (33.8)	.79[a]
Medication for dermatology disease treatment (n=397)	128 (32.2)	54 (34.4)	74 (30.8)	.46[a]
Treatment experiences from people who had undergone dermatology disease treatment (n=397)	80 (20.2)	28 (17.8)	52 (21.7)	.35[a]
Others (n=396)	8 (2.0)	3 (1.9)	5 (2.1)	.91[a]
Credibility score regarding dermatological information sources on social media, mean (SD)				
Family members (n=397)	6.9 (2.3)	7.1 (2.1)	6.8	.33[b]
Friends/relatives (n=392)	6.5 (2.1)	6.5 (2.1)	6.5	.60[b]
Celebrities (including famous medical professionals) (n=387)	5.7 (2.4)	5.7 (2.4)	5.7	.66[b]
Television programs/magazines (n=399)	6.9 (2.3)	7.1 (2.1)	6.8	.19[b]
Dermatological product retailers (n=386)	4.8 (2.3)	4.9 (2.3)	4.8	.65[b]
Dermatology companies (n=390)	5.2 (2.4)	5.1 (2.3)	5.2	.92[b]

[a]Chi-squared test.

[b]Mann-Whitney test.

Table 3 outlines the social media engagement by dermatology patients. Actively searching for, actively sharing, and actively applying dermatological information were reported by 95.2% (380/399), 81.4% (323/397), and 85.4% (339/397) of the patients, respectively. Dermatological information on social media was perceived as useful or very useful by 57% (229/399) of the patients. The mean engagement score was moderate (mean 8.4, SD 2.4). The social media engagement score was significantly different between male and female patients (*P*<.001).

Table 3. Engagement with social media among dermatology patients, with comparisons between genders.

Characteristics	Total sample	Men	Women	*P* value
Actively searching for dermatological information on social media, n (%) (n=399)				
No	19 (4.8)	10 (6.3)	9 (3.8)	.24[a]
Yes	380 (95.2)	149 (93.7)	231 (96.3)	
Actively sharing dermatological information on social media, n (%) (n=397)				
No	74 (18.6)	36 (22.8)	38 (15.9)	.09[a]
Yes	323 (81.4)	122 (77.2)	201 (84.1)	
Actively applying dermatological information found on social media, n (%) (n=397)				
No	58 (14.6)	30 (18.9)	28 (11.8)	.05[a]
Yes	339 (85.4)	129 (81.1)	210 (88.2)	
Perceived usefulness of dermatological information on social media, n (%) (n=399)				
Very useful	47 (11.8)	17 (10.8)	30 (12.4)	.39[a]
Useful	182 (45.6)	73 (46.2)	109 (45.2)	
Neutral	154 (38.6)	58 (36.7)	96 (39.8)	
Not useful	14 (3.5)	9 (5.7)	5 (2.1)	
Completely not useful	2 (0.5)	1 (0.6)	1 (0.4)	
Social media engagement score, mean (SD) (n=399)	8.4 (2.5)	8.0 (2.7)	8.7 (2.2)	.00[b]

[a]Chi-squared test.

[b]Mann-Whitney test.

The results of three multivariable regression models are displayed in Table 4. Among dermatology patients, women were more likely to use social media (odds ratio [OR] 2.23, 95% CI 1.23-4.06), while older patients were less likely to use social media. Compared with male patients, female patients were also more likely to be interested in dermatological information on social media (OR 3.09, 95% CI 1.35-7.09) and have higher social media engagement scores (coefficient 0.68, 95% CI 0.17-1.18).

Respondents who were married/had a partner had a higher likelihood of being interested in dermatology information (OR 2.37, 95% CI 1.01-5.53). Regarding social media engagement, higher scores were present for patients using Instagram and who rated the credibility of "family members" and "dermatology companies" higher. Meanwhile, lower social media engagement scores were related with higher credibility scores for dermatological product retailers.

Table 4. Factors associated with social media use and engagement in multivariable regression models.

Characteristics	Uses social media			Interest in any dermatological information on social media			Social media engagement score		
	OR[a]	95% CI	*P* value	OR	95% CI	*P* value	Coefficient	95% CI	*P* value
Gender									
Male	ref[b]	—[c]	—	ref	—	—	ref	—	—
Female	2.23	1.23-4.06	.008	3.09	1.35-7.09	.008	0.68	0.17-1.18	.009
Age									
18-30 years	ref	—	—	—	—	—	—	—	—
31-40 years	0.45	0.16-1.27	.132	—	—	—	—	—	—
41-50 years	0.07	0.03-0.19	.000	—	—	—	—	—	—
51-60 years	0.02	0.01-0.06	.000	—	—	—	—	—	—
>60 years	0.01	0.00-0.04	.000	—	—	—	—	—	—
Occupation									
Unemployed	ref	—	—	—	—	—	—	—	—
Freelancer	1.48	0.16-13.61	.729	—	—	—	—	—	—
White-collar worker	1.68	0.18-15.73	.648	—	—	—	—	—	—
Blue-collar worker	0.40	0.04-3.81	.428	—	—	—	—	—	—
Student	0.85	0.07-9.81	.894	—	—	—	—	—	—
Other	1.74	0.16-18.57	.648	—	—	—	—	—	—
Location of residence									
Urban	—	—	—	ref	—	—	—	—	—
Rural	—	—	—	2.24	0.74-6.83	.156	—	—	—
Marital status									
Single	—	—	—	ref	—	—	—	—	—
Married	—	—	—	2.37	1.01-5.53	.047	—	—	—
Uses Facebook									
No	—	—	—	ref	—	—	ref	—	—
Yes	—	—	—	2.82	0.85-9.37	.090	0.64	–0.26-1.55	.163
Uses Instagram									
No	—	—	—	—	—	—	ref	—	—
Yes	—	—	—	—	—	—	0.58	0.00-1.15	.049
Credibility score regarding dermatological information sources on social media									
Family members	—	—	—	—	—	—	0.15	0.03-0.26	.012
Dermatological product retailers	—	—	—	—	—	—	–0.19	–0.38-0.00	.049
Dermatology companies	—	—	—	—	—	—	0.22	0.04-0.39	.016

[a]Odds ratio.

[b]Reference group.

[c]Not applicable.

Discussion

Principal Findings

Our study found that, despite social media use by a high proportion of dermatology patients, utilizing this platform as a source of credible information for dermatological issues remains modest. Women were more likely to be interested in dermatological information on social media and be engaged with social media. The findings suggest that increased dermatologist involvement in contributing to online dermatological content and more effort to develop targeted, individualized information should be considered to take advantage of social media platforms.

Previous studies have documented the modest use of social media to find or share health-related content and particularly dermatology-related information. Despite reportedly high general social media engagement (85.0-99.3% of the participants reported regular access of at least one social media platform), only 19.0-31.7% of the participants reported accessing dermatology-related information [29,48]. We found that younger patients (aged 18-30 years) were significantly more likely to use social media. Young people in Asia are influenced more by social media than young people in Western countries because young people in Asia have a higher rate of smartphone use [49].

The higher percentage of use found in our study may reflect the increased popularity of social media in health care, due to technological advances and recent changes in the public perception of social media [50]. Our findings support the argument that there has been a desire among patients to use social media as an additional medium to traditional platforms for obtaining medical information [48]. Thus, social networking sites can be utilized as a platform to distribute educational information regarding dermatological issues for a wider reach of the population and at a potentially lower cost, especially in resource-poor settings in developing countries [51,52].

Regarding the sources of dermatological information on social media sites, our findings showed that the highest credibility scores were given to information received from family members, friends, televisions programs, and magazines. This popularity of informal information sources further highlights the lack of active contribution from dermatological health care providers and dermatologists to health information online. Dermatologists have expressed concern that patients might be misled by other social media indicators (eg, number of followers) without checking the educational background and clinical experience of information providers [53]. Increasing the involvement of medical professionals is crucial, as contributions by those with certified expertise would enhance the accuracy and reliability of information available online, reducing the possibility of incidents occurring as a result of misleading, inaccurate information [29,54]. Indeed, concerns over the quality of dermatology-related knowledge obtained online are a main barrier to enhancing the use of social media as a source of health information for health care service users [29]. Such concerns among service users may explain the medium level of engagement with social media for dermatological content reported in our study. Another possible reason for such low engagement may be participant concern about the privacy and security of personal data shared online [55,56]. Taking necessary measures to ensure the confidentiality of patient information over online platforms would also be important when attempting to boost the utilization of social media sites.

In addition, the sociodemographic characteristics of our participants were associated with their level of concern regarding dermatological information on social media and social media engagement. Women, married respondents, and Facebook users were more likely to be interested in dermatological issues on social media. These findings suggest that Facebook, in particular, could serve as the primary social media platform for disseminating dermatological information to targeted groups of online users. For example, this information could focus on dermatological issues that are most relevant to women and married individuals. Previous studies have argued the potential of Facebook for knowledge distribution, owing to its large user base, versatility in providing information in various forms, and capacity to allow for interactions and connections between users [57,58]. The positive association between engagement and the credibility score given to family members and dermatology companies as sources of social media information may also be partially explained by the ability to facilitate communications between sources and receivers of information: the more credible the sources, the more those sources would be used.

One of the implications that can be drawn from our findings is that the presence of dermatologists on social media platforms to provide official, scientific, evidence-based dermatological information should be increased. To facilitate this, the marketing capabilities of dermatology health facilities should be enhanced, so they can reach a wider population. And, patient-physician communication should be encouraged through social networking sites, notably Facebook, with careful consideration of privacy protection measures. The adoption of the Law on Cybersecurity in Vietnam provided stricter regulations on the content and transfer of data online and can be expected to impact the extent of online channel use by both patients and physicians. This should be taken into consideration when designing communication and education campaigns and programs. Regarding content, dermatological information should be created and distributed in an individually customized manner, targeting specific groups with relevant information.

Limitations

This study has certain limitations. First, the self-reported nature of the questionnaire may have introduced recall bias. Second, although effort was made to enhance the diversity of participants by conducting research at a central dermatological hospital, the adoption of a convenient sampling technique and the fact that the study was conducted at a single hospital could affect the generalizability of our study. In addition, although the instrument we used to measure social media engagement has a theoretical background and provides valuable insights on the topic, it has not been officially validated. There are also several possible research considerations and directions not yet covered in our study that may be recommended for further studies. Further research may benefit from studying other online media platforms such as Google and YouTube that have considerable influence on dermatology patients in developed countries [59,60] or exploring the relationship between social media and cutaneous concerns associated with stigmatized medical conditions (eg, substance abuse). Moreover, further research may consider examining the effect of dermatological conditions on family quality of life, such as atopic dermatitis [61], as well as the impact of social media on caregivers of dermatology patients [62].

Conclusion

In conclusion, this study found high levels of social media use among dermatology patients, but only a moderate level of utilization and credibility regarding the use of social media as a source of dermatological information. Sociodemographic characteristics were associated with dermatology-related social media use and engagement. The results of this study recommend enhancing the involvement of dermatologists on social media platforms, in terms of knowledge contribution through social media for both patients and the general public. In addition, more efforts should be given in developing individualized information that targets specific groups of dermatology patients.

Acknowledgments

Our thanks to Vietnam National Hospital of Dermatology and Venereology that gave us permission and support to conduct this study. In addition, we are grateful to all the patients who gave us their time and willingness to participate in this study.

References

1. Karimkhani C, Dellavalle RP, Coffeng LE, Flohr C, Hay RJ, Langan SM, et al. Global Skin Disease Morbidity and Mortality: An Update From the Global Burden of Disease Study 2013. JAMA Dermatol 2017 May 01;153(5):406-412 [FREE Full text] [doi: 10.1001/jamadermatol.2016.5538] [Medline: 28249066]
2. Schofield J, Fleming D, Grindlay D, Williams H. Skin conditions are the commonest new reason people present to general practitioners in England and Wales. Br J Dermatol 2011 Nov;165(5):1044-1050. [doi: 10.1111/j.1365-2133.2011.10464.x] [Medline: 21692764]
3. Awadalla F, Rosenbaum DA, Camacho F, Fleischer AB, Feldman SR. Dermatologic disease in family medicine. Fam Med 2008;40(7):507-511. [Medline: 18928078]
4. Kerr O, Tidman M, Walker J, Aldridge R, Benton E. The profile of dermatological problems in primary care. Clin Exp Dermatol 2010 Jun;35(4):380-383. [doi: 10.1111/j.1365-2230.2009.03586.x] [Medline: 19874334]
5. Hong J, Koo B, Koo J. The psychosocial and occupational impact of chronic skin disease. Dermatol Ther 2008;21(1):54-59. [doi: 10.1111/j.1529-8019.2008.00170.x] [Medline: 18318886]
6. Fortune DG, Richards HL, Main CJ, Griffiths CE. What patients with psoriasis believe about their condition. Journal of the American Academy of Dermatology 1998 Aug;39(2):196-201. [doi: 10.1016/s0190-9622(98)70074-x]
7. Zhang M, Cheow E, Ho CS, Ng BY, Ho R, Cheok CCS. Application of low-cost methodologies for mobile phone app development. JMIR Mhealth Uhealth 2014;2(4):e55 [FREE Full text] [doi: 10.2196/mhealth.3549] [Medline: 25491323]
8. Zhang MW, Ho RC, Loh A, Wing T, Wynne O, Chan SWC, et al. Current status of postnatal depression smartphone applications available on application stores: an information quality analysis. BMJ Open 2017 Nov 14;7(11):e015655 [FREE Full text] [doi: 10.1136/bmjopen-2016-015655] [Medline: 29138195]
9. Rajagopalan A, Shah P, Zhang MW, Ho RC. Digital Platforms in the Assessment and Monitoring of Patients with Bipolar Disorder. Brain Sci 2017 Nov 12;7(11) [FREE Full text] [doi: 10.3390/brainsci7110150] [Medline: 29137156]
10. Zhang MWB, Ho RCM, Cassin SE, Hawa R, Sockalingam S. Online and smartphone based cognitive behavioral therapy for bariatric surgery patients: Initial pilot study. Technol Health Care 2015;23(6):737-744. [doi: 10.3233/THC-151026] [Medline: 26409514]
11. Zhang MWB, Fang P, Ho RCM. Global outreach and user preferences of a smartphone application developed for drinkers. Technol Health Care 2016 Jul 27;24(4):495-501 [FREE Full text] [doi: 10.3233/THC-161143] [Medline: 26890229]
12. Tran BX, Le XTT, Nguyen PN, Le QNH, Mai HT, Nguyen HLT, et al. Feasibility of e-Health Interventions on Smoking Cessation among Vietnamese Active Internet Users. Int J Environ Res Public Health 2018 Dec 20;15(1) [FREE Full text] [doi: 10.3390/ijerph15010165] [Medline: 29361694]
13. Zhang MWB, Ho RCM. Harnessing the potential of the Kinect sensor for psychiatric rehabilitation for stroke survivors. Technol Health Care 2016 Dec 04;24(4):599-602 [FREE Full text] [doi: 10.3233/THC-161147] [Medline: 27061386]
14. Zhang MWB, Ho CSH, Fang P, Lu Y, Ho RCM. Methodology of developing a smartphone application for crisis research and its clinical application. Technol Health Care 2014;22(4):547-559. [doi: 10.3233/THC-140819] [Medline: 24898865]
15. Leow MQH, Chan SWC. Evaluation of a video, telephone follow-ups, and an online forum as components of a psychoeducational intervention for caregivers of persons with advanced cancer. Palliat Support Care 2016 Dec;14(5):474-478 [FREE Full text] [doi: 10.1017/S1478951516000225] [Medline: 27071801]

16. Zhang MWB, Chan S, Wynne O, Jeong S, Hunter S, Wilson A, et al. Conceptualization of an evidence-based smartphone innovation for caregivers and persons living with dementia. Technol Health Care 2016 Sep 14;24(5):769-773. [doi: 10.3233/THC-161165] [Medline: 27129032]
17. Ho K, Peter WWP. Harnessing the social web for health and wellness: issues for research and knowledge translation. J Med Internet Res 2014;16(2):e34 [FREE Full text] [doi: 10.2196/jmir.2969] [Medline: 24518432]
18. Eysenbach G. Medicine 2.0: social networking, collaboration, participation, apomediation, and openness. J Med Internet Res 2008;10(3):e22 [FREE Full text] [doi: 10.2196/jmir.1030] [Medline: 18725354]
19. George DR, Rovniak LS, Kraschnewski JL. Dangers and opportunities for social media in medicine. Clin Obstet Gynecol 2013 Sep;56(3):453-462 [FREE Full text] [doi: 10.1097/GRF.0b013e318297dc38] [Medline: 23903375]
20. Ventola CL. Social media and health care professionals: benefits, risks, and best practices. P T 2014 Jul;39(7):491-520 [FREE Full text] [Medline: 25083128]
21. Househ M, Borycki E, Kushniruk A. Empowering patients through social media: the benefits and challenges. Health Informatics J 2014 Mar;20(1):50-58. [doi: 10.1177/1460458213476969] [Medline: 24550564]
22. Grajales FJ, Sheps S, Ho K, Novak-Lauscher H, Eysenbach G. Social media: a review and tutorial of applications in medicine and health care. J Med Internet Res 2014;16(2):e13 [FREE Full text] [doi: 10.2196/jmir.2912] [Medline: 24518354]
23. We Are Social. 2018 Nov 19. Digital in 2018: World's Internet Users Pass the 4 Billion Mark URL: https://wearesocial.com/uk/blog/2018/01/global-digital-report-2018 [accessed 2020-02-02]
24. Travers RL. Social media in dermatology: moving to Web 2.0. Semin Cutan Med Surg 2012 Sep;31(3):168-173 [FREE Full text] [doi: 10.1016/j.sder.2012.06.003] [Medline: 22929354]
25. Rupert DJ, Moultrie RR, Read JG, Amoozegar JB, Bornkessel AS, O'Donoghue AC, et al. Perceived healthcare provider reactions to patient and caregiver use of online health communities. Patient Educ Couns 2014 Sep;96(3):320-326. [doi: 10.1016/j.pec.2014.05.015] [Medline: 24923652]
26. Ho Y, O'Connor BH, Mulvaney SA. Features of online health communities for adolescents with type 1 diabetes. West J Nurs Res 2014 Oct;36(9):1183-1198. [doi: 10.1177/0193945913520414] [Medline: 24473058]
27. Smailhodzic E, Hooijsma W, Boonstra A, Langley DJ. Social media use in healthcare: A systematic review of effects on patients and on their relationship with healthcare professionals. BMC Health Serv Res 2016 Aug 26;16:442 [FREE Full text] [doi: 10.1186/s12913-016-1691-0] [Medline: 27562728]
28. Hawn C. Take two aspirin and tweet me in the morning: how Twitter, Facebook, and other social media are reshaping health care. Health Aff (Millwood) 2009;28(2):361-368 [FREE Full text] [doi: 10.1377/hlthaff.28.2.361] [Medline: 19275991]
29. Antheunis ML, Tates K, Nieboer TE. Patients' and health professionals' use of social media in health care: motives, barriers and expectations. Patient Educ Couns 2013 Sep;92(3):426-431. [doi: 10.1016/j.pec.2013.06.020] [Medline: 23899831]
30. Hardiker NR, Grant MJ. Factors that influence public engagement with eHealth: A literature review. Int J Med Inform 2011 Jan;80(1):1-12. [doi: 10.1016/j.ijmedinf.2010.10.017] [Medline: 21112244]
31. Bosslet GT, Torke AM, Hickman SE, Terry CL, Helft PR. The patient-doctor relationship and online social networks: results of a national survey. J Gen Intern Med 2011 Oct;26(10):1168-1174 [FREE Full text] [doi: 10.1007/s11606-011-1761-2] [Medline: 21706268]
32. D'Souza K, Henningham L, Zou R, Huang J, O'Sullivan E, Last J, et al. Attitudes of Health Professional Educators Toward the Use of Social Media as a Teaching Tool: Global Cross-Sectional Study. JMIR Med Educ 2017 Aug 04;3(2):e13 [FREE Full text] [doi: 10.2196/mededu.6429] [Medline: 28778841]
33. Frisch NC, Borycki EM, Mickelson G, Atherton P, Novak-Lauscher H, Hooker D, et al. Use of social media and web 2.0 technologies to increase knowledge and skills of british columbia nurses. NI 2012 (2012) 2012;2012:117 [FREE Full text] [Medline: 24199067]
34. Wang JV, O'Donnell M, Albornoz CA, Keller M, Saedi N. Resident experiences with social media: modernizing dermatology training. Int J Dermatol 2018 Dec;57(12):e169-e170 [FREE Full text] [doi: 10.1111/ijd.14182] [Medline: 30101440]
35. Zhang MWB, Ho RCM, Hawa R, Sockalingam S. Analysis of the Information Quality of Bariatric Surgery Smartphone Applications Using the Silberg Scale. Obes Surg 2016 Jan;26(1):163-168. [doi: 10.1007/s11695-015-1890-5] [Medline: 26424704]
36. DeBord LC, Patel V, Braun TL, Dao H. Social media in dermatology: clinical relevance, academic value, and trends across platforms. J Dermatolog Treat 2018 Sep 28:1-30 [FREE Full text] [doi: 10.1080/09546634.2018.1530444] [Medline: 30265614]
37. Tran BX, Huong LT, Hinh ND, Nguyen LH, Le BN, Nong VM, et al. A study on the influence of internet addiction and online interpersonal influences on health-related quality of life in young Vietnamese. BMC Public Health 2017 Jan 31;17(1):138 [FREE Full text] [doi: 10.1186/s12889-016-3983-z] [Medline: 28143462]
38. Tran BX, Mai HT, Nguyen LH, Nguyen CT, Latkin CA, Zhang MWB, et al. Vietnamese validation of the short version of Internet Addiction Test. Addict Behav Rep 2017 Dec;6:45-50 [FREE Full text] [doi: 10.1016/j.abrep.2017.07.001] [Medline: 29450235]
39. Karimkhani C, Connett J, Boyers L, Quest T, Dellavalle RP. Dermatology on instagram. Dermatol Online J 2014 Jul 15;20(7) [FREE Full text] [Medline: 25046455]
40. Amir M, Sampson BP, Endly D, Tamai JM, Henley J, Brewer AC, et al. Social networking sites: emerging and essential tools for communication in dermatology. JAMA Dermatol 2014 Jan;150(1):56-60. [doi: 10.1001/jamadermatol.2013.6340]

[Medline: 24196212]
41. Benabio J. The value of social media for dermatologists. Cutis 2013 Jun;91(6):269-270. [Medline: 23837146]
42. Patel RR, Yazd NKK, Dellavalle RP. Dermatology on Snapchat. Dermatol Online J 2017 Jul 15;23(7) [FREE Full text] [Medline: 29469694]
43. Falzone AE, Brindis CD, Chren M, Junn A, Pagoto S, Wehner M, et al. Teens, Tweets, and Tanning Beds: Rethinking the Use of Social Media for Skin Cancer Prevention. Am J Prev Med 2017 Sep;53(3S1):S86-S94 [FREE Full text] [doi: 10.1016/j.amepre.2017.04.027] [Medline: 28818251]
44. Balieva F, Kupfer J, Lien L, Gieler U, Finlay AY, Tomás-Aragonés L, et al. The burden of common skin diseases assessed with the EQ5D™ : a European multicentre study in 13 countries. Br J Dermatol 2017 May;176(5):1170-1178. [doi: 10.1111/bjd.15280] [Medline: 28032340]
45. Nguyen SH, Dang AK, Vu GT, Nguyen CT, Le THT, Truong NT, et al. Lack of Knowledge about Sexually Transmitted Diseases (STDs): Implications for STDs Prevention and Care among Dermatology Patients in an Urban City in Vietnam. Int J Environ Res Public Health 2019 Mar 26;16(6) [FREE Full text] [doi: 10.3390/ijerph16061080] [Medline: 30917565]
46. Di Gangi PM, Wasko M. Social Media Engagement Theory: Exploring the Influence of User Engagement on Social Media Usage. JOEUC 2016;28(2):53-73. [doi: 10.4018/joeuc.2016040104]
47. Voorveld HAM, van Noort G, Muntinga DG, Bronner F. Engagement with Social Media and Social Media Advertising: The Differentiating Role of Platform Type. Journal of Advertising 2018 Feb 13;47(1):38-54. [doi: 10.1080/00913367.2017.1405754]
48. Ross NA, Todd Q, Saedi N. Patient seeking behaviors and online personas: social media's role in cosmetic dermatology. Dermatol Surg 2015 Feb;41(2):269-276 [FREE Full text] [doi: 10.1097/DSS.0000000000000267] [Medline: 25654198]
49. Mak K, Lai C, Watanabe H, Kim D, Bahar N, Ramos M, et al. Epidemiology of internet behaviors and addiction among adolescents in six Asian countries. Cyberpsychol Behav Soc Netw 2014 Nov;17(11):720-728. [doi: 10.1089/cyber.2014.0139] [Medline: 25405785]
50. Russell J. Hootsuite Social Media Management. 2017 Jan 31. Social Media in Health Care: The Benefits, Challenges, and Opportunities URL: http://www.marketinghub.today/social-media-in-health-care-the-benefits-challenges-and-opportunities/ [accessed 2020-02-02]
51. Hanson AH, Krause LK, Simmons RN, Ellis JI, Gamble RG, Jensen JD, et al. Dermatology education and the Internet: traditional and cutting-edge resources. J Am Acad Dermatol 2011 Oct;65(4):836-842 [FREE Full text] [doi: 10.1016/j.jaad.2010.05.049] [Medline: 21820206]
52. Hay AA, Gamble RG, Huff LS, Dellavalle RP. Internet social networking sites and the future of dermatology journals: promises and perils. J Am Acad Dermatol 2011 Sep;65(3):e81-e83 [FREE Full text] [doi: 10.1016/j.jaad.2011.04.028] [Medline: 21839304]
53. Galadari HI. Social media and modern dermatology. Int J Dermatol 2018 Dec;57(1):110-111 [FREE Full text] [doi: 10.1111/ijd.13821] [Medline: 29090452]
54. George DD, Wainwright BD. Dermatology resources on the internet. Semin Cutan Med Surg 2012 Sep;31(3):183-190. [doi: 10.1016/j.sder.2012.06.002] [Medline: 22929356]
55. Thompson LA, Dawson K, Ferdig R, Black EW, Boyer J, Coutts J, et al. The intersection of online social networking with medical professionalism. J Gen Intern Med 2008 Jul;23(7):954-957 [FREE Full text] [doi: 10.1007/s11606-008-0538-8] [Medline: 18612723]
56. Thompson MA, Younes A, Miller RS. Using social media in oncology for education and patient engagement. Oncology (Williston Park) 2012 Sep;26(9):782, 784-785, 791 [FREE Full text] [Medline: 23061330]
57. Kim WB, Marinas JEC, Vender RB. Public Engagement with Dermatology Contents on Facebook. J Cutan Med Surg 2015;19(3):304-308 [FREE Full text] [doi: 10.2310/7750.2014.14119] [Medline: 25775650]
58. Kim W, Vender R. Use of facebook as a tool for knowledge dissemination in dermatology. J Cutan Med Surg 2014 Oct;18(5):341-344 [FREE Full text] [doi: 10.2310/7750.2014.14022] [Medline: 25186996]
59. Hill MK, Patel RR, Anand P, Dellavalle RP. Dermatology on Google. Dermatol Online J 2018 Apr 15;24(4) [FREE Full text] [Medline: 29906016]
60. Boyers LN, Quest T, Karimkhani C, Connett J, Dellavalle RP. Dermatology on YouTube. Dermatol Online J 2014 Jun 15;20(6) [FREE Full text] [Medline: 24945641]
61. Chernyshov PV, Ho RC, Monti F, Jirakova A, Velitchko SS, Hercogova J, et al. An International Multi-center Study on Self-assessed and Family Quality of Life in Children with Atopic Dermatitis. Acta Dermatovenerol Croat 2015;23(4):247-253. [Medline: 26724875]
62. Ho RCM, Giam YC, Ng TP, Mak A, Goh D, Zhang MWB, et al. The influence of childhood atopic dermatitis on health of mothers, and its impact on Asian families. Pediatr Allergy Immunol 2010 May;21(3):501-507 [FREE Full text] [doi: 10.1111/j.1399-3038.2009.00972.x] [Medline: 20546527]

Abbreviations

NHDV: National Hospital of Dermatology and Venereology.
OR: odds ratio.

7

Assessing YouTube as an Educational Tool for Shingles

Teevit Dunnsiri[1], BS; Takumi Kawashita[1], BS; Sharon C Lee[1], BS; Aaron Kumar Monga[1], BS; Benjamin K P Woo[2], MD

[1]Western University of Health Sciences, Pomona, CA, United States
[2]Olive View-UCLA Medical Center, Sylmar, CA, United States

Corresponding Author:
Teevit Dunnsiri, BS
Western University of Health Sciences
309 E 2nd St
Pomona, CA
United States

Email: teevit@g.ucla.edu

Abstract

Background: YouTube is a popular platform with many videos, which have potential educational value for medical students. Due to the lack of peer review, other surrogates are necessary to determine the content quality of such educational videos. Few studies have analyzed the research background or academic affiliation of the physicians associated with the production of YouTube videos for medical education. The research background or academic affiliations of those physicians may be a reflection of the content quality of these educational videos.

Objective: This study identifies physicians associated with the production of educational YouTube videos about shingles and analyzes those physicians based on their research background or academic affiliation, which may be good surrogates for video content quality.

Methods: Using the YouTube search engine with default settings, the term "shingles" was searched on May 8, 2020. A cross-sectional study was performed using the first 50 search results. A search on Scopus for each identified physician was performed, and data regarding their research background and academic affiliation were recorded.

Results: Of the 50 YouTube videos, 35 (70%) were categorized as academic. Of the 35 academic videos, 24 (71%) videos featured physicians, totaling 25 physicians overall. Out of these 25 physicians, 5 (20%) had at least 1 shingles-related publication and 8 (32%) had an h-index >10. A total of 21 (84%) physicians held an academic affiliation.

Conclusions: These results ensure to a certain degree the quality of the content in academic videos on YouTube for medical education. However, further evaluation is needed for this growing platform.

KEYWORDS

YouTube; medical education; online; shingles; herpes zoster; peer review; dermatology; research background; content quality; views

Introduction

Shingles, also referred to as herpes zoster, classically presents as a painful vesicular rash distributed along a dermatomal pattern. Symptoms typically last for 2-4 weeks. However, pain can persist even after the rash resolves in a complication known as postherpetic neuralgia. Shingles is caused by reactivation of the varicella-zoster virus, which lies dormant in nerve tissue after resolution of the initial infection known as chickenpox. Reactivation is typically due to stress or a weakened immunity. Approximately 1 million cases of shingles occur each year in the United States [1]. Despite the introduction of a shingles vaccine in 2006, recent studies have found no significant decline in the incidence of cases [2].

As online media platforms become more pervasive in our society, medical students are finding different methods to incorporate these resources into their education [3]. YouTube is a popular platform with many videos, which have potential educational value [4-6]. However, a study on YouTube videos as an educational resource on psoriasis found that misleading videos had a similar number of views to high-quality videos [7]. Although other studies have supported the educational value of YouTube videos, they have also acknowledged the need for more evaluation, particularly via peer-review [8,9].

A different study on psoriasis content on YouTube found that only 7.1% of the reviewed videos were associated with a medical institution or physician. The study concluded that this emphasized the need for more medical professionals to participate on YouTube in order to raise the quality of information [10]. However, few studies have thoroughly analyzed the physicians associated with the production of YouTube videos for dermatological medical education. Due to the lack of peer-review for YouTube videos, some studies have postulated that the research background of physicians featured in these videos for medical education could be a surrogate for content quality [9]. This study identifies physicians associated with the production of academic YouTube videos about shingles and analyzes their research background and academic affiliation, which may be good surrogates for video content quality.

Methods

Using the YouTube search engine with default settings, the term "shingles" was searched on May 8, 2020. A cross-sectional study was conducted using the first 50 search results, which were sorted by relevance. Recorded data on the YouTube videos included the category (academic, video blog or "vlog", patient interview, or miscellaneous), number of views, type of health professional associated with the video, and the name of the physician if available. Videos categorized as miscellaneous included commercials and local news reports. An academic video was defined as a video having scientifically correct information about the causes, symptoms, treatment, or prevention of the disease. The accuracy of information from a video was verified by medical students using UpToDate, an evidence-based medical resource. If the presence of a health professional was not clearly discernible in the video, the YouTube channel descriptions of the video producers were investigated.

Scopus is a large abstract and citation database for research. A search on each identified physician was performed on Scopus. Data was recorded from Scopus regarding the searched physicians' area of specialty, h-index, number of publications, academic affiliations, and number of shingles-related publications. The h-index is a measure of the research output and citation impact of an author [11]. The h-index was categorized as either 0-10 or >10.

Physician variables such as having a shingles-related publication, h-index >10, or academic affiliation were recorded. Difference in the average number of views between videos associated with a physician who had a shingles-related publication, an h-index >10, or an academic affiliation was analyzed. Welch's unpaired *t* test was utilized due to unequal sample sizes between different groups.

Results

From the first 50 "shingles" search results on YouTube, there were 35 academic videos, 6 patient interviews, 3 vlogs, and 6 miscellaneous videos. From the 35 academic videos, there were 25 physicians, 1 nurse practitioner, 1 pharmacist, 1 dentist, and 1 medical student identified. A total of 7 academic videos were produced by educational media outlets without an identified health professional. A physician was featured in 2 different academic videos, and 2 academic videos had more than one physician featured. From the 25 physicians identified from academic videos, there were 4 internists, 4 ophthalmologists, 4 family physicians, 3 infectious disease physicians, 3 anesthesiologists, 2 dermatologists, 2 obstetrician-gynecologists, 1 plastic surgeon, 1 urologist, and 1 rheumatologist.

The average number of publications for these 25 physicians was 62 (SD 130). The number of publications ranged from 0 to 529. Among these 25 physicians, 5(20%) had at least 1 shingles-related publication and 8 (32%) had an h-index >10. The h-index had an average of 13 (SD 22) and a range of 0 to 86. A total of 84% (21/25) of the physicians had an academic affiliation (Table 1).

Table 1. Physicians sorted by qualities.

Physician quality	n (%), N=25
Shingles-related publication	5 (20)
H-index >10	8 (32)
Academic affiliation	21 (84)

For academic YouTube videos associated with a verified physician, the average number of views was 9676 (SD 16,888) if there was a shingles-related publication, 59,439 (SD 118,706) if there was an academic affiliation, and 42,191 (SD 184,823) if there was an h-index >10. The difference in the average number of views compared to those of videos without these characteristics was not significant (Table 2). Only 4 videos featured physicians who authored a shingles-related publication and only 3 videos featured physicians without an academic affiliation. The total number of views for the 24 academic videos with a verified physician was 1,325,693. The number of views had a median of 20,554 and an average of 55,237 (SD 111,890). The numbers of views ranged from 231 to 537,390. The video with the most views was associated with an MD-PhD dermatologist who held an academic affiliation. This video alone accounted for 41% of the total number of views for academic videos with a verified physician.

Table 2. Comparison of the average number of views by physician characteristics.

Physician quality	No. of videos	Average no. of views, Mean (SD)	*P* value
Shingles-related publication			.07
Yes	4	9676 (16,888)	
No	20	64,349 (120,771)	
Academic affiliation			.36
Yes	21	59,439 (118,706)	
No	3	25,826 (39,739)	
h-index			.57
0-10	16	42,191 (52,065)	
>10	8	81,329 (184,823)	

Discussion

YouTube is one of the world's most popular online media platforms, which many medical students utilize as a resource to supplement their education. Prior studies have suggested the potential benefit that YouTube has for improving medical education. However, those studies also mentioned the need for more evaluations in order to ensure the quality of YouTube videos [8,9]. The aim of this study was to analyze the physicians associated with the production of YouTube videos that could be incorporated into medical education. This study was performed around shingles because the unique presentation of this infection makes it well-suited to be studied on online media platforms.

A significant majority of identified physicians had an affiliation with a renowned academic institution with many having produced publications. The substantial research background and academic affiliations of these physicians ensure to a certain degree the accuracy of information in educational YouTube videos about shingles. However, these surrogates for content quality cannot replace the critical analysis that peer-review provides. Preferably, an external rating system should be developed to enable critical analysis by physicians and avoid the limitations that traditional forms of peer-review would impose.

The quality of academic content in a YouTube video may contribute to its popularity. In fact, the video with the most views (537,390) was associated with an MD-PhD dermatologist who has an academic affiliation. This may provide reassurance to viewers given that the associated physician is trained in a specialty that manages patients with shingles. Although videos with physicians who held an academic affiliation or an h-index >10 did trend towards more views, this study did not find a significant difference between the number of views and research background of the physicians associated with a video. This suggests that there may be other more significant factors that contribute to the popularity of a video such as the length of time since the video was posted and the number of subscribers of the YouTube channel.

This study has a few limitations that should be considered. The most significant limitation is that the study was unable to characterize the audience of these YouTube videos. Therefore, the proportion of views that could be attributed to medical students could not be gauged. Future studies should utilize YouTube Analytics to survey the audience [12]. Other limitations which also prevented characterization of the audience include YouTube channels turning off the feedback and commenting feature. Moreover, the small sample size in certain categories was a limitation in this study. This limitation was weighed against the decreased relevance of videos as the overall sample size of the study increased. Outside of the first 50 search results were less relevant videos about other topics such as rooftop shingles.

Although this study to a certain degree supports the quality of YouTube videos on shingles for medical education, more evaluation is needed for this growing platform. Future studies should examine how medical students may utilize social media platforms to share such videos. Some studies have suggested that platforms such as WhatsApp and Instagram were highly efficacious in the dissemination of educational information linked to YouTube videos [13,14].

YouTube is an efficient and accessible resource for medical students to supplement their learning. Half of the videos reviewed were associated with verified physicians most of which had an academic affiliation. This study supports to a certain degree the academic quality of YouTube videos about shingles produced for medical education. This provides reassurance to viewers that the information they are receiving is accurate. However, more studies in the future will be needed to assess the utility of YouTube as a tool for medical education.

References

1. Insinga RP, Itzler RF, Pellissier JM, Saddier P, Nikas AA. The incidence of herpes zoster in a United States administrative database. J Gen Intern Med 2005 Aug;20(8):748-753 [FREE Full text] [doi: 10.1111/j.1525-1497.2005.0150.x] [Medline: 16050886]

2. Johnson BH, Palmer L, Gatwood J, Lenhart G, Kawai K, Acosta CJ. Annual incidence rates of herpes zoster among an immunocompetent population in the United States. BMC Infect Dis 2015 Nov 06;15:502 [FREE Full text] [doi: 10.1186/s12879-015-1262-8] [Medline: 26546419]
3. Koya KD, Bhatia KR, Hsu JTS, Bhatia AC. YouTube and the expanding role of videos in dermatologic surgery education. Semin Cutan Med Surg 2012 Sep;31(3):163-167 [FREE Full text] [doi: 10.1016/j.sder.2012.06.006] [Medline: 22929353]
4. Lam NHT, Tsiang JT, Woo BKP. Exploring the Role of YouTube in Disseminating Psychoeducation. Acad Psychiatry 2017 Dec;41(6):819-822 [FREE Full text] [doi: 10.1007/s40596-017-0835-9] [Medline: 29022242]
5. Lam NHT, Woo BKP. YouTube as a New Medium for Dementia Education Among Chinese Americans. Community Ment Health J 2020 Apr;56(3):435-439 [FREE Full text] [doi: 10.1007/s10597-019-00493-7] [Medline: 31641910]
6. Guo JZ, Chong KPL, Woo BKP. Utilizing YouTube as platform for psychiatric emergency patient outreach in Chinese Americans. Asian J Psychiatr 2020 Apr;50:101960 [FREE Full text] [doi: 10.1016/j.ajp.2020.101960] [Medline: 32086173]
7. Qi J, Trang T, Doong J, Kang S, Chien AL. Misinformation is prevalent in psoriasis-related YouTube videos. Dermatol Online J 2016 Nov 15;22(11). [Medline: 28329562]
8. Sunderland N, Camm CF, Glover K, Watts A, Warwick G. A quality assessment of respiratory auscultation material on YouTube. Clin Med (Lond) 2014 Aug;14(4):391-395 [FREE Full text] [doi: 10.7861/clinmedicine.14-4-391] [Medline: 25099841]
9. Shires CB, Wilson CD, Sebelik M. Thyroid surgery YouTube videos: estimating quality by surgeon characteristics and view rate. Gland Surg 2019 Jun;8(3):207-211 [FREE Full text] [doi: 10.21037/gs.2018.10.01] [Medline: 31328098]
10. Lenczowski E, Dahiya M. Psoriasis and the Digital Landscape: YouTube as an Information Source for Patients and Medical Professionals. J Clin Aesthet Dermatol 2018 Mar;11(3):36-38 [FREE Full text] [Medline: 29606999]
11. Gray R, Hassanein E, Thompson DR. Journal editors and their h-index. J Adv Nurs 2017 Sep;73(9):2031-2034 [FREE Full text] [doi: 10.1111/jan.13070] [Medline: 27400154]
12. Woo BKP, Chung JOP. Using YouTube analytics to evaluate a Chinese video-based lecture regarding Parkinson's disease. J Clin Neurosci 2018 Apr;50:300 [FREE Full text] [doi: 10.1016/j.jocn.2018.01.001] [Medline: 29361404]
13. Shu S, Woo BKP. The Roles of YouTube and WhatsApp in Dementia Education for the Older Chinese American Population: Longitudinal Analysis. JMIR Aging 2020 Apr 13;3(1):e18179 [FREE Full text] [doi: 10.2196/18179] [Medline: 32281940]
14. Lam NH, Woo BK. Efficacy of Instagram in Promoting Psychoeducation in the Chinese-Speaking Population. Health Equity 2020;4(1):114-116 [FREE Full text] [doi: 10.1089/heq.2019.0078] [Medline: 32258963]

8

Associations Between Emotions, Social Media Use and Sun Exposure Among Young Women: Ecological Momentary Assessment Study

Jessica Fitts Willoughby[1], PhD; Jessica Gall Myrick[2], PhD; Stephanie Gibbons[1], MA; Clark Kogan[3], PhD

[1]The Edward R Murrow College of Communication, Washington State University, Pullman, WA, United States

[2]Donald P Bellisario College of Communications, Pennsylvania State University, University Park, PA, United States

[3]Center for Interdisciplinary Statistical Education and Research, Washington State University, Pullman, WA, United States

Corresponding Author:
Jessica Fitts Willoughby, PhD
The Edward R Murrow College of Communication
Washington State University
208 Goertzen Hall
PO Box 642520
Pullman, WA, 99164-2520
United States

Email: jessica.willoughby@wsu.edu

Abstract

Background: Research has pointed to a connection between social media use, emotions, and tanning behaviors. However, less is known about the role specific emotions may play in influencing social media use and how emotions and social media use may each be associated with outdoor tanning.

Objective: This paper aims to examine the connection between emotions, social media use, and outdoor tanning behaviors among young women, a group particularly important for skin cancer prevention efforts.

Methods: We used ecological momentary assessment to collect data from 197 women aged 18 to 25 years 3 times a day for 7 days in July 2018. We collected data from women in 2 states.

Results: We found that boredom was associated with increased time spent on social media and that increased time spent on social media was associated with increased time spent outdoors without sun protection.

Conclusions: Our results highlight that social media may be a particularly important channel for skin cancer prevention efforts targeting young women, as more social media use was associated with increased time spent outdoors with skin exposed. Researchers should consider the role of emotions in motivating social media use and subsequent tanning behaviors. Additionally, as boredom was associated with social media use, intervention developers would benefit from developing digital and social media interventions that entertain as well as educate.

KEYWORDS

social media; skin cancer; emotions; cancer prevention; health communication; ecological momentary assessment

Introduction

Background

It is estimated that more than 100,000 new cases of melanoma, the deadliest type of skin cancer, will be diagnosed in the United States in 2020 [1], and melanoma is one of the most prevalent cancers in young women [2]. Younger skin is particularly vulnerable to the effects of ultraviolet light and the skin damage it may cause [3]. Despite the health implications of exposure to ultraviolet light, young women often express a desire to have tan skin and believe having a tan makes them look healthier [4]. Taken together, these statistics and preferences point to an increased risk of skin cancer among young women.

As such, researchers are eager to better understand the psychosocial and behavioral factors that predict risky skin behaviors like tanning. Previous research has found that emotions are associated with indoor tanning behaviors in young women [5], as is young women's use of social media [6]. Additionally, research has found that intentional outdoor tanning is significantly greater among girls who spend more time on their cell phones [7].

One psychosocial predictor that may help predict tanning is emotions, which may be particularly important for understanding both media use and tanning behaviors for a number of reasons. Appraisal theory suggests that specific emotions may be linked with action tendencies based on automatic subjective evaluations [8]. For example, a person experiences happiness when they have gained something they desire. The action tendencies associated with happiness include moving toward the happiness-inducing event, sharing positive outcomes, and celebration [8,9]. However, there is a lack of understanding about the role different emotions might play in motivating social media use and outdoor tanning, a risk behavior related to skin cancer.

In this manuscript, we examine the associations among emotions and social media use, emotions and risky outdoor skin behaviors, and social media use and outdoor tanning behavior using ecological momentary assessment. This method allows us to see how emotions, media use, and tanning behavior interrelate in real time throughout the course of a week. This may be important, as previous research has found that emotions vary throughout the day in response to stressors (eg, minor hassles that happen throughout the day in people's lives) [10]. Therefore, capturing emotion data at a single point in time may substantially increase the noise, thereby reducing the power. Additionally, digital media use is often frequent and dynamic, leading to challenges in determining how to best measure media exposure [11]. Previous research in other topic areas has found that retrospective self-report in communication may be difficult [12]. As the use of ecological momentary assessment is beneficial for collecting data and may better assess complex or dynamic data [13], we used 3 daily surveys over the course of a week to assess social media use, emotions, and related outcomes among young women.

Emotions and Social Media

Research has unearthed both positive and negative consequences of using social media, warranting a perpetual need to understand the evolving media platform [14]. A great deal of social media research has focused on the linear effect that social media may have on one's emotions [15,16]. This includes outcomes such as increased depression, anxiety, need of belonging, empathy, social desirability, social support, and others. However, the relationship between social media use and one's emotions is often cyclical, with certain emotions and personality types perpetuating social media consumption [14].

For example, rather than observing how social media use leads to loneliness, it is important to also observe that users turn to social media as a substitute for social interaction [16]. Certain personality traits and emotions, such as extroversion and levels of instability, are associated with social media use and willingness to interact [17]. Forgas [18] argues that emotions influence every aspect of an individual's life and stimulate each behavior in some aspect. As such, emotions influence social media use, too. Motives for social media use are unique, since they encompass "a diverse and complex set of (often unconscious) decision-making activities, influenced by a large number of individual, collective, and environmental factors" [14]. Positive outcomes of social media use include entertainment or connectivity, while negative emotional outcomes may include users' feelings that they are wasting time or distracting themselves from more meaningful social interaction [14]. These emotional experiences have been shown to predict social media use, especially with regard to information sharing, entertainment, and convenience [19-21]. Research has found that young adults use social media for a variety of reasons, including information [22], entertainment and leisure [23], socialization [24], and keeping in contact with others [23]. The previously discussed research leads to our first research question (research question 1): Which emotions are associated with the increased use of social media among young women?

Emotions and Tanning

Many individuals have positive emotional associations with the sun [25]. In fact, researchers have identified a physiological link between exposure to UV light and the feel-good chemicals released by our bodies, called endorphins [26]. As such, it may not be surprising that ultraviolet exposure can make people feel good. Expectations or beliefs that tanning will result in a positive emotional state have been consistently found to predict both indoor and outdoor tanning [27-29]. Conversely, individuals who have negative emotional associations with tanning (eg, they think they will be uncomfortable while doing it or are anxious about the health risks) are less likely to perform the behavior [30].

According to the broaden-and-build theory, positive emotions exist to motivate individuals to broaden the scopes of their attention and skills while also building resources and relationships to help them cope with future negative situations [31]. Tanning is often a social activity done with friends and reported to be an enjoyable, positive experience [25]. However, positive emotions can also reinforce behaviors that elicit them, even if individuals know the behavior is risky [32]. As such, the positive emotional association that individuals build with tanning behaviors may continue to motivate them to pursue this cancer-causing behavior to maintain a positive emotional state or alleviate a negative one.

This supposition is also in line with mood management theory, which argues that people often seek stimuli (be it a behavior or a media message) that help them achieve a more positive mood [33,34]. For example, recent work using the National Cancer Institute's Family Life, Activity, Sun, Health, and Eating (FLASHE) cross-sectional survey found that adolescents who reported being frequent outdoor tanners were more likely to experience loneliness than adolescents who reported they did not tan outdoors [7]. Although more research is needed to understand this relationship, it could be that adolescents in the survey tanned outdoors in order to reap the positive emotional benefits that could help them cope with feelings of loneliness. This lack of clear consensus around the role of positive emotions and tanning behaviors led to the following research question (research question 2): Are more positive emotions associated with increased time spent outdoors without sun protection among young women?

Social Media and Tanning

Although there is some understanding of how social media may influence well-being, researchers have called for more research to be conducted related to digital natives and social media's impact on behavior, health, and society [23]. Research has found that media use is connected to a variety of tanning behaviors [4,6,35,36]. Of particular note, young women may desire to look like people in the media [37]. In US culture, tan skin is a commonly held beauty standard, and women often engage in outdoor or indoor tanning to achieve this standard. Although previous research has observed how media sources such as television [38] and magazines [35,36] influence tanning behaviors, a recent focus has been on social media [6,7]. Social media expands on traditional media platforms, as there are greater opportunities to interact within the media and exchange images. Additionally, social media is a channel frequently used by young women [39]. Social media has been found to have an indirect but positive relationship with indoor tanning use among young women, while traditional mass media has not [5]. Such research purports that social media may perpetuate the desire to engage in tanning behaviors [5,40].

A theoretical rationale for the effects of social media on tanning behaviors comes from social cognitive theory [41,42], which posits that people can learn from behaviors modeled in media. Although media may not always directly model tanning behavior, people who are rewarded or viewed positively and are tan could influence young women to aim to achieve a similar look. Social media has been found to be related to the belief that indoor tanning leads to positive outcomes, such as improved appearance, greater mood, and improved health, while simultaneously being negatively associated with health and social consequences [5].

In part, this relationship may also have to do with the connections and relationships that can occur around tanning. Researchers have found tanning to be a social experience, as indoor tanners are likely to discuss tanning with friends [43]. In a study that looked at different platforms and their connections to tanning behaviors, Willoughby and Myrick [6] found that image-based social media platforms, such as Snapchat, Instagram, and Pinterest, were all positively associated with sunbathing, suggesting that the inclusion of images of tanned or tanning people may encourage young women to spend time sunbathing. Based on the previously discussed literature, we propose the following hypothesis: Increased social media use will be associated with increased time spent outdoors without sun protection among young women.

Methods

Study Design

We conducted an ecological momentary assessment (EMA) of young women's emotions, social media use, and outdoor tanning behaviors over a 7-day period in July 2018. EMA is a data collection method that allows for real-time data collection. It uses mobile devices to ask participants to report on moods or behaviors at specific points in time close to when the events occurred. Consequently, EMA has potential advantages over traditional data collection methods, including its usefulness for measuring mood and behavior [44].

Recruitment

Participants were recruited from 2 universities in the United States, one in the Pacific Northwest and one in the Northeast. A mix of in-person and online methods were used to recruit young adult college women at the participating universities. If they were interested and met inclusion criteria (ie, identified as a woman and were aged 18-29 years), participants signed up via a text message program to receive study updates. All participants received the EMA over the same 7-day period in July 2018.

Procedures

Participants received 3 messages a day. The first assessment was sent at 10 AM and asked participants about their current emotions. The second assessment was sent at 4 PM and asked about social media use over the past 6 hours, time spent outdoors, and current emotions. The third assessment was sent at 8 PM and asked about social media use over the past 4 hours, current emotions, time spent outdoors, and the weather. We selected the timing of the surveys to fall around peak UV exposure, which occurs between 10 AM and 4 PM [45], with an end time of 8 PM to avoid having the surveys sent too late in the evening for some participants. At the end of the week, participants were asked to complete a longer survey that asked about demographics, attitudes, and behaviors. For completing at least half of the EMA surveys and the posttest, participants received US $50 in cash. Prior to conducting the research, the first author's institutional review board approved all procedures.

Measures

Individual emotions were measured at 3 time points by asking participants to "rate how much of each emotion describes how you are feeling" on a 5-point Likert-type scale from "none of this emotion at all" to "a great deal of this emotion." The emotions assessed included the following: content, excited, sad, envious, anxious, and bored. We selected these specific emotions based on previous research that examined emotions and tanning [27,46,47]. We examined both the discrete emotions and a composite measure of positivity. Composite measures of positivity have been used in previous research [48]. We created the composite measure to indicate whether a person was experiencing a greater level of positive emotions by adding together contentment and excitement and then subtracting sadness, envy, anxiety, and boredom. The emotions data were summarized to obtain the average of each emotional state over all 7 days and over all 3 time points. The creation of the composite measure is similar to composite creation measures in other work on emotion regulation [49].

Social media was measured at 2 time points daily (second and third survey) with the question "How often have you used the following social media since the last survey?" on a slider scale with half-hour increments marked. The options were Instagram, Facebook, Twitter, Snapchat, and text messaging. As we were focused on the role of social media collectively for this study, we added together the amount of time participants reported spending on Instagram, Facebook, Twitter, and Snapchat. We calculated the sum of the hours spent on social media over the day divided by the proportion of the daily hours that were observed via survey response. For instance, if only morning social media usage was recorded, then the total amount of time on social media was divided by 0.6, as the time period represents 60% of the time participants reported social media use. If participants responded to both surveys, then it would be the total number of hours observed that day.

Sun exposure was measured with the question "How much time did you spend outdoors with your skin exposed?" on a slider scale with half-hour increments marked at both 4 PM and 8 PM. If there was an observation at 8 PM but no observation at 4 PM (missing data), we used the amount of time outdoors divided by 0.4 (as the 4 PM to 8 PM time period represents 40% of the overall time they were questioned about outdoor tanning). If data were available at both times, we summed the amount of time to determine total time outdoors. The time periods used were selected because they encompass the peak sun hours in which participants could have spent time outdoors. The item is similar to items used in previous research that considered time spent outside without sun protection as a measure of sun exposure [50,51], but it included specific time frames to take advantage of the multiple measurements in EMA.

Perceived weather was measured with 3 items that asked participants to "please indicate how strongly you disagree or agree with the following statements regarding the weather today" on a 5-point Likert-type scale: "It was sunny outside," "It was warm outside," and "The weather was nice." We averaged the 3 weather variables to obtain a new weather variable that indicated whether the weather was nice (Cronbach α=.853).

Analysis Strategy

We collected data from 197 individuals, but due to missing data, we had 192 participants in the data frame that was used to address research question 1 and 179 participants in the data frame that was used to address research question 2.

To assess research question 1, which asked which specific emotions were associated with increased use of social media, we fit a linear model relating the logarithm of the average daily amount of time (out of the 10 hours assessed) that participants used social media to the average emotional state of an individual. Emotions were included in the regression using natural cubic splines in order to allow for a nonlinear relationship between the emotional scale and the log of the social media usage. We computed an adjusted generalization of the Spearman rank correlation to motivate the number of knots to use for each cubic spline. Correlations between each emotion and overall social media use were small for all variables except boredom. We therefore considered a restricted cubic spline for boredom (with 3 knots) and included all other terms as linear. Between 3 and 5 knots is typically found to be sufficient for a spline, and as our correlation between boredom and social media use was only moderate, 3 knots was selected [52]. We constructed residual plots to assess the plausibility of the normality and variance homogeneity assumption and found little evidence to suggest major deviation. Wald *F* statistics were computed to summarize the effect of each emotion on social media use.

To assess research question 2, which asked if increased positive emotions were associated with increased time spent outdoors without sun protection, and hypothesis 1, which posited that increased use of social media would be associated with increased time spent outdoors without sun protection, we performed a generalized least squares regression to relate daily time outdoors to positivity and social media use after adjusting for weather and accounting for correlation within individuals via the use of a compound symmetric correlation structure. As all correlations between variables were very small, we considered only linear terms in our regression analysis. We prefer generalized least squares to mixed-effects modeling, as it has a certain elegance for continuous responses [52]. We used the square root transformation for the time spent outdoors to help improve the plausibility of residual normality. Residuals were assessed for the plausibility of normality and variance homogeneity. Mild deviations from normality were found, but they were not substantial enough to warrant further transformations or a change in the distributional assumptions. Furthermore, there was little evidence to suggest more than minor deviations from variance homogeneity. We conducted Wald tests to assess the overall effect of positivity, weather, and social media on time spent outdoors.

Results

Sample

We collected demographic information at the end with a posttest survey (N=149). Some people did not respond to all surveys; as such, we examined the sample descriptive statistics by each analysis frame for comparison, finding minimal differences. We report on the descriptive data for individuals who completed the posttest survey.

On average, participants were aged 20.5 (SD 6.81) years. A total of 69.8% (104/149) of participants were from Washington state, and 26.2% (39/149) of participants were from Pennsylvania; 4.0% (6/149) reported being from another state. Nearly two-thirds (110/149, 73.8%) of participants reported being White or Caucasian. The majority of participants reported spending time outdoors in the sun a few times per week (65/149, 43.6%) or once per week (31/149, 20.8%). In addition, 36.2% (54/149) of participants had indoor tanned at some time in their life. Table 1 presents additional demographic information.

Table 1. Demographic information of study participants.

Variable	Participants, n (%)[a]
Race	
White or Caucasian	110 (74)
Asian or Pacific Islander	19 (13)
Hispanic or Latina	16 (11)
Black or African American	9 (6)
American Indian or Native American	4 (3)
Other	1 (1)
Grade	
Freshman	37 (25)
Sophomore	19 (13)
Junior	42 (28)
Senior	39 (27)
Other or not applicable	12 (7)
Not diagnosed with skin cancer	149 (100)
Someone close ever diagnosed with skin cancer (yes)	64 (43)
Area in which they live	
Rural (eg, in the country)	44 (30)
Urban (eg, in the city)	20 (13)
Suburban (eg, near a city, outside a city)	79 (53)
Indoor tan ever (yes)	54 (36)

[a]Descriptive data included 149 individuals, as some participants did not complete the posttest questionnaire.

Research Questions and Hypothesis Testing

For research question 1, we found evidence suggesting an association between one or more emotions and social media use ($F_{7,184}$=5.94; *P*<.001). Specifically, boredom was associated with increased social media use ($F_{2,7}$=14.70; *P*<.001). To interpret the effect size of boredom, we fit a simplified model in which boredom was reduced to a linear effect. We found an estimated increase of 67% (95% CI 37%-103%) in social media usage for every 1-unit increase in boredom (Figure 1). We assessed the evidence that the effect of boredom on social media use was nonlinear and found no evidence against linearity (*P*=.10). We did not find evidence that levels of contentment, excitement, sadness, envy, or anxiousness were associated with social media use with the current sample (Table 2).

Figure 1. Average daily social media use (in hours) plotted against average boredom. The blue line shows the model predictions after back transformation across different boredom ratings, computed at the mean value for all other emotions.

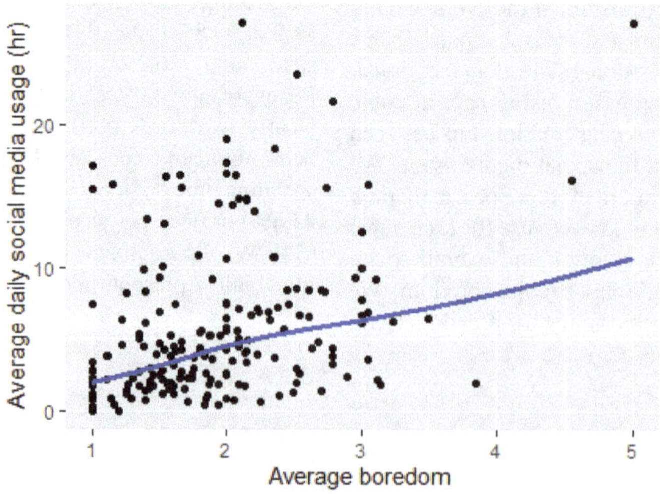

Table 2. Social media use analysis of variance.

Emotion	Partial sum of squares	Mean squares	*F* value (*df*)	*P* value
Bored	23.80	11.90	14.70[a] (2)	<.001
Content	0.53	0.53	0.66 (1)	.42
Excited	0.94	0.94	1.16 (1)	.28
Sad	0.38	0.38	0.46 (1)	.50
Envious	1.42	1.42	1.76 (1)	.19
Anxious	0.34	0.34	0.41 (1)	.52

[a]Significant at the *P*<.001 level.

For research question 2, there was evidence suggesting some association between time spent outdoors and the explanatory variables of positivity, weather, and social media (N=184; χ^2_3=17.9; *P*<.001). Further Wald tests found slight evidence of an effect of positivity (*P*=.08) and strong evidence for a modest effect of social media (*P*<.001) on time spent outdoors without sun protection, providing support for hypothesis 1 (Figure 2 and Table 3).

Figure 2. Average daily time outdoors (in hours) plotted against average daily social media use. The blue line shows the model predictions after back transformation across different social media usage levels, computed at the mean value for positivity and weather.

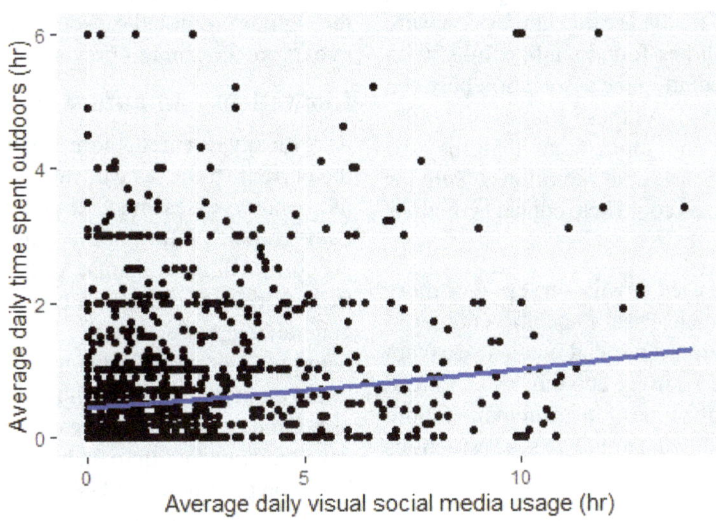

Table 3. Results of Wald analysis of variance on increased amount of time spent outdoors.

Factor	Chi-square (*df*)	*P* value
Positivity	3.1 (1)	.08
Weather	3.7 (1)	.06
Social media	13.9 (1)	<.001

Discussion

Principal Findings

This research used an EMA study conducted with young women over the course of a week in July to assess the relationships between emotions, social media use, and time spent outdoors. Of the emotions we assessed, we found only boredom associated with increased use of social media, with increased reports of boredom associated with increased time spent on social media. The magnitude of the effect was substantial, with boredom at greater levels nearly doubling social media use. Additionally, increased use of social media was significantly associated with increased time spent outdoors without sun protection. Below, we discuss these findings in greater depth.

Boredom, a low-arousal negative emotional state, occurs when an individual is unable or unwilling to dedicate their attention to whatever is currently in front of them [53]. Another definition of boredom is monotony combined with frustration [54]. Individuals experiencing boredom have been found to visit more websites during an internet search task than overstimulated, stressed individuals [55]. In our study, increased levels of boredom were associated with increased social media use, highlighting how individuals may use social media as a distraction or way to entertain themselves [23]. If bored individuals turn to social media that portray tan celebrities and peers, it could then motivate them to tan as another means of shifting their emotional state to something more pleasant.

Of the other emotions we assessed, including contentment, excitement, envy, anxiety, and sadness, none were significantly associated with social media use in our analyses. There may be a few different reasons for this. First, according to the appraisal theory of emotions, different emotions predispose people to take certain actions (called action tendencies) [8]. However, those action tendencies are typically directed at the underlying cause of that emotion. For example, if an individual is afraid of skin cancer, the action tendency is to avoid the threat somehow (possibly by not tanning). Since we measured emotions more generally (ie, not directly related to tanning), they may have predicted a number of potential actions more generally too. Future work could collect emotional responses with a specific target.

Second, previous research has found that the use of specific social media sites (ie, Facebook) for surveillance was associated with depression, with envy mediating the relationship. However, no direct effects between social media use and depression were found [56]. Additional research has found similar links, with envy and social comparison mediating the association between Facebook use and depression [57]. As these studies highlight, there are potential mediators and moderators that may be associated with social media use and emotions. Perhaps different, unaccounted for variables could help connect emotions to social media.

Lastly, it is possible that, as we used 3 daily surveys 4 or more hours apart, our time measurement wasn't specific enough to see the resulting impact of emotions on social media use except with boredom, which provided a strong enough result to lead to increased social media use at the time of measurement. Future research could benefit from varying the timing to see if emotions then impact resulting social media use.

In addition to finding an association between boredom and subsequent social media use, we found that increased use of social media was associated with increased time spent outdoors without sun protection. This supports previous research, which has found a connection between social media and tanning behaviors [5-7]. Americans frequently use social media, with young adults (aged 18-24 years) using a variety of platforms and most of them (71%) visiting the platforms multiple times each day [39]. Nearly 3 out of 4 young people use Instagram, a highly visual form of social media, with young women often reporting frequent use. The content to which young women are exposed could be showcasing the benefits of tanning behaviors. In line with social cognitive theory [42], when individuals see behaviors that are modeled and rewarded, they may be more likely to engage in such behaviors. Additionally, as peers and socialization may impact tanning behaviors [43,58], social media may play an especially important role. This supports other research that has highlighted the possibility of using social media for skin cancer prevention efforts [59].

Taken together, these findings have implications for skin cancer prevention strategies among young women. In particular, social media is a well-suited platform for prevention efforts, as individuals who spend time in the sun without sun protection are also likely to use social media. Additionally, as young women turn to social media when bored, strategies that employ some form of entertainment may be particularly well suited to engaging the audience and garnering attention toward prevention efforts. Strategies such as entertainment education, which is the inclusion of educational content in entertaining formats [60], have been found to be effective for a variety of health topics related to risky behaviors [61,62]. Entertainment education efforts targeting young women in digital media have been found to be effective at influencing elements of narrative that may lead to behavior change, such as transportation and engagement [63,64]. As young women may be turning to social media when bored, including prevention efforts that entertain while also educating may help by first garnering attention, which can be difficult in the crowded social media environment. A recent meta-analysis of narrative game-based health behavior interventions found that such interventions had a large effect on improving knowledge, a medium effect on self-efficacy, and small effects on increasing enjoyment and encouraging health behaviors [65]. Narrative game-based interventions provided through or promoted on social media could be a useful option to explore for tanning prevention efforts.

Limitations and Future Directions

As with any research, there are limitations to keep in mind with the current study. As we waited until the end of the ecological momentary assessment to elicit demographic information, demographic information was not available for a small proportion of participants. Additionally, while the sample came from 2 locations, it was a convenience sample that cannot be generalized more broadly. Additionally, we assessed only 6 emotions that participants may have felt, which were selected based on previous research related to tanning and social media use. Other emotions that were not captured in this study may have motivated participant behaviors. We also selected our time based on peak hours of UV exposure, so it is possible that there was social media use that occurred outside of our window of assessment, which could further impact findings associated with the role of emotions and social media use in particular. Perhaps emotions are stronger drivers of social media use only at certain times of day. We tried to mitigate the effects of a lack of data at certain time points in our creation of the composite variable, but we recognize that some instances of social media use were likely not captured, such as use during times that were outside our data collection efforts (eg, 11 PM) or on platforms that were not included (eg, Pinterest). However, the study does help advance the research in this area by using a different form of measurement through the use of ecological momentary assessment, allowing participants to report on media use, emotions, and behaviors closer in time to when they occurred, which should help reduce some of the potential difficulties of assessing dynamic constructs and issues with retrospective recall. However, although the analyses we conducted allowed us to assess the proposed research questions and hypotheses in a manner comparable to other research that has examined emotions, social media, and tanning in between-subject analyses [5,7,47], this analytical decision did not allow us to look at within-person differences. Future work could benefit from the addition of within-person analyses to further address the connections between emotions, social media use, and tanning.

Future research would also benefit from looking at younger audiences, as research suggests adolescents may also be impacted by social media in regard to indoor tanning behaviors [5]. Examining more specific social media channels and their associations with tanning behaviors, as well as the content presented in social media, would also be beneficial. Previous research has found different associations with tanning behaviors based on specific platforms [6]. A greater understanding of the specific content to which young people are exposed could help further explain effects beyond mere exposure, as previous research in other topic areas has found that perceptions of media messages may be influential among young people [66,67]. Future research also should continue to explore the relationship between social media and tanning behaviors among young women to further parse out the mechanisms through which effects occur and to continue to bolster prevention efforts. Additionally, more work in measurement, specifically for use in EMA studies, would be beneficial.

Conclusion

Our week-long ecological momentary assessment study of young women found that boredom, more than other emotional predictors, was associated with increased use of social media and that increased use of social media was associated with time spent outdoors without sun protection. This means that social media such as Snapchat, Instagram, Twitter, and Facebook may be prime channels for intervention and present an opportunity for reaching young women who have an increased risk of engaging in risky sun behaviors. Additionally, interventions developed for these channels should aim to be entertaining and engaging, as boredom was associated with social media use in our sample. By creating interventions that can entertain and educate, attention may be increased, potentially leading to greater intervention effects.

References

1. Key statistics for melanoma skin cancer. American Cancer Society. URL: https://www.cancer.org/cancer/melanoma-skin-cancer/about/key-statistics.html [accessed 2020-11-20]
2. Bleyer A, O'Leary M, Barr M, Ries L. Cancer epidemiology in older adolescents and young adults 15 to 29 years of age, including SEER incidence and survival: 1975-2000. National Cancer Institute Surveillance, Epidemiology, and End Results Program. 2006. URL: https://seer.cancer.gov/archive/publications/aya/ [accessed 2020-11-20]
3. Volkmer B, Greinert R. UV and children's skin. Prog Biophys Mol Biol 2011 Dec;107(3):386-388. [doi: 10.1016/j.pbiomolbio.2011.08.011] [Medline: 21907231]
4. Dennis LK, Lowe JB, Snetselaar LG. Tanning behavior among young frequent tanners is related to attitudes and not lack of knowledge about the dangers. Health Educ J 2009 Sep;68(3):232-243 [FREE Full text] [doi: 10.1177/0017896909345195] [Medline: 22707763]
5. Myrick JG, Noar SM, Kelley D, Zeitany AE. The relationships between female adolescents' media use, indoor tanning outcome expectations, and behavioral intentions. Health Educ Behav 2016 Sep 02;44(3):403-410. [doi: 10.1177/1090198116667251] [Medline: 27590838]
6. Willoughby JF, Myrick JG. Entertainment, social media use and young women's tanning behaviours. Health Educ J 2018 Dec 23;78(3):352-365. [doi: 10.1177/0017896918819643]
7. Niu Z, Parmar V, Xu B, Coups EJ, Stapleton JL. Prevalence and correlates of intentional outdoor and indoor tanning among adolescents in the United States: Findings from the FLASHE survey. Prev Med Rep 2018 Sep;11:187-190. [doi: 10.1016/j.pmedr.2018.06.014] [Medline: 29992085]
8. Lazarus RS. Progress on a cognitive-motivational-relational theory of emotion. Am Psychol 1991 Aug;46(8):819-834. [doi: 10.1037//0003-066x.46.8.819] [Medline: 1928936]
9. Roseman IJ. Emotional behaviors, emotivational goals, emotion strategies: multiple levels of organization integrate variable and consistent responses. Emotion Rev 2011 Sep 20;3(4):434-443. [doi: 10.1177/1754073911410744]
10. Stawski RS, Sliwinski MJ, Almeida DM, Smyth JM. Reported exposure and emotional reactivity to daily stressors: the roles of adult age and global perceived stress. Psychol Aging 2008;23(1):52-61. [doi: 10.1037/0882-7974.23.1.52] [Medline: 18361654]
11. Niederdeppe J. Meeting the challenge of measuring communication exposure in the digital age. Commun Methods Meas 2016 Apr 20;10(2-3):170-172. [doi: 10.1080/19312458.2016.1150970]
12. Eveland WP, Hutchens MJ, Shen F. Exposure, attention, or "use" of news? Assessing aspects of the reliability and validity of a central concept in political communication research. Commun Methods Meas 2009 Dec 09;3(4):223-244. [doi: 10.1080/19312450903378925]
13. Smyth JM, Stone AA. Ecological momentary assessment research in behavioral medicine. J Happiness Stud 2003;4(1):35-52. [doi: 10.1023/A:1023657221954]
14. Widén G, Lindström J, Brännback M, Huvila I, Nyström AG. Mixed emotions in active social media use - fun and convenient or shameful and embarrassing? 2015 Presented at: iConference 2015; March 24-27, 2015; Newport Beach, CA.
15. Escobar-Viera CG, Shensa A, Bowman ND, Sidani JE, Knight J, James AE, et al. Passive and active social media use and depressive symptoms among United States adults. Cyberpsychol Behav Soc Netw 2018 Jul;21(7):437-443. [doi: 10.1089/cyber.2017.0668] [Medline: 29995530]

16. Berryman C, Ferguson CJ, Negy C. Social media use and mental health among young adults. Psychiatr Q 2018 Jun;89(2):307-314. [doi: 10.1007/s11126-017-9535-6] [Medline: 29090428]
17. Correa T, Hinsley AW, de Zúñiga HG. Who interacts on the web?: the intersection of users' personality and social media use. Comput Hum Behav 2010 Mar;26(2):247-253. [doi: 10.1016/j.chb.2009.09.003]
18. Forgas JP. Affect in social thinking and behavior. New York, NY: Psychology Press; 2006.
19. Choi M, Toma CL. Social sharing through interpersonal media: patterns and effects on emotional well-being. Comput Hum Behav 2014 Jul;36:530-541. [doi: 10.1016/j.chb.2014.04.026]
20. Stieglitz S, Dang-Xuan L. Emotions and information diffusion in social media—sentiment of microblogs and sharing behavior. J Manage Inf Syst 2013 Jun 7;29(4):217-248. [doi: 10.2753/MIS0742-1222290408]
21. Williams DL, Crittenden VL, Keo T, McCarty P. The use of social media: an exploratory study of usage among digital natives. J Public Aff 2012 Mar 06;12(2):127-136. [doi: 10.1002/pa.1414]
22. Kim K, Yoo-Lee E, Joanna Sin S. Social media as information source: undergraduates' use and evaluation behavior. 2011 Presented at: ASIST 2011: Annual Meeting of The American Society for Information Science and Technology; Oct 7-12, 2011; New Orleans, LA. [doi: 10.1002/meet.2011.14504801283]
23. Bolton RN, Parasuraman A, Hoefnagels A, Migchels N, Kabadayi S, Gruber T, et al. Understanding Generation Y and their use of social media: a review and research agenda. J Serv Manage 2013 Jun 14;24(3):245-267. [doi: 10.1108/09564231311326987]
24. Valkenburg PM, Peter J, Schouten AP. Friend networking sites and their relationship to adolescents' well-being and social self-esteem. Cyberpsychol Behav 2006 Oct;9(5):584-590. [doi: 10.1089/cpb.2006.9.584] [Medline: 17034326]
25. Potente S, Coppa K, Williams A, Engels R. Legally brown: using ethnographic methods to understand sun protection attitudes and behaviours among young Australians 'I didn't mean to get burnt--it just happened!'. Health Educ Res 2010 Nov 08;26(1):39-52. [doi: 10.1093/her/cyq066] [Medline: 21059798]
26. Feldman SR, Liguori A, Kucenic M, Rapp SR, Fleischer AB, Lang W, et al. Ultraviolet exposure is a reinforcing stimulus in frequent indoor tanners. J Am Acad Dermatol 2004 Jul;51(1):45-51. [doi: 10.1016/j.jaad.2004.01.053] [Medline: 15243523]
27. Myrick JG, Noar SM, Kelley D, Zeitany AE, Morales-Pico BM, Thomas NE. A longitudinal test of the Comprehensive Indoor Tanning Expectations Scale: the importance of affective beliefs in predicting indoor tanning behavior. J Health Psychol 2016 Jul 10;22(1):3-15. [doi: 10.1177/1359105315595116] [Medline: 26231616]
28. Yoo J, Hur W. Body-tanning attitudes among female college students. Psychol Rep 2014 Apr;114(2):585-596. [doi: 10.2466/06.07.pr0.114k21w5] [Medline: 24897909]
29. Carcioppolo N, Orrego Dunleavy V, Myrick JG. A closer look at descriptive norms and indoor tanning: investigating the intermediary role of positive and negative outcome expectations. Health Commun 2018 Sep 10;34(13):1619-1627. [doi: 10.1080/10410236.2018.1517632] [Medline: 30198759]
30. Noar SM, Myrick JG, Morales-Pico B, Thomas NE. Development and validation of the Comprehensive Indoor Tanning Expectations Scale. JAMA Dermatol 2014 May 01;150(5):512-521. [doi: 10.1001/jamadermatol.2013.9086] [Medline: 24500373]
31. Fredrickson BL. The role of positive emotions in positive psychology. The broaden-and-build theory of positive emotions. Am Psychol 2001 Mar;56(3):218-226 [FREE Full text] [Medline: 11315248]
32. Kourosh AS, Harrington CR, Adinoff B. Tanning as a behavioral addiction. Am J Drug Alcohol Abuse 2010 Jun 15;36(5):284-290. [doi: 10.3109/00952990.2010.491883] [Medline: 20545604]
33. Zillmann D. Mood management through communication choices. Am Behav Sci 2016 Jul 27;31(3):327-340. [doi: 10.1177/000276488031003005]
34. Knobloch-Westerwick S. Mood management: theory, evidence, and advancements. In: Bryant J, Vorderer P, editors. Psychology of Entertainment. Mahwah, NJ: Lawrence Erlbaum Associates; 2006:239-254.
35. Dixon HG, Warne CD, Scully ML, Wakefield MA, Dobbinson SJ. Does the portrayal of tanning in Australian women's magazines relate to real women's tanning beliefs and behavior? Health Educ Behav 2011 Jan 24;38(2):132-142. [doi: 10.1177/1090198110369057] [Medline: 21263062]
36. Cho H, Lee S, Wilson K. Magazine exposure, tanned women stereotypes, and tanning attitudes. Body Image 2010 Sep;7(4):364-367. [doi: 10.1016/j.bodyim.2010.04.002] [Medline: 20573553]
37. Cafri G, Thompson JK, Roehrig M, Rojas A, Sperry S, Jacobsen PB, et al. Appearance motives to tan and not tan: evidence for validity and reliability of a new scale. Ann Behav Med 2008 Mar 21;35(2):209-220. [doi: 10.1007/s12160-008-9022-2] [Medline: 18365298]
38. Fogel J, Krausz F. Watching reality television beauty shows is associated with tanning lamp use and outdoor tanning among college students. J Am Acad Dermatol 2013 May;68(5):784-789. [doi: 10.1016/j.jaad.2012.09.055] [Medline: 23261546]
39. Social Media Use in 2018. Pew Research Center. URL: https://www.pewresearch.org/internet/2018/03/01/social-media-use-in-2018/ [accessed 2020-11-20]
40. Noar SM, Myrick JG, Zeitany A, Kelley D, Morales-Pico B, Thomas NE. Testing a social cognitive theory-based model of indoor tanning: implications for skin cancer prevention messages. Health Commun 2015;30(2):164-174. [doi: 10.1080/10410236.2014.974125] [Medline: 25470441]

41. Bandura A. Self-efficacy: toward a unifying theory of behavioral change. Psychol Rev 1977 Mar;84(2):191-215. [Medline: 847061]
42. Bandura A. Social Foundations of Thought and Action. Upper Saddle River, NJ: Prentice-Hall; 1986.
43. Rodríguez VM, Daniel CL, Welles BF, Geller AC, Hay JL. Friendly tanning: young adults' engagement with friends around indoor tanning. J Behav Med 2017 Feb 8;40(4):631-640. [doi: 10.1007/s10865-017-9832-4] [Medline: 28181003]
44. Moskowitz DS, Young SN. Ecological momentary assessment: what it is and why it is a method of the future in clinical psychopharmacology. J Psychiatry Neurosci 2006 Jan;31(1):13-20 [FREE Full text] [Medline: 16496031]
45. Sun safety. American Skin Association. URL: https://www.americanskin.org/resource/safety.php [accessed 2020-11-20]
46. Myrick JG, Holton AE, Himelboim I, Love B. #Stupidcancer: exploring a typology of social support and the role of emotional expression in a social media community. Health Commun 2015 Oct 09;31(5):596-605. [doi: 10.1080/10410236.2014.981664]
47. Myrick J, Willoughby J. Beyond demographics: The relationship of young women's emotional states with skin damaging and skin safety behaviors. 2017 Presented at: Annual Meeting of the National Communication Association; Nov 16-19, 2017; Dallas, TX.
48. Kraus A, Myrick JG. Feeling bad about feel-good ads: the emotional and body-image ramifications of body-positive media. Commun Res Rep 2017 Oct 17;35(2):101-111. [doi: 10.1080/08824096.2017.1383233]
49. Miyamoto Y, Ma X. Dampening or savoring positive emotions: a dialectical cultural script guides emotion regulation. Emotion 2011 Dec;11(6):1346-1357. [doi: 10.1037/a0025135] [Medline: 21910543]
50. Hanwell H, Vieth R, Cole D, Scillitani A, Modoni S, Frusciante V, et al. Sun exposure questionnaire predicts circulating 25-hydroxyvitamin D concentrations in Caucasian hospital workers in southern Italy. J Steroid Biochem Mol Biol 2010 Jul;121(1-2):334-337. [doi: 10.1016/j.jsbmb.2010.03.023] [Medline: 20298782]
51. Diffey B, Norridge Z. Reported sun exposure, attitudes to sun protection and perceptions of skin cancer risk: a survey of visitors to Cancer Research UK's SunSmart campaign website. Br J Dermatol 2009 Jun;160(6):1292-1298. [doi: 10.1111/j.1365-2133.2009.09149.x] [Medline: 19416235]
52. Harrell F. Regression modeling strategies: With application to linear models, logistic and ordinal regression, and survival analysis. New York, NY: Springer International Publishing; 2015.
53. Eastwood JD, Frischen A, Fenske MJ, Smilek D. The unengaged mind: defining boredom in terms of attention. Perspect Psychol Sci 2012 Sep;7(5):482-495. [doi: 10.1177/1745691612456044] [Medline: 26168505]
54. Hill A, Perkins R. Towards a model of boredom. Br J Psychol 1985 May;76(2):235-240. [doi: 10.1111/j.2044-8295.1985.tb01947.x] [Medline: 4027489]
55. Mastro DE, Eastin MS, Tamborini R. Internet search behaviors and mood alterations: a selective exposure approach. Media Psychol 2002 May;4(2):157-172. [doi: 10.1207/s1532785xmep0402_03]
56. Tandoc EC, Ferrucci P, Duffy M. Facebook use, envy, and depression among college students: is facebooking depressing? Comput Hum Behav 2015 Feb;43:139-146. [doi: 10.1016/j.chb.2014.10.053]
57. Appel H, Gerlach A, Crusius J. The interplay between Facebook use, social comparison, envy, and depression. Curr Opinion Psychol 2016 Jun;9:44-49 [FREE Full text] [doi: 10.1016/j.copsyc.2015.10.006]
58. Holman DM, Watson M. Correlates of intentional tanning among adolescents in the United States: a systematic review of the literature. J Adolesc Health 2013 May;52(5 Suppl):S52-S59 [FREE Full text] [doi: 10.1016/j.jadohealth.2012.09.021] [Medline: 23601612]
59. Falzone AE, Brindis CD, Chren M, Junn A, Pagoto S, Wehner M, et al. Teens, tweets, and tanning beds: rethinking the use of social media for skin cancer prevention. Am J Prev Med 2017 Sep;53(3S1):S86-S94 [FREE Full text] [doi: 10.1016/j.amepre.2017.04.027] [Medline: 28818251]
60. Singhal A, Rogers E. Entertainment-education: A communication strategy for social change. New York, NY: Routledge; 2012.
61. Kim K, Lee M, Macias W. An alcohol message beneath the surface of ER: how implicit memory influences viewers' health attitudes and intentions using entertainment-education. J Health Commun 2014;19(8):876-892. [doi: 10.1080/10810730.2013.837556] [Medline: 24479746]
62. van Leeuwen L, Renes RJ, Leeuwis C. Televised entertainment-education to prevent adolescent alcohol use: perceived realism, enjoyment, and impact. Health Educ Behav 2013 Apr;40(2):193-205. [doi: 10.1177/1090198112445906] [Medline: 22773596]
63. Willoughby JF, Liu S. Do pictures help tell the story? An experimental test of narrative and emojis in a health text message intervention. Comput Hum Behav 2018 Feb;79:75-82. [doi: 10.1016/j.chb.2017.10.031]
64. Willoughby JF, Niu Z, Liu S. Assessing the potential use of narrative and the entertainment education strategy in an mHealth text-message intervention. J Health Commun 2018;23(1):20-27. [doi: 10.1080/10810730.2017.1396628] [Medline: 29252131]
65. Zhou C, Occa A, Kim S, Morgan S. A meta-analysis of narrative game-based interventions for promoting healthy behaviors. J Health Commun 2020;25(1):54-65. [doi: 10.1080/10810730.2019.1701586] [Medline: 31829829]
66. Rodgers KB, Hust SJT, Willoughby JF, Wheeler J, Li J. Adolescents' sex-related alcohol expectancies and alcohol advertisements in magazines: the role of wishful identification, realism, and beliefs about women's enjoyment of sexualization. J Health Commun 2019;24(4):395-404. [doi: 10.1080/10810730.2019.1630523] [Medline: 31215356]
67. Willoughby JF, Hust SJT, Li J, Couto L. Social media, marijuana and sex: an exploratory study of adolescents' intentions

to use and college students' use of marijuana. J Sex Res 2020 Oct 09:1-13. [doi: 10.1080/00224499.2020.1827217] [Medline: 33034543]

Abbreviations

EMA: ecological momentary assessment
FLASHE: Family Life, Activity, Sun, Health, and Eating

9

Tanning Misinformation Posted by Businesses on Social Media and Related Perceptions of Adolescent and Young Adult White Non-Hispanic Women: Mixed Methods Study

Megan Andreas Moreno[1], MD, MSEd, MPH; Marina C Jenkins[1], BS; DeAnn Lazovich[2], PhD

[1]Department of Pediatrics, University of Wisconsin-Madison, Madison, WI, United States

[2]Department of Epidemiology and Community Health, University of Minnesota, Minneapolis, MN, United States

Corresponding Author:
Megan Andreas Moreno, MD, MSEd, MPH
Department of Pediatrics
University of Wisconsin-Madison
2870 University Ave
Suite 200
Madison, WI, 53705
United States

Email: mamoreno@pediatrics.wisc.edu

Abstract

Background: Indoor ultraviolet (UV) tanning is common and consequential, increasing the risk for cancers including melanoma and basal cell carcinoma. At-risk groups include adolescents and young adults, who often report beliefs about benefits of tanning. Adolescent and young adults are also among the most ubiquitous social media users. As previous studies support that content about tanning is common on social media, this may be a way that young women are exposed to influential content promoting tanning, including health misinformation.

Objective: The purpose of this study was to evaluate health misinformation promoted by indoor tanning businesses via social media and to understand young women's perceptions of this misinformation.

Methods: This mixed methods study included (1) retrospective observational content analysis of indoor tanning salons' content on Facebook over 1 year and (2) qualitative interviews with a purposeful national sample of 46 White non-Hispanic women, age 16 to 23 years, who had recently tanned indoors. We assessed experiences with tanning businesses' posted content on social media through interviews. We used the constant comparative approach for qualitative analyses.

Results: Content analysis findings included data from indoor tanning businesses (n=147) across 50 states, yielding 4956 total posts. Among 9 health misinformation topics identified, the most common was the promotion of UV tanning as a safe way to get Vitamin D (n=73, 1.5%). An example post was "Stop by Body and Sol to get your daily dose of Vitamin D." Another misinformation topic was promoting tanning for health benefits (n=31, 0.62%), an example post was "the flu is not a season, it's an inability to adapt due to decreased sun exposure…" A total of 46 participants completed interviews (age: mean 20 years, SD 2). Almost all participants (45/46, 98%) used Facebook, and 43.5% (20/46) followed an indoor tanning business on social media. Approximately half of participants reported seeing social media posts from tanning salons about Vitamin D, an example of a participant comment was "I have [seen that] a few times..." Among the participants, approximately half believed it was safe to get Vitamin D from indoor UV tanning; a participant stated: "I think it is a valid benefit to UV tanning."

Conclusions: Despite the low frequency (range 0.5%-1.5%) of social media posts promoting health misinformation, participants commonly reported viewing these posts, and their perceptions aligned with health misinformation. Health education campaigns, possibly using social media to target at-risk populations, may be an innovative approach for tanning prevention messages.

KEYWORDS

adolescent; social media; tanning; technology; media

Introduction

In 2009, the World Health Organization classified ultraviolet (UV) radiation-emitting tanning devices as Class I carcinogens [1]. Indoor UV tanning has been shown to increase the risk of developing squamous and basal cell carcinoma and melanoma, particularly among people who start at an early age or tan frequently [1-5]. Fortunately, indoor tanning has declined over the past decade among adolescents and young adults, who have traditionally represented a population with a high prevalence of this behavior [6,7]. However, among the highest adolescent risk group of White non-Hispanic females, indoor tanning rates remained above 10% in 2017, which is nearly twice the overall rate of tanning among adolescents [8,9].

Previous studies have identified several factors that influence an adolescent or young adult's decision to pursue indoor tanning. These include beliefs about tanning contributing to beauty [10], social factors such as peer tanning behaviors [11], and positive attitudes and intentions toward tanning [12,13]. The role of media in promoting positive attitudes and intentions toward indoor tanning remains understudied. Previous studies have examined traditional media and found that watching reality television was associated with tanning [14] and that exposure to tan models in magazines promoted positive attitudes toward tanning [15]

In today's digital world, messages promoting indoor tanning may be shared through social media [16], which has nearly ubiquitous use among adolescent and young adults [17]. Previous studies [18,19] support social media as a platform in which comparison to others' appearances is positively associated with body dissatisfaction and even as a risk factor for eating disorders. Social media content related to tanning behavior is common, a previous study [20] examined Twitter and found 7.7 mentions of indoor tanning per minute, with only a small percentage mentioning health risks. While studies such as this have illustrated how users generate and share content about tanning on social media, less is known about the content shared by tanning businesses. Researchers in related fields, such as alcohol research, have hypothesized that the engagement and interaction that can occur with businesses via social media influence how marketing effects progress from awareness to encouraging behavior [21].

The spread of misinformation through social media can be particularly influential, as it is tied to emotions, identity, and one's social network. For this study we define misinformation as inaccurate or false information. Indoor tanning salons' business profiles on social media may increase exposure to misinformation among adolescent and young adults. The purpose of this mixed methods study was to evaluate health misinformation promoted by indoor UV tanning salons via social media and to understand adolescent and young adult's perceptions of this misinformation.

Methods

Overview

This mixed methods study included social media content analysis and qualitative interviews. Content analysis was conducted on the social media platform Facebook between the dates May 1, 2015 and April 30, 2016. This data collection received an exemption for observation of public information from the Seattle Children's institutional review board (15506 exempt).

Participant interviews were conducted after content analysis was complete in order to include observations from content analysis in the interview. These data were collected between May 8, 2017 and July 7, 2017. This data collection was approved by the Seattle Children's institutional review board (15710).

Social Media Content Analysis

Design

At the time of this study, Facebook was among the most popular sites used by the adolescent and young adult population [22]. Facebook also offered business profiles that allowed development of a free-standing multimedia profile with capacity to connect to and interact with users. Given its popularity among our target population and the robust content available for coding, this platform was selected for evaluation for this study.

Purposeful Sampling

The focus of this study was content posted on social media by businesses that provide indoor UV tanning. Our goal was to identify social media profiles created and maintained by indoor tanning salons. We focused on profiles that were popular among users and had both current and historical content to evaluate. Our goal was to evaluate 1 year of content retrospectively. For each of the 50 states, we evaluated 3 tanning business profiles to capture range and variation across businesses. We used purposeful sampling to identify profiles, a strategy used for description and investigation into social processes of particular groups.

Search Strategy

To identify potential profiles for evaluation, we conducted a search on Facebook for each of the 50 states using search terms in the form *"tanning salon" + [state]*, where *[state]* was replaced by each state name; we set the search criteria to deliver responses by relevance.

From the list of search results, we reviewed the first 10 business profiles listed, and from those profiles, we selected the 3 business profiles that had the largest number of followers.

We then evaluated each of the 3 profiles to ensure that they were publicly available profiles and that they prioritized UV tanning services. To confirm that the business prioritized UV tanning services, the business profile needed to meet a minimum of 2 of the 3 criteria: (1) include the word "tanning" in name of the business or business category selected on Facebook was "tanning salon," (2) describe the provision of UV tanning services in the About Me section of the profile, and (3) have 25% or more of the posts by the profile owner in the past month refer to UV tanning. Additional inclusion criteria were that the business must have had the profile for at least 1 year (in order for us to be able to evaluate a full year of content) and that the business must have made at least 1 post during 2015 (to ensure that the profile was active during the coding period).

Facebook profiles that were labeled as unofficial pages were excluded: Facebook profiles have the option to indicate whether they are an official page sponsored by a busines or an unofficial page, which often represents an individual who is a fan or supporter of the business. Furthermore, because of our state-based approach to coding, tanning salon chains that extended to multiple states were excluded, though tanning chains located within single states were included.

If inclusion criteria were not met by a given profile, we selected the profile with the next highest number of followers. We developed a list of all salons that met inclusion criteria and the link to the Facebook page (so that the pages could be returned to later for coding).

Codebook Development and Variables

Through a previous study [23], we have created various codebooks containing keywords and image interpretation used in evaluating Facebook profiles for references to other health risk behaviors such as substance use and risky sexual behavior. Through a review of the literature [13,23,24] and pilot coding, we developed and tested a codebook focused on tanning-related health misinformation. We also recorded basic information about the tanning business, including the name, location, and number of followers.

Interrater Reliability

We conducted interrater agreement assessments at the beginning and end of the coding process. Interrater agreement ranged from 84% to 99% at the beginning to 91% to 100% at the end of coding across the health misinformation variables.

Procedure

Trained coders reviewed 1 year of content on each business social media profile. Assessing a full year of content allowed us to capture data to represent events (ie, spring break) and seasons. Pilot data collection illustrated that most tanning business profiles posted multiple times per day and frequently duplicated the same post during a given day or across a given month. Thus, our content analysis strategy was to evaluate 1 post per day, selected as the final post of that day, every third day of the month. This strategy allowed us to ensure that both weekdays and weekends were included in each month's evaluations and to vary the day of the week evaluated over time. Furthermore, if that post was identical to the post evaluated from a previous day, that post was skipped and the prior post for that day was evaluated. This allowed us to diversify the content evaluated.

We recorded data for each selected post as follows: for text posts, we recorded verbatim text; for user-generated photos, we recorded a thorough description of the photo; and for popular public images, such as memes or other downloadable icons, we copied and pasted the image into the data set. We also recorded the date that the post was uploaded to the social media profile. Each social media post was considered the unit of analysis and was thus categorized and coded based on which constructs were represented in that post. Data were extracted to a customized database (FileMaker, Claris International) and saved into a secure data file that was password protected.

Qualitative Interviews

Design

A qualitative approach was best suited to investigating young women's experiences and perspectives [25]. The goal of this inquiry was to understand individual experiences and allow participants privacy in their responses to questions. Thus, individual interviewing was selected as the method.

Participant Sample and Recruitment

Given the qualitative approach, the goal sample size was 40 participants with experience with both indoor tanning and engagement with a tanning salon on social media. With purposeful sampling and this sample size, we estimated we could achieve theoretical saturation. We conducted purposeful recruitment to target participants who were among the demographic most likely to engage in tanning: White non-Hispanic females ages 16 through 23 years [26]. Our purposeful sampling also included focused recruitment efforts on participants who were likely to have engaged with indoor tanning salon content on social media. Thus, we recruited participants via Facebook advertisements. A Facebook advertisement was created and targeted to a national sample of women ages 16 through 23 years. The advertisement was posted for a total of 3 weeks. The advertisement described an interview study about indoor UV tanning experiences. Interested participants were directed to a website to complete eligibility screening to ensure they met inclusion criteria (experienced indoor tanning in the past year and were in our target demographic). These potentially eligible participants then underwent phone screening to confirm eligibility and complete informed consent. We obtained informed consent from participants over the age of 18 years and the parents of minors; We obtained informed assent from participants under the age of 18 years.

Interview Guide Development and Training

During interviews, we asked about perceptions and experiences viewing content from indoor tanning businesses on social media. Questions were designed to invite sharing of perspectives without judgment. Interview questions were designed to be semistructured and open-ended, allowing participants to expand their comments with follow-up prompts. Interview questions included asking participants about their indoor tanning experiences as well as their social media usage. Example questions included "In what ways do indoor tanning salons use social media?" Interviewers then provided a brief overview of the study findings regarding observations of health misinformation on social media. Participants were asked about thoughts, experiences, and reactions to this shared information.

Interviewer training involved reading training materials, observing standardized interviews, and conducting a minimum of 1 pilot interview prior to conducting interviews for this study. There were 2 interviewers for this study.

Data Collection

Interviews were conducted by phone. The interviewer confirmed that the participant was in a private and comfortable location prior to beginning the interview. Data were recorded in a customized online platform (FileMaker Pro) during the interviews. Interviews lasted between 20 and 40 minutes. Participants received a US $40 incentive upon completing the interview.

Analysis

Three investigators with experience in qualitative analysis were involved in the analysis process. The investigators utilized a constant comparative approach to categorize responses [25]. Two of the 3 investigators first individually reviewed all transcripts and then met to discuss data categorization. The goal of the first cycle was to collaboratively develop and apply a coding schema. The 2 investigators then independently coded 5 interviews (blinded to one another's coding). After coding the transcripts, they reviewed the codes unblinded. All 3 investigators then met and discussed and reached consensus for any additions or revisions to coding categories. The third senior investigator served to resolve unclear areas or disagreements between investigators. The coding process was then applied to a second set of interviews with 2 investigators. The purpose of this second review was to evaluate reliability and validity of the initial classification criteria. After coding review, discussion and achieving consensus on the coding categories, the coding approach was applied to the remaining interviews using the same constant comparative approach.

Results

Social Media Content Analysis

Of a total of 147 indoor tanning business Facebook pages that were evaluated across 50 states, 3 businesses closed prior to coding initiation. This sample of indoor tanning business Facebook pages yielded 4956 posts. Among 8 health misinformation topics identified, the most common were posts promoting misinformation about Vitamin D (n=73, 1.3%). This misinformation typically focused on tanning as a safe and healthy way to get Vitamin D. The American Academy of Dermatology notes that tanning beds are not a safe way to get Vitamin D given the cancer risk [27]. Furthermore, since bulbs in tanning beds mostly emit UVA light, vitamin D can only be generated via UVB light. Thus, tanning beds do not provide sufficient exposure to create adequate doses of Vitamin D [27]. An example post was

> *Stop by Body and Sol to get your daily dose of Vitamin D.*

Most indoor tanning businesses that displayed misinformation about Vitamin D did so infrequently. Many businesses had only 1 Vitamin D–related post within the 1-year sample, though 3 businesses had 5 or more of this category of posts.

A second category was misinformation about tanning as a medical treatment (n=31 posts, 0.6%), for example,

> *...the flu is not a season, it's an inability to adapt due to decreased sun exposure...*

Some of these posts were consistent with described inaccuracies in an investigative report provided to the US House of Representatives. These inaccuracies mainly center on promoting tanning as having health benefits or as a health treatment, there is no evidence to support tanning as a safe health treatment for illness including mental illness, inflammatory diseases, sleep problems or pain disorders [28]. Most businesses that displayed misinformation about tanning as a medical treatment had only 1 of these posts within the 1-year sample; there were no businesses with more than 3 posts of this type in the 1-year sample.

Another category of misinformation was promoting misinformation about the benefits of a "base tan" (n=29 posts, 0.5%) The posts often argued that a base tan would prevent sunburn or was a protective measure to take prior to a vacation. There is no evidence that a base tan is protective against sunburn or against cancer risks from sun exposure [27]. Most tanning businesses displayed only 1 of these posts in the 1-year sample, and many were posted in late winter, prior to spring break season. Table 1 displays the 8 categories of health misinformation, and Table 2 displays example social media posts.

Table 1. Health misinformation displayed on Facebook posts (N=4956) by businesses across 50 states over a 1-year period.

Misinformation category and number of posts	Businesses (N=147), n
About Vitamin D (n=73)	37
1	26
2	6
3	2
5	1
9	1
15	1
Tanning as a medical treatment (n=31)	26
1	22
2	3
3	1
Indoor tanning is equivalent to sunshine (n=31)	18
1	11
2	4
3	2
9	1
About base tan (n=29)	14
1	10
2	3
13	1
Indoor tanning as safer than outdoor tanning (n=3)	3
1	3
About health benefits of tanning (n=7)	6
1	5
2	1
About skin appearance (n=40)	21
1	15
2	4
3	1
14	1
About cancer (n=7)	5
1	4
2	1

Table 2. Example posts.

Misinformation category	Posts
About Vitamin D	• "Best supplementation of UV next to an IV" • #VitaminD • "D is for doping: Vitamin D"
Tanning as a medical treatment	• "UVB from tanning is a safe treatment for acne, eczema and seasonal depression" • "Link to article describing tanning as prevention for cancer, autism and depression"
Indoor tanning is equivalent to sunshine	• "Tanning=sunshine" • "Now serving sunshine"
About base tan	• "A base tan will keep you safe from UV rays" • "Start working on that base tan so you don't burn at the beach"
Indoor tanning as safer than outdoor tanning	• "Tanning indoor is taking responsibility for your tan. Prevent sunburn and using an indoor tanning lotion for best results!"
About health benefits of tanning	• "Women who avoid sunbathing during the summer are twice as likely to die as those who sunbathe every day" • "Getting enough sun optimizes 10% of our genes"
About skin appearance	• "Tanning lotions will tighten your skin" • "Tanning as 'age rewinding'"
About cancer	• "A great peer-reviewed journal article…but a little nerdy :) from the US National Library of Medicine and the National Institute of Health, showing that a continuous pattern of sun exposure appears NOT to increase risk of melanoma." • "According to a recent study the risk of skin cancer, particularly melanoma, decreases with proper tanning bed use"

Qualitative Interviews

A total of 46 interviews were conducted (age: mean 20 years, SD 2) and 26 states were represented in our sample. Among our participants, 45 (97.8%) used Facebook, and 20 (43.5%) followed an indoor tanning salon on social media. Most participants (38/46, 82.6%) mentioned viewing indoor tanning salon posts on social media to find out about sales or special offers; fewer (3/46, 6.5%) noted that they learned tips related to tanning from these posts.

Approximately half (21/46, 45.5%) of participants acknowledged that indoor tanning businesses likely used social media to "draw people in" and influence tanning behavior. Some participants who followed tanning businesses on social media specifically noted that social media posts may normalize tanning behaviors or "promote tanning benefits." Table 3 includes the most common topics that participants described viewing on indoor tanning salons' social media pages.

Just over half (25/46, 54.3%) of participants expressed that social media influenced their friends, or people in general, to go tanning more often, and 52.2% (24/46) mentioned that social media influenced them personally to tan more. Some participants (4/46, 8.7%) stated that posts on social media by indoor tanning salons led them to see tanning as safer than the sun or the business as trustworthy.

As Vitamin D was the most common category of social media misinformation posts, we asked participants whether they had seen indoor tanning businesses post on social media about Vitamin D. Approximately half (20/46, 43%) of participants reported seeing social media posts from tanning salons about Vitamin D:

> *I have [seen that] a few times…* [Participant]

Among those participants, approximately half (25/46, 54%) believed it was safe to get Vitamin D from indoor tanning stating, for example,

> *I think it is a valid benefit to UV tanning.* [Participant]

Table 3. Qualitative interviews with White non-Hispanic adolescent and young adult women about indoor tanning and social media (n=46).

Topic	Participants (n=46), n (%)	Example quotations
Type of content posted by indoor tanning salons on social media reported by participants		
Deals and sales	38 (82.6)	"They post $4 tan weeks, come tan for $5, promotions and deals mainly"
Lotions	12 (26.0)	"They post sales on lotion and promotions trying to get new people to come in, on Twitter for retweets they give away free lotion and tanning minutes"
Tanning tips	3 (6.5)	"...they also give tips for what is good for your skin and what isn't"
How tanning salons use social media		
Attract new customers	20 (45.5)	"They are trying to get customers or potential customers"
Showcase deals or promotions	18 (40.9)	"To promote brand recognition and specials they are running that month...They also promote employment for that salon. If you work at the salon, you get free tanning."
Remind and/or motivate people to tan	7 (15.9)	"There is also the psychological aspect to it where they post motivations like, "everyone looks good tan" to try to get more people to start tan"
Sell lotions	6 (13.6)	"Advertising their prices and different lotions they have for their clients"
Promote tanning benefits	4 (9.1)	"They probably want to decrease the stigma in tanning to make it look more beneficial"
Target young people	3 (6.8)	"To reach their target market or to target those who are younger"
What role does social media play in you or your friends tanning		
Influences people to tan more	25 (54.3)	"I think it would make us tan more than we actually do want to or intend to"
Influence the participant to tan more	24 (52.2)	"It has made me want to tan. I used to be against, but then Facebook drew me into it and now I'm doing it"
Motivate to go tanning by deals	18 (38.1)	"If there's a deal more people will be inclined to do it, even people that don't regularly tan will go to take advantage of the deal"
Seeing friends post about tanning, not tanning salons, is influence to them	14 (30.4)	"When you see your friends on Facebook and they're tan it makes you want to be tan as well"
Motivate to go tanning by pictures of tan people	13 (28.3)	"I definitely see that it affects it. When you see people that are tan on social media you wish you were that tan"
Normalizes tanning	7 (15.2)	"I definitely thinking that seeing it a lot on social media makes it very normal. Since you see everyone else on social media, it makes it very acceptable"
Influences viewers to see tanning as safe	4 (8.7)	"Makes it seem like a safe thing to do. You don't think about the risks"

Discussion

General

This mixed methods study included social media content analysis and qualitative participant interviews. We found an overall low frequency of social media posts promoting health misinformation (range 0.5%-1.5%); however, many (20/46,43.5%) of our participants actively followed tanning businesses on social media, and participants commonly reported remembering misinformation posts such as those promoting tanning as a safe way to get Vitamin D.

Our first finding was that social media posts related to health misinformation were uncommon. Most of the content posted by tanning businesses was related to other topics, such as deals or sales as described by our participants. These findings are consistent with a previous study examining hashtags related to tanning that found that most tanning salon posts were related to price reductions [29]. We found that the most common category of misinformation—indoor tanning as a safe way to get Vitamin D—comprised less than 2% of posts recorded across the year. It is important to clarify that our data did not represent that UV tanning could provide Vitamin D, but that posts described UV tanning as a safe way to achieve Vitamin D, which identifies these statements as clear misinformation as there is no evidence that the body can achieve adequate Vitamin D levels safely (given cancer risks) or adequately [27]. Furthermore, in many categories of health misinformation, most tanning businesses displayed only 1 post in that category across our 1-year evaluation period. Given these findings, it is even more striking that many participants reported recalling these posts. This finding suggests that these health misinformation posts, while uncommon, were memorable and may have been influential. Our findings from participant comments clearly support that the practice of following social media tanning businesses contributed to reminders to participants to go tanning, through deals and specials, and reminders about motivations to tan. It is also important to note that a social media platform is interactive, whereby users and businesses can interact bidirectionally. Thus, while the frequency of these health misinformation posts displayed by tanning businesses was uncommon, these posts can be shared or distributed across an individual's own social media.

Our second finding was that, among our purposeful sample focused on those who engage in indoor tanning as well as social media, participants commonly engaged with social media related to tanning. As nearly half (20/46, 43.5%) participants followed a tanning business on social media, this supports the potential reach and influence that tanning salons have among young social media users. Participants described that indoor tanning salons' social media pages provided them reminders, nudges, and information about special deals and sales. Participants described the influence of tanning-related social media on their own tanning attitudes, as well as on their behaviors. This finding suggests that, of the approximately 10% of young White females who continue to engage in indoor tanning, social media may be a viable platform to reach this at-risk population with education or intervention approaches.

Limitations

Our study is not without limitations. This study focused on tanning businesses that were present on Facebook, and we did not examine other platforms such as Snapchat or Instagram. We were interested in how popular tanning businesses utilized social media to engage with customers. Thus, our purposeful sampling strategy prioritized selection of tanning businesses that were popular on social media (ie, by number of followers). We excluded tanning salon chains that extended across states, which allowed us to focus on individual businesses within states. However, tanning salons within chains may reach more viewers compared to individual businesses. Furthermore, our Facebook data were from 2015; however, the role of Facebook as a platform to connect to businesses remains relevant today, and no new laws or regulations governing tanning business content on social media have arisen since that time. Finally, our qualitative interviews were purposeful in order to target the at-risk population for indoor tanning, thus evaluating external validity of our sample was not appropriate for this study.

Implications

Despite these limitations, our study has implications in the area of health misinformation. While the overall reduction in indoor tanning behaviors among women and adolescents [6,7] is a public health triumph, a significant at-risk group of White young women remain engaged in this health risk behavior [8,9]. Our study findings suggest that some of these women who tan are also connected to indoor tanning salons on social media. While misinformation may not be common or a significant motivator for adolescent and young adult tanning, social media connections between businesses and adolescents and young adults are very common and may provide ongoing engagement with and encouragement of tanning behavior, that is, this social media connection may foster ongoing relationships with tanning businesses and behavioral nudges to go tanning through deals and reminders about motivations to tan.

An initial strategy to prevent adolescents from following these businesses on social media may be to consider requiring *age-gating* for indoor tanning businesses. Age-gating would block access to indoor tanning social media pages for youth under age 18. The age-gating approach is currently used by alcohol companies on social media, and youth are supportive of applying this restriction to other businesses on social media [30]. Additional strategies may include creating regulations about health misinformation directed at indoor tanning businesses, similar to strategies used to limit health misinformation about tobacco and marijuana. Finally, strategies to reach at-risk women may include placing targeted educational campaigns on social media, similar to the Facebook advertisements that we used to recruit for this study, which were successful in identifying the population at risk for consequences of indoor tanning.

Our study focused on health misinformation messages shared on social media by tanning salons. However, the implications of our findings may contribute to a critical conversation about how health misinformation shared via social media may reach vulnerable populations and potential prevention strategies. First, age-gating may present a valid approach to limit youth access to content from businesses based on minimum age limits, such as alcohol, tobacco, e-cigarettes, marijuana, and tanning. Second, regulations that clearly define allowable messages on any medium (print, online, or social media) are critical to consider. Enhancing efforts around surveillance of social media would be an important part of such regulations. It is possible that funds from tax revenues related to these sale of these products could support regular and ongoing monitoring of industry compliance. Challenges to monitoring social media content include its potentially ephemeral nature, as well as the ability in social media to target content behaviorally, geographically, and temporally. While surveillance may not capture all businesses that post misinformation, for example, many of the businesses that posted Vitamin D misinformation did so only once during our data collection time period. However, ongoing surveillance may be likely to identify businesses that repeatedly post misinformation. For example, we found that 1 tanning business displayed 13 posts promoting misinformation about benefits of a base tan. Finally, our study illustrates that it is possible to create a sampling strategy to evaluate posts over time and to develop a codebook to identify content and achieve interrater reliability for such content. The content and keywords identified in this study may inform other social media surveillance methods using machine learning or automated text analysis for more widespread evaluation. It is also possible that partnering with adolescents and young adults who are often at the forefront of the learning curve for digital media may lead to creative prevention approaches.

Acknowledgments

The authors would like to thank contributors Nikita Midamba and Adrienne Ton. This study was funded by the National Cancer Institute (grant R03 CA201953-01); the funders had no involvement in study processes or writing.

References

1. El Ghissassi F, Baan R, Straif K, Grosse Y, Secretan B, Bouvard V, WHO International Agency for Research on Cancer Monograph Working Group. A review of human carcinogens--part D: radiation. Lancet Oncol 2009 Aug;10(8):751-752. [doi: 10.1016/s1470-2045(09)70213-x] [Medline: 19655431]
2. International Agency for Research on Cancer Working Group on artificial ultraviolet (UV) lightskin cancer. The association of use of sunbeds with cutaneous malignant melanoma and other skin cancers: a systematic review. Int J Cancer 2007 Mar 01;120(5):1116-1122 [FREE Full text] [doi: 10.1002/ijc.22453] [Medline: 17131335]
3. Ferrucci L. M., Indoor tanning and risk of early-onset basal cell carcinoma. J Am Acad Dermatol 2012;67(4):552-562. [doi: 10.1158/1538-7445.am2012-635] [Medline: 22153793]
4. Lazovich D, Vogel RI, Berwick M, Weinstock MA, Anderson KE, Warshaw EM. Indoor tanning and risk of melanoma: a case-control study in a highly exposed population. Cancer Epidemiol Biomarkers Prev 2010 Jun;19(6):1557-1568 [FREE Full text] [doi: 10.1158/1055-9965.EPI-09-1249] [Medline: 20507845]
5. Colantonio S, Bracken MB, Beecker J. The association of indoor tanning and melanoma in adults: systematic review and meta-analysis. J Am Acad Dermatol 2014 May;70(5):847-57.e1. [doi: 10.1016/j.jaad.2013.11.050] [Medline: 24629998]
6. Guy GP, Watson M, Seidenberg AB, Hartman AM, Holman DM, Perna F. Trends in indoor tanning and its association with sunburn among US adults. J Am Acad Dermatol 2017 Jun;76(6):1191-1193 [FREE Full text] [doi: 10.1016/j.jaad.2017.01.022] [Medline: 28522044]
7. Holman DM, Jones SE, Qin J, Richardson LC. Prevalence of indoor tanning among U.S. high school students from 2009 to 2017. J Community Health 2019 Dec 22;44(6):1086-1089 [FREE Full text] [doi: 10.1007/s10900-019-00685-y] [Medline: 31230221]
8. Guy GP, Berkowitz Z, Tai E, Holman DM, Everett Jones S, Richardson LC. Indoor tanning among high school students in the United States, 2009 and 2011. JAMA Dermatol 2014 May 01;150(5):501-511 [FREE Full text] [doi: 10.1001/jamadermatol.2013.7124] [Medline: 24577222]
9. Skin cancer prevention progress report. Centers for Disease Control and Prevention. 2019. URL: https://www.cdc.gov/cancer/skin/pdf/SkinCancerPreventionProgressReport-2019-508.pdf [accessed 2020-12-20]
10. Mosher CE, Danoff-Burg S. Addiction to indoor tanning: relation to anxiety, depression, and substance use. Arch Dermatol 2010 Apr 01;146(4):412-417 [FREE Full text] [doi: 10.1001/archdermatol.2009.385] [Medline: 20404230]
11. Mosher CE, Danoff-Burg S. Social predictors of sunscreen and self-tanning product use. J Am Coll Health 2005 Nov;54(3):166-168. [doi: 10.3200/jach.54.3.166-168] [Medline: 16335316]
12. Mayer JA, Woodruff SI, Slymen DJ, Sallis JF, Forster JL, Clapp EJ, et al. Adolescents' use of indoor tanning: a large-scale evaluation of psychosocial, environmental, and policy-level correlates. Am J Public Health 2011 May;101(5):930-938 [FREE Full text] [doi: 10.2105/AJPH.2010.300079] [Medline: 21421947]
13. Lazovich D, Forster J, Sorensen G, Emmons K, Stryker J, Demierre M, et al. Characteristics associated with use or intention to use indoor tanning among adolescents. Arch Pediatr Adolesc Med 2004 Sep 01;158(9):918-924. [doi: 10.1001/archpedi.158.9.918] [Medline: 15351760]
14. Fogel J, Krausz F. Watching reality television beauty shows is associated with tanning lamp use and outdoor tanning among college students. J Am Acad Dermatol 2013 May;68(5):784-789. [doi: 10.1016/j.jaad.2012.09.055] [Medline: 23261546]
15. Dixon HG, Warne CD, Scully ML, Wakefield MA, Dobbinson SJ. Does the portrayal of tanning in Australian women's magazines relate to real women's tanning beliefs and behavior? Health Educ Behav 2011 Apr 24;38(2):132-142. [doi: 10.1177/1090198110369057] [Medline: 21263062]
16. Hossler EW, Conroy MP. YouTube as a source of information on tanning bed use. Arch Dermatol 2008 Oct 20;144(10):1395-1396. [doi: 10.1001/archderm.144.10.1395] [Medline: 18936411]
17. Smith A, Anderson M. Social media use in 2018. Pew Research Center. 2018. URL: http://www.pewinternet.org/2018/03/01/social-media-use-in-2018/ [accessed 2020-12-20]
18. Cohen R, Blaszczynski A. Comparative effects of Facebook and conventional media on body image dissatisfaction. J Eat Disord 2015 Jul 2;3(1):23-15-0061-3 [FREE Full text] [doi: 10.1186/s40337-015-0061-3] [Medline: 26140215]
19. Lee H, Lee HE, Choi J, Kim JH, Han HL. Social media use, body image, and psychological well-being: a cross-cultural comparison of Korea and the United States. J Health Commun 2014 Dec 09;19(12):1343-1358. [doi: 10.1080/10810730.2014.904022] [Medline: 24814665]
20. Seidenberg AB, Pagoto SL, Vickey TA, Linos E, Wehner MR, Costa RD, et al. Tanning bed burns reported on Twitter: over 15,000 in 2013. Transl Behav Med 2016 Jun 18;6(2):271-276 [FREE Full text] [doi: 10.1007/s13142-016-0388-6] [Medline: 27356997]
21. McClure AC, Tanski SE, Li Z, Jackson K, Morgenstern M, Li Z, et al. Internet alcohol marketing and underage alcohol use. Pediatrics 2016 Feb;137(2):e20152149 [FREE Full text] [doi: 10.1542/peds.2015-2149] [Medline: 26738886]
22. Lenhart A. Pew Research Center. URL: https://www.pewresearch.org/internet/2015/04/09/teens-social-media-technology-2015/ [accessed 2021-05-03]
23. Moreno MA, Parks MR, Zimmerman FJ, Brito TE, Christakis DA. Display of health risk behaviors on MySpace by adolescents: prevalence and associations. Arch Pediatr Adolesc Med 2009 Jan 05;163(1):27-34. [doi: 10.1001/archpediatrics.2008.528] [Medline: 19124700]

24. Bagdasarov Z, Banerjee S, Greene K, Campo S. Indoor tanning and problem behavior. J Am Coll Health 2010 Aug 06;56(5):555-562. [doi: 10.3200/jach.56.5.555-562]
25. Glesne C. Becoming Qualitative Researchers. 2nd ed. Reading, MA: Longman; 1999:34-65.
26. Guy GP, Berkowitz Z, Everett Jones S, Holman DM, Garnett E, Watson M. Trends in indoor tanning among US high school students, 2009-2013. JAMA Dermatol 2015 Apr 01;151(4):448-450 [FREE Full text] [doi: 10.1001/jamadermatol.2014.4677] [Medline: 25535810]
27. 10 surprising facts about indoor tanning. American Academy of Dermatology Association. URL: https://tinyurl.com/xpbm3kpa [accessed 2021-05-01]
28. False and misleading health information provided to teens by the indoor tanning industry investigative report. Dermatology Nurses' Association. Washington, DC: U.S. House of Representatives Committee on Energy and Commerce URL: https://www.dnanurse.org/sites/default/files/downloads/2012/Tanning%20Investigation%20Report%202.1.12.pdf [accessed 2021-05-01]
29. Ricklefs CA, Asdigian NL, Kalra HL, Mayer JA, Dellavalle RP, Holman DM, et al. Indoor tanning promotions on social media in six US cities #UVTanning #tanning. Transl Behav Med 2016 Jun 26;6(2):260-270 [FREE Full text] [doi: 10.1007/s13142-015-0378-0] [Medline: 27356996]
30. Moreno MA, Gower AD, Jenkins MC, Kerr B, Gritton J. Marijuana promotions on social media: adolescents' views on prevention strategies. Subst Abuse Treat Prev Policy 2018 Jul 02;13(1):23-24 [FREE Full text] [doi: 10.1186/s13011-018-0152-7] [Medline: 29961426]

Abbreviations

UV: ultraviolet

10

Tetrahydrocannabinol and Skin Cancer: Analysis of YouTube Videos

Andrina Mamo[1], BS; Mindy D Szeto[1], MS; Roya Mirhossaini[2], MD; Andrew Fortugno[3], MD; Robert P Dellavalle[1], MD, PhD, MSPH

[1]Department of Dermatology, University of Colorado Anschutz Medical Campus, Aurora, CO, United States

[2]Department of Medicine, Riverside Community Hospital, Riverside, CA, United States

[3]Department of Medicine, University of Tennessee Health Sciences Center, Memphis, TN, United States

Corresponding Author:
Mindy D Szeto, MS
Department of Dermatology
University of Colorado Anschutz Medical Campus
1665 Aurora Court, 3rd Floor
Mailstop F703
Aurora, CO, 80045
United States

Email: mindy.szeto@cuanschutz.edu

Abstract

Background: Cannabis oil is being used topically by patients with skin cancer as a homeopathic remedy, and has been promoted and popularized on social media, including YouTube. Although topical cannabinoids, especially tetrahydrocannabinol (THC), may have antitumor effects, results from a sparse number of clinical trials and peer-reviewed studies detailing safety and efficacy are still under investigation.

Objective: We sought to assess the accuracy, quality, and reliability of THC oil and skin cancer information available on YouTube.

Methods: The 10 most-viewed videos on THC oil and skin cancer were analyzed with the Global Quality Scale (GQS), DISCERN score, and useful/misleading criteria based on presentation of erroneous and scientifically unproven information. The videos were also inspected for source, length, and audience likes/dislikes. Top comments were additionally examined based on whether they were favorable, unfavorable, or neutral regarding the video content.

Results: All analyzed videos (10/10, 100%) received a GQS score of 1, corresponding to poor quality of content, and 9/10 (90%) videos received a DISCERN score of 0, indicating poor reliability of information presented. All 10 videos were also found to be misleading and not useful according to established criteria. Top comments were largely either favorable (13/27, 48%) or neutral (13/27, 48%) toward the content of the videos, compared to unfavorable (1/27, 4%).

Conclusions: Dermatologists should be aware that the spread of inaccurate information on skin cancer treatment currently exists on popular social media platforms and may lead to detrimental consequences for patients interested in pursuing alternative or homeopathic approaches.

KEYWORDS

THC; tetrahydrocannabinol; skin cancer; YouTube; cannabis; social media; internet

Introduction

Cannabis oil as a homeopathic remedy for skin cancer was most popularized by Rick Simpson, a Canadian medical marijuana activist. In 2003, Rick Simpson claimed that he was able to cure his basal cell carcinoma with his specially extracted "Rick Simpson Oil," an illegally produced high-tetrahydrocannabinol (THC) oil made from *Cannabis indica* [1]. An online documentary called Healing Cancer with Cannabis: The Rick Simpson Story [2] currently has over 150,000 views on YouTube and documents Rick Simpson's journey to curing both his skin cancer and that of others, including basal cell carcinoma and melanoma. Given the increasing importance of social media and YouTube in disseminating information about health care and dermatology [3], we sought to characterize the quality of information patients attain from popular YouTube videos concerning THC and skin cancer.

Methods

On June 5, 2020, we searched YouTube using the phrase "THC skin cancer." The ranking option of "view count" was selected. The search resulted in a total of 32 videos; however, only nonduplicate videos with over 1000 views were analyzed in order to obtain accurate representation and capture the most popular videos that had reached the largest YouTube audiences. Two independent reviewers viewed and evaluated all videos, and any discrepancies between reviewers were discussed and resolved in a consensus meeting. All reviewers were experienced in skin cancer pathogenesis, clinical presentation, and treatment. Various predetermined attributes were surveyed, and videos were scored for quality and usefulness with the 5-point Likert scale Global Quality Scale (GQS) as described in Textbox 1 [3,4].

Textbox 1. Global Quality Scale 5-point scale description.

1. Poor quality, poor flow of the video, most information missing, not at all useful for patients. I would highly discourage a patient with skin cancer from watching this video.
2. Generally poor quality and poor flow. Some information listed but many important topics missing. Of very limited use to patients. I would discourage a patient with skin cancer from watching this video.
3. Moderate quality, suboptimal flow. Some important information is adequately discussed but other information is poorly discussed. Somewhat useful for patients. I would neither encourage nor discourage a patient with skin cancer from watching this video.
4. Good quality and generally good flow. Most of the relevant information is listed, but some topics not covered. Useful for patients. I would encourage a patient with skin cancer to watch this video.
5. Excellent quality and flow, very useful for patients. I would highly encourage a patient with skin cancer to watch this video.

Videos were additionally rated on an adapted DISCERN 5-point reliability scale, an assessment of health information quality used in previous studies [3,5]. Scoring of content accounted for the breadth of skin cancer information discussed, including epidemiology, pathogenesis, clinical features, and treatment. One DISCERN point was earned for each criteria fulfilled, for a maximum of 5 points (Textbox 2).

Textbox 2. Adapted DISCERN content reliability score description.

Reliability of information (0 points for no, 1 point for yes)

1. Are the aims clear and achieved?
2. Are reliable sources of information used? (ie, speaker is a dermatologist, publications were cited)
3. Is the information presented balanced and unbiased?
4. Are additional sources of information listed for patient reference?
5. Are areas of uncertainty mentioned?

Videos were further classified as useful or misleading based on the following yes/no criteria established in prior literature [6-10]:

1. Useful, if they contained scientifically sound information about any aspect of skin cancer.
2. Misleading, if they contained scientifically erroneous or unproven information about any aspect of skin cancer.

For each video, the top 3 comments determined by YouTube according to the number of "thumbs up" ratings were additionally assessed for whether the comment was favorable, neutral, or unfavorable toward the video content. The source and date of the comment were also recorded.

Results

The 10 videos surveyed (Multimedia Appendix 1) had a total view count of 645,821 views, with an average of 64,582 views per video. Video length ranged from around 2 minutes to over 107 minutes. Sources of videos were varied, and included cannabis companies, Rick Simpson affiliates, and patient perspectives. The surveyed videos had positive social engagement, with a cumulative "thumbs up" score of 4923, and a "thumbs down" score of 183.

Overall, 10/10 videos (100%) had a GQS score of 1, corresponding to "poor quality, poor flow of the video, most information missing, not at all useful for patients." Just 1 of 10 (10%) videos received a score of 1 of a possible 5 points on the DISCERN scale, corresponding to poor content reliability, while 9/10 (90%) videos received a score of 0. All 10 videos received a "no" rating according to the useful criteria, and a "yes" rating for misleading.

Summaries of video content and top comments for each video are shown in Multimedia Appendix 2. The commenting feature was turned off for one video. Overall, comments were all posted by individual YouTube users, and were largely favorable or neutral toward the video content, with 13/27 comments (48%)

classified as favorable, 13/27 (48%) neutral, and 1/27 (4%) unfavorable.

Discussion

Principal Findings

Patients are increasingly interested in and selecting nontraditional and alternative therapies for a variety of health conditions. Cannabis oil has achieved great popularity in the past few decades for the treatment of both nonmelanoma and melanoma skin cancers, despite the current lack of evidence; no clinical trials have yet to test their safety and efficacy in humans. Although early preclinical studies have shown that cannabinoids and cannabinoid derivatives may potentially have antitumor effects on keratinocyte carcinoma and melanoma [11], other studies have demonstrated that cannabinoids can be potent proinflammatory chemotactic agents in cell culture models [12].

The body's endocannabinoid system regulates cell growth through primary endocannabinoids, such as arachidonoyl ethanolamide (AEA) and 2-arachidonoyl glycerol (2-AG), and their metabolism by fatty acid amide hydrolase (FAAH). As detailed in previous reports [13], cannabinoid receptors CB1 and CB2 are found to be expressed on both nonmelanoma and melanoma skin cancers, with the former being largely expressed in the synaptic terminal in order to regulate neurotransmission, and the latter playing a role in activation of psychoactive properties [13].

Melanoma has largely been attributed to chronic sun damage (CSD) as well as non-CSD causes due to mutations in the cell regulatory pathway [14]. A study conducted by Armstrong et al [15] on melanoma cells treated with the cannabinoid THC displayed antitumor properties through the activation of autophagy and apoptotic pathways in vivo and in vitro. Similarly, cannabinoids have displayed antitumor effects in several other studies, focusing on CB2's anti-inflammatory properties and inhibition of Akt, a key element in the survival pathway of melanomas [16,17].

Cannabinoids have also demonstrated antitumor effects in nonmelanoma skin cancers. Squamous cell carcinomas (SCCs) are some of the most common cancers in humans and have been linked to risk factors including, but not limited to, UV exposure, chemical carcinogens, and viral infections [18]. Induction of apoptosis and tumor regression as an established effect of cannabinoid application has become evident through depression of angiogenic factors, such as vascular endothelial growth factor (VEGF) and angiopoietin-2 (Ang2), as well as decreasing activation of epidermal growth factor receptors (EGF-R) [19].

Although promising research on the treatment of skin cancers with cannabinoids is currently being conducted, the spread of information rooted in evidence-based medicine remains minimal on social media sites such as YouTube. Analysis of video content by two separate reviewers with health care experience and an educational background in skin cancer resulted in assessment of the information presented as uniformly misleading to viewers, along with a GQS of 1 assigned to all videos, demonstrating the pervasiveness of poor-quality information, and also largely unreliable content according to DISCERN criteria. It is concerning that top comments in response to these videos were overwhelmingly either favorable or neutral, highlighting the possibility that fake or secondary individual user accounts could be commenting to generate the outward appearance of validity and support for the video content. With the increasing use of social media, viral content, and thus the immense audience that can be reached via different platforms, including YouTube, inaccurate information can easily be spread to viewers who may be searching for solutions to skin-related problems. It is important for dermatologists to be aware that social media use may subsequently encourage patients to rely on information not provided by trained physicians and health care teams. Potentially harmful side effects or adverse consequences could be experienced by patients due to the dissemination of incorrect or poorly understood information. An increase in the presence of board-certified dermatologists on social media platforms would allow for improved patient education and propagation of medically accurate information to audiences seeking knowledge on skin cancer treatment with cannabinoids.

Conclusion

This study reiterates the importance of accessible, trustworthy, and engaging educational content curated by medical professionals for patients seeking information about skin cancer treatment online. In the surveyed YouTube data, no videos were curated by medical professionals tackling the popular issue of THC for the treatment of skin cancer, thus highlighting an opportunity for future engagement on social media to improve health education.

References

1. Li JY, Kampp JT. Review of Common Alternative Herbal "Remedies" for Skin Cancer. Dermatol Surg 2019;45(1):58-67. [doi: 10.1097/dss.0000000000001622]
2. Harrigan C. Healing Cancer with Cannabis: The Rick Simpson Story. 2017 May 12. URL: https://www.youtube.com/watch?v=Ak3Zo7-hNO0) [accessed 2020-09-21]
3. Qi J, Trang T, Doong J, Kang S, Chien A. Misinformation is prevalent in psoriasis-related YouTube videos. Dermatol Online J 2016 Nov 15;22(11):13030/qt7qc9z2m5. [Medline: 28329562]
4. Bernard A, Langille M, Hughes S, Rose C, Leddin D, Veldhuyzen van Zanten S. A systematic review of patient inflammatory bowel disease information resources on the World Wide Web. Am J Gastroenterol 2007 Sep;102(9):2070-2077. [doi: 10.1111/j.1572-0241.2007.01325.x] [Medline: 17511753]

5. Charnock D, Shepperd S, Needham G, Gann R. DISCERN: an instrument for judging the quality of written consumer health information on treatment choices. J Epidemiol Community Health 1999 Feb 01;53(2):105-111 [FREE Full text] [doi: 10.1136/jech.53.2.105] [Medline: 10396471]
6. Pandey A, Patni N, Singh M, Sood A, Singh G. YouTube as a source of information on the H1N1 influenza pandemic. Am J Prev Med 2010 Mar;38(3):e1-e3. [doi: 10.1016/j.amepre.2009.11.007] [Medline: 20171526]
7. Murugiah K, Vallakati A, Rajput K, Sood A, Challa NR. YouTube as a source of information on cardiopulmonary resuscitation. Resuscitation 2011 Mar;82(3):332-334. [doi: 10.1016/j.resuscitation.2010.11.015] [Medline: 21185643]
8. Singh AG, Singh S, Singh PP. YouTube for information on rheumatoid arthritis--a wakeup call? J Rheumatol 2012 May 01;39(5):899-903. [doi: 10.3899/jrheum.111114] [Medline: 22467934]
9. Sood A, Sarangi S, Pandey A, Murugiah K. YouTube as a source of information on kidney stone disease. Urology 2011 Mar;77(3):558-562. [doi: 10.1016/j.urology.2010.07.536] [Medline: 21131027]
10. Delli K, Livas C, Vissink A, Spijkervet F. Is YouTube useful as a source of information for Sjögren's syndrome? Oral Dis 2016 Apr 11;22(3):196-201. [doi: 10.1111/odi.12404] [Medline: 26602325]
11. Mounessa JS, Siegel JA, Dunnick CA, Dellavalle RP. The role of cannabinoids in dermatology. J Am Acad Dermatol 2017 Jul;77(1):188-190. [doi: 10.1016/j.jaad.2017.02.056] [Medline: 28416341]
12. Klein TW. Cannabinoid-based drugs as anti-inflammatory therapeutics. Nat Rev Immunol 2005 May;5(5):400-411. [doi: 10.1038/nri1602] [Medline: 15864274]
13. Scheau C, Badarau IA, Mihai L, Scheau A, Costache DO, Constantin C, et al. Cannabinoids in the Pathophysiology of Skin Inflammation. Molecules 2020 Feb 04;25(3):652 [FREE Full text] [doi: 10.3390/molecules25030652] [Medline: 32033005]
14. Turner N, Ware O, Bosenberg M. Genetics of metastasis: melanoma and other cancers. Clin Exp Metastasis 2018 Aug 2;35(5-6):379-391. [doi: 10.1007/s10585-018-9893-y] [Medline: 29722002]
15. Armstrong JL, Hill DS, McKee CS, Hernandez-Tiedra S, Lorente M, Lopez-Valero I, et al. Exploiting cannabinoid-induced cytotoxic autophagy to drive melanoma cell death. J Invest Dermatol 2015 Jun;135(6):1629-1637 [FREE Full text] [doi: 10.1038/jid.2015.45] [Medline: 25674907]
16. Kis B, Ifrim FC, Buda V, Avram S, Pavel IZ, Antal D, et al. Cannabidiol-from Plant to Human Body: A Promising Bioactive Molecule with Multi-Target Effects in Cancer. Int J Mol Sci 2019 Nov 25;20(23):5905 [FREE Full text] [doi: 10.3390/ijms20235905] [Medline: 31775230]
17. Blázquez C, Carracedo A, Barrado L, Real PJ, Fernández-Luna JL, Velasco G, et al. Cannabinoid receptors as novel targets for the treatment of melanoma. FASEB J 2006 Dec 25;20(14):2633-2635. [doi: 10.1096/fj.06-6638fje] [Medline: 17065222]
18. Dotto G, Rustgi A. Squamous Cell Cancers: A Unified Perspective on Biology and Genetics. Cancer Cell 2016 May 09;29(5):622-637 [FREE Full text] [doi: 10.1016/j.ccell.2016.04.004] [Medline: 27165741]
19. Casanova ML, Blázquez C, Martínez-Palacio J, Villanueva C, Fernández-Aceñero MJ, Huffman JW, et al. Inhibition of skin tumor growth and angiogenesis in vivo by activation of cannabinoid receptors. J Clin Invest 2003 Jan 1;111(1):43-50. [doi: 10.1172/jci200316116]

Abbreviations

2-AG: 2-arachidonoyl glycerol
AEA: arachidonoyl ethanolamide
AP-2: angiopoietin-2
CSD: chronic sun damage
EGF-R: epidermal growth factor receptor
FAAH: fatty acid amide hydrolase
GQS: Global Quality Scale
SCC: squamous cell carcinoma
THC: tetrahydrocannabinol
VEGF: vascular endothelial growth factor

Content in YouTube Videos for Rosacea

Corey H Basch[1], MPH, EdD; Priscila E Laforet[2], MPH; Grace C Hillyer[3], MPH, EdD; Erica J Seidel[4], PsyD; Christie Jaime[1], MS

[1]Department of Public Health, William Paterson University, Wayne, NJ, United States

[2]Division of Hematology/Oncology, Department of Medicine, Columbia University Irving Medical Center, New York, NY, United States

[3]Department of Epidemiology, Mailman School of Public Health, Columbia University, New York, NY, United States

[4]Department of Student Life/Counseling Center, Borough of Manhattan Community College, New York, NY, United States

Corresponding Author:
Corey H Basch, MPH, EdD
Department of Public Health
William Paterson University
300 Pompton Rd
Wayne, NJ, 07470
United States

Email: baschc@wpunj.edu

Abstract

Background: Rosacea is an inflammatory skin disease that is chronic in nature. In addition to the physical symptoms, there are substantial quality of life issues that patients with rosacea experience, largely due to the visible nature in which rosacea manifests.

Objective: The purpose of this study was to describe the content related to rosacea in highly viewed English- and Spanish-language videos on YouTube.

Methods: We coded identifying information for each video and categories including characteristics of rosacea, clinical solutions, and alternative solutions. The 100 YouTube videos examined were viewed 18.5 million times between 2006 and 2020, and 57.3% (10,652,665/18,592,742) of these views were of consumer videos.

Results: Videos posted by consumers more often promoted or were trying to sell a product or procedure (32/55, 58% of consumers vs 10/31, 32% of medical professionals and 4/14, 29% of television, internet, news, or entertainment sources; $P=.03$) and more frequently mentioned the use of makeup or other ways to cover up rosacea (30/55, 55% of consumers vs 6/31, 19% of medical professionals and 2/14, 14% of television, internet, news, or entertainment sources; $P<.001$). Videos sourced from medical professionals more often mentioned medication (17/31, 55%) than videos uploaded by consumers (14/55, 25%) or TV, internet, news, or entertainment sources (3/14, 21%) ($P=.01$).

Conclusions: Given that rosacea is experienced differently for each person, consumer advice that works for one individual may not work for another. There is a need for reliable videos on rosacea to emphasize this and clarify misconceptions.

KEYWORDS

rosacea; YouTube; social media; skin disease; skin; chronic; dermatology

Introduction

Rosacea is an inflammatory skin disease that is chronic in nature [1]. The cause of rosacea is unknown and the pathophysiology is inadequately comprehended [1]. Current statistics indicate that this is a prevalent problem, with an estimated 416 million adults affected [2] worldwide and an estimated 16 million individuals with rosacea in the United States [3]. Recent research has led to improved understanding of the common triggers and symptomology of this widely experienced issue. Triggers of rosacea include genetic and environmental factors [1], and patients are often encouraged to monitor environmental triggers closely to avoid the onset of symptoms.

The most commonly identifiable symptom of rosacea includes redness or flushing in the face, but the range of symptoms can be variable and are broken down into subtypes. The American Academy of Dermatology has identified 4 subtypes: (1) subtype 1, which is characterized by visible redness, flushing, and blood vessels; (2) subtype 2, in which acne-like breakouts are common; (3) subtype 3, which is rare and involves thickening skin that can result in rhinophyma, a thickened and bulbous nose; and (4) subtype 4, which affects the eyes with issues ranging from burning and stinging to the development of cysts [4]. It is possible to experience more than one subtype at a time. Naturally, because subtypes are varied and may overlap, treatments are dependent upon related symptoms and patient experiences [5]. These treatments include but are not limited to topical therapies [6-9], antibiotics [10], laser and pulsed light therapies [11-15], and reconstructive surgery [16,17].

In addition to the physical symptoms, there are substantial quality of life issues that patients with rosacea experience, largely due to the visible nature in which rosacea manifests [4]. Much has been written and researched about the medical aspects of rosacea, such as causes, prognosis, and treatment, but the psychological impact of the condition is infrequently discussed and of great importance to those with this condition. With limited ability to control triggers and the lack of a cure, patients are challenged with a lifelong chronic condition that alters their facial appearance, which often impacts their self-esteem and quality of life, especially when the rosacea is severe [18-21].

Current research suggests that 90% of Americans use the internet [22], and many consumers search the web for information related to their health. YouTube is a highly popular medium for sharing information through videos, with an estimated 2 billion unique users [23]. Studies of YouTube are prevalent on a variety of health issues and issues concerning the skin specifically [24-27]. The purpose of this study was to describe the content related to rosacea in highly viewed English- and Spanish-language videos on YouTube.

Methods

The 100 videos with the most views on YouTube were identified using the keyword "rosacea" on May 31, 2020, and were recorded and coded. Videos in English and Spanish were included in the study. Six videos were not reviewed, as they were in a language other than English or Spanish, and they were replaced with the next 6 videos in English or Spanish.

Metadata were identified for each video, including the URL, source of video upload (consumer, medical professional, television- or internet-based news, or entertainment television), number of views, length of video in minutes and seconds, date of upload, language in which the video was recorded, and whether the video featured a medical doctor. A fact sheet from the American Academy of Dermatology was used to create coding categories for content [4]. Categories included characteristics of rosacea, clinical solutions, and alternative solutions.

Characteristics of rosacea included a general description of the condition, triggers and flare-ups of rosacea, the fact that rosacea is more common among women, and the impact of rosacea on the quality of life, such as feelings of frustration, embarrassment, worry, low self-esteem, anxiety, and depression. Mentions by subtype were noted. Specific details of the symptom subtype are noted below. Clinical solutions included mentions of surgery for thickened skin, laser treatment, medication, measures to protect against the sun, a potential cure, and the promotion of products or procedures. Skin care tips and mentions of makeup to cover the skin were included in the alternative solutions category. Responses were coded as "yes" or "no" for whether the video mentioned each of the above characteristics or solutions.

Frequencies and percentages of all categorical variables were calculated, and means, standard deviations, and ranges were determined for the number of views and video length. Video source was recoded as consumer, medical professional, or combined television-based news and entertainment television. Chi-square tests and analysis of variance were used to assess possible associations between video source and the characteristics and content of the videos. Authors EJS and CJ each coded half the videos and then coded a random 10% subset to ascertain interrater reliability. Using Cohen κ (κ=0.92), interrater reliability was shown to be excellent. Because human subjects were not involved in this study, this protocol was not reviewed by an institutional review board, per the policies at William Paterson University and Columbia University.

Results

The 100 YouTube videos examined were viewed 18.5 million times between 2006 and 2020, and 57.3% (10,652,665/18,592,742) of these views were of consumer videos (Table 1).

Table 1. Characteristics of YouTube videos (N=100) about rosacea by video upload source.

Characteristic	Total (N=100)	Consumer (n=55)	Medical professional (n=31)	Television- or internet-based news and entertainment television (n=14)	*P* value
Video characteristics					
Views, n (%)	18,592,742 (100)	10,652,665 (57.3)	5,527,057 (29.2)	2,513,020 (13.5)	N/A[a]
Views, mean (SD)	185,927 (205,020)	193,685 (205,962)	175,066 (210,611)	179,501 (202,362)	.45
Views, range	33,076-1,407,672	40,254-1,407,672	42,443-1,003,575	33,076-782,574	N/A
Video length (min), mean (SD)	10.53 (8.92)	11.45 (8.60)	9.20 (7.53)	9.93 (12.60)	.42
Video length (min), range	0.82-46.17	0.83-46.17	0.82-25.93	1.60-43.32	N/A
Video upload date, n (%)					.15
2006-2010	6 (6.0)	3 (5.5)	2 (6.5)	1 (7.1)	
2011-2015	35 (35.0)	16 (29.1)	10 (32.3)	9 (64.3)	
2016-2020	59 (59.0)	26 (47.3)	19 (61.3)	4 (28.6)	
Language of video, n (%)					.03
English	78 (78.0)	40 (72.7)	29 (93.5)	9 (64.3)	
Spanish	22 (22.0)	15 (27.3)	2 (6.5)	5 (35.7)	
Features a medical professional, n (%)	33 (33.0)	1 (1.8)	27 (87.1)	5 (35.7)	<.001
Characteristics of rosacea, n (%)					
Included general description of rosacea	65 (65.0)	31 (56.4)	22 (71.0)	12 (85.7)	.09
Mentions triggers and flare-ups	52 (52.0)	23 (41.8)	19 (61.3)	10 (71.4)	.07
Mentions rosacea is more common in women	9 (9.0)	5 (9.1)	1 (3.2)	3 (21.4)	.14
Mentions impact on quality of life	30 (30.0)	19 (34.5)	7 (22.6)	4 (28.6)	.51
Mentions subtype 1 signs and symptoms[b]	65 (65.0)	31 (56.4)	22 (71.0)	12 (85.7)	.09
Mentions subtype 2 signs and symptoms[c]	65 (65.0)	30 (54.5)	23 (74.2)	12 (85.7)	.04
Mentions subtype 3 signs and symptoms[d]	33 (33.0)	12 (21.8)	14 (45.2)	7 (50.0)	.03
Mentions subtype 4 signs and symptoms[e]	14 (14.0)	6 (10.9)	3 (9.7)	5 (35.7)	.04
Clinical solutions, n (%)					
Mentions surgery for thickened skin	3 (3.0)	1 (1.8)	0 (0.0)	2 (14.3)	.03
Mentions laser treatment	22 (22.0)	8 (14.5)	11 (35.5)	3 (21.4)	.08
Mentions medication	34 (34.0)	14 (25.5)	17 (54.8)	3 (21.4)	.01
Mentions sun protection	40 (40.0)	17 (30.9)	18 (58.1)	5 (35.7)	.05
Mentions a cure	8 (8.0)	5 (9.1)	1 (3.2)	2 (14.3)	.41
Promotes or sells a product or procedure	46 (46.0)	32 (58.2)	10 (32.3)	4 (28.6)	.03
Alternative solutions, n (%)					
Promotes an alternative treatment	31 (31.0)	17 (30.9)	8 (25.8)	6 (42.9)	.52
Mentions skin care tips	54 (54.0)	32 (58.2)	17 (54.8)	5 (35.7)	.32
Mentions makeup or other ways to cover up rosacea	38 (38.0)	30 (54.5)	6 (19.4)	2 (14.3)	<.001

[a]N/A: not applicable.

[b]Subtype 1 signs and symptoms: flushing and redness, particularly in the center of the face; visible broken blood vessels and spider veins; skin that is swollen, very sensitive, or may sting and burn; rough, dry, or scaling skin; and skin that tends to flush or blush easily.

[c]Subtype 2 signs and symptoms: acne-like breakouts that tend to come and go and are found in the areas where the skin is very red, oily skin or skin that is very sensitive or may sting and burn, visible broken blood vessels and spider veins, and plaques with raised patches of skin.

[d]Subtype 3 signs and symptoms: bumpy skin or skin that begins to thicken, particularly on the nose, chin, forehead, cheeks, and ears; visible broken blood vessels and spider veins; oily skin; and large pores.

[e]Subtype 4 signs and symptoms: rosacea in the eyes where the eyes appear watery or bloodshot, feel gritty, burn or sting, itch, or are dry and sensitive to light; blurry or decreased vision; and visible broken blood vessels or a cyst on the eyelid.

The mean number of views was 185,927 (SD 205,020), and the mean length of the videos was 10.53 minutes (SD 8.92 minutes). Most videos were uploaded between 2016 and 2020 (59/100, 59.0%), recorded in English (78/100, 78.0%), and did not feature a medical professional (67/100, 67.0%).

Consumer videos less often mentioned signs and symptoms of subtypes 2 and 3 (subtype 2: 30/55, 55% of consumers vs 23/31, 74% of medical professionals and 12/14, 86% of television or internet; P=.04; subtype 3: 12/55, 22% of consumers vs 14/31, 45% of medical professionals and 7/14, 50% of television or internet; P=.03). Videos posted by consumers, however, more often promoted or were trying to sell a product or procedure (32/55, 58% of consumers vs 10/31, 32% of medical professionals and 4/14, 29% of television, internet, news, or entertainment; P=.03) and more frequently mentioned the use of makeup or other ways to cover up rosacea (30/55, 55% of consumers vs 6/31, 19% of medical professionals and 2/14, 14% of television, internet, news, or entertainment; P<.001). Videos sourced from medical professionals more often mentioned medication (17/31, 55%) than videos uploaded by consumers (14/55, 25%) or television, internet, news, or entertainment sources (3/14, 21%) (P=.01). Videos uploaded from a television, internet, news, or entertainment source more often mentioned subtype 4 (5/14, 36% vs 6/55, 11% of consumers and 3/31, 10% of medical professionals; P=.04) and surgical treatments for thickened skin (2/14, 14%) compared with consumer (1/55, 2%) and medical professional (0/0, 0%) videos (P=.03).

Discussion

To our knowledge, this is the first study to examine the content of both English and Spanish rosacea videos on YouTube. The majority of the 100 most popular rosacea YouTube videos were uploaded by consumers. Thus, medical professionals should be aware that consumer opinions and thoughts on rosacea are accessed more often than professional materials. The type of information presented in the videos analyzed also varied depending on the source. Videos sourced from medical professionals were most likely to mention information on medication and the use of sun protection as treatments for rosacea, while videos sourced from consumers were most likely to mention information on alternative treatments like the use of makeup to cover up rosacea. Research indicates that cosmetics can exacerbate rosacea [28-30], and as such, the prevalent makeup tutorials related to covering rosacea could be promoting products that cause flares. In addition, rather than focusing on avoiding triggers, this content focused on hiding symptoms.

Within the context of the connection between self-esteem and body image [31], research is delving further into rosacea's social and emotional fallout. Patients may avoid social situations, retreat from relationships, or think negatively about themselves as a result of their symptoms. An increase in symptoms of depression and anxiety related to the severity of the rosacea have been reported [19]. Women are more likely to be diagnosed with rosacea, exacerbating the gaps in self-esteem that already exist between men and women [32], suggesting that, for women, a holistic approach to treating the condition may be warranted to affect both the psychological and physical manifestations of the disease [33].

Further, the videos sourced from consumers were also found to be the most likely to include information to sell a product. This discovery highlights that consumers may have various underlying motivations to upload videos on rosacea, such as commercial sponsorship, which might result in the communication of misinformation to increase sales of a sponsored product to treat rosacea. Analysis of the videos revealed that the accuracy and reliability of the information found in the videos varied greatly. This is best highlighted by the videos that included information on a cure despite the fact that there is no cure for rosacea. The findings of this study are similar to a prior study of rosacea on a variety of internet sources, including YouTube videos, which concluded that internet sources could contain peer-generated content that was harmful or misleading [34].

This study has limitations that warrant mention. The cross-sectional design indicates that data were only collected at one point in time, and given the fact that content on the internet is in flux, the most popular videos could change over time. Additionally, this study only included videos in English and Spanish despite videos being available in an array of languages. Further, there is no way to delineate who viewed each video and the reason they did so. Therefore, the study strictly offers insight on the content and coverage of information in the widely viewed videos on YouTube.

Nonetheless, this study offers insight into the content available on YouTube about rosacea. Given that rosacea is experienced differently for each person, consumer advice that works for one individual may not work for another. There is a need for reliable videos on rosacea to emphasize this and clarify misconceptions. Further study is needed on the accuracy and reliability of information on rosacea in videos sourced by consumers, as well as on the factors that influence consumers to create and upload videos on rosacea for YouTube.

References

1. Buddenkotte J, Steinhoff M. Recent advances in understanding and managing rosacea. F1000Res 2018;7:1885 [FREE Full text] [doi: 10.12688/f1000research.16537.1] [Medline: 30631431]
2. Gether L, Overgaard L, Egeberg A, Thyssen J. Incidence and prevalence of rosacea: a systematic review and meta-analysis.

Br J Dermatol 2018 Aug;179(2):282-289. [doi: 10.1111/bjd.16481] [Medline: 29478264]

3. National Rosacea Society. Rosacea now estmated to affect at least 16 million Americans. Rosacea Review. 2010. URL: https://www.rosacea.org/rosacea-review/2010/winter/rosacea-now-estimated-to-affect-at-least-16-million-americans [accessed 2020-09-15]
4. Rosacea: signs and symptoms. American Academy of Dermatology Association. 2020. URL: https://www.aad.org/public/diseases/rosacea/what-is/symptoms [accessed 2020-09-21]
5. Johnson SM, Berg A, Barr C. Managing Rosacea in the Clinic: From Pathophysiology to Treatment-A Review of the Literature. J Clin Aesthet Dermatol 2020 Apr;13(Suppl 4):S17-S22 [FREE Full text] [Medline: 32802248]
6. Stein L, Kircik L, Fowler J, Tan J, Draelos Z, Fleischer A, et al. Efficacy and safety of ivermectin 1% cream in treatment of papulopustular rosacea: results of two randomized, double-blind, vehicle-controlled pivotal studies. J Drugs Dermatol 2014 Mar;13(3):316-323. [Medline: 24595578]
7. Taieb A, Khemis A, Ruzicka T, Barańska-Rybak W, Berth-Jones J, Schauber J, Ivermectin Phase III Study Group. Maintenance of remission following successful treatment of papulopustular rosacea with ivermectin 1% cream vs. metronidazole 0.75% cream: 36-week extension of the ATTRACT randomized study. J Eur Acad Dermatol Venereol 2016 May;30(5):829-836. [doi: 10.1111/jdv.13537] [Medline: 26691278]
8. Fowler J, Jarratt M, Moore A, Meadows K, Pollack A, Steinhoff M, Brimonidine Phase II Study Group. Once-daily topical brimonidine tartrate gel 0·5% is a novel treatment for moderate to severe facial erythema of rosacea: results of two multicentre, randomized and vehicle-controlled studies. Br J Dermatol 2012 Mar;166(3):633-641 [FREE Full text] [doi: 10.1111/j.1365-2133.2011.10716.x] [Medline: 22050040]
9. Del Rosso JQ. Topical a-Agonist Therapy for Persistent Facial Erythema of Rosacea and the Addition of Oxmetazoline to the Treatment Armamentarium: Where Are We Now? J Clin Aesthet Dermatol 2017 Jul;10(7):28-32 [FREE Full text] [Medline: 29104721]
10. Del Rosso JQ, Leyden JJ, Thiboutot D, Webster GF. Antibiotic use in acne vulgaris and rosacea: clinical considerations and resistance issues of significance to dermatologists. Cutis 2008 Aug;82(2 Suppl 2):5-12. [Medline: 18924545]
11. Al-Niaimi F, Glagoleva E, Araviiskaia E. Pulsed dye laser followed by intradermal botulinum toxin type-A in the treatment of rosacea-associated erythema and flushing. Dermatol Ther 2020 Nov;33(6):e13976. [doi: 10.1111/dth.13976] [Medline: 32633449]
12. Papageorgiou P, Clayton W, Norwood S, Chopra S, Rustin M. Treatment of rosacea with intense pulsed light: significant improvement and long-lasting results. Br J Dermatol 2008 Sep;159(3):628-632. [doi: 10.1111/j.1365-2133.2008.08702.x] [Medline: 18565174]
13. Larson AA, Goldman MP. Recalcitrant rosacea successfully treated with multiplexed pulsed dye laser. J Drugs Dermatol 2007 Aug;6(8):843-845. [Medline: 17763618]
14. Tirico M, Jensen D, Green C, Ross E. Short pulse intense pulsed light versus pulsed dye laser for the treatment of facial redness. J Cosmet Laser Ther 2020 Mar 17;22(2):60-64. [doi: 10.1080/14764172.2020.1717540] [Medline: 32041440]
15. Kawana S, Ochiai H, Tachihara R. Objective evaluation of the effect of intense pulsed light on rosacea and solar lentigines by spectrophotometric analysis of skin color. Dermatol Surg 2007 Apr;33(4):449-454. [doi: 10.1111/j.1524-4725.2007.33092.x] [Medline: 17430379]
16. Saad M, Matteucci P. A very severe case of rhinophyma requiring a three-stage reconstruction with a forehead flap. Ann R Coll Surg Engl 2020 Oct;102(8):e219-e222. [doi: 10.1308/rcsann.2020.0164] [Medline: 32808811]
17. Kang JK, Lee JS, Choi JH, Shin MS, Yun BM. Surgical treatment of rhinophyma using an ordinary bur. Arch Craniofac Surg 2020 Aug;21(4):264-267 [FREE Full text] [doi: 10.7181/acfs.2020.00199] [Medline: 32867419]
18. Baldwin HE, Harper J, Baradaran S, Patel V. Erythema of Rosacea Affects Health-Related Quality of Life: Results of a Survey Conducted in Collaboration with the National Rosacea Society. Dermatol Ther (Heidelb) 2019 Dec;9(4):725-734 [FREE Full text] [doi: 10.1007/s13555-019-00322-5] [Medline: 31512178]
19. Egeberg A, Hansen PR, Gislason GH, Thyssen JP. Patients with Rosacea Have Increased Risk of Depression and Anxiety Disorders: A Danish Nationwide Cohort Study. Dermatology 2016;232(2):208-213. [doi: 10.1159/000444082] [Medline: 26954304]
20. Bewley A, Fowler J, Schöfer H, Kerrouche N, Rives V. Erythema of Rosacea Impairs Health-Related Quality of Life: Results of a Meta-analysis. Dermatol Ther (Heidelb) 2016 Jun;6(2):237-247 [FREE Full text] [doi: 10.1007/s13555-016-0106-9] [Medline: 26983751]
21. Bewley A, Fowler J, Schöfer H, Kerrouche N, Rives V. Erythema of Rosacea Impairs Health-Related Quality of Life: Results of a Meta-analysis. Dermatol Ther (Heidelb) 2016 Jun;6(2):237-247 [FREE Full text] [doi: 10.1007/s13555-016-0106-9] [Medline: 26983751]
22. Anderson M, Perrin A, Jiang J, Kumar M. 10% of Americans don't use the internet. Who are they? Pew Research Center. 2019 Apr 22. URL: https://www.pewresearch.org/fact-tank/2019/04/22/some-americans-dont-use-the-internet-who-are-they/ [accessed 2020-09-16]
23. YouTube for Press. YouTube. URL: https://www.youtube.com/about/press/ [accessed 2020-08-23]
24. Basch CH, Basch CE, Hillyer GC, Reeves R. YouTube Videos Related to Skin Cancer: A Missed Opportunity for Cancer Prevention and Control. JMIR Cancer 2015 Mar 02;1(1):e1 [FREE Full text] [doi: 10.2196/cancer.4204] [Medline: 28410167]

25. Basch CH, Brown AA, Fullwood MD, Clark A, Fung IC, Yin J. YouTube as a source of information on skin bleaching: a content analysis. Clin Exp Dermatol 2018 Jun;43(4):399-403. [doi: 10.1111/ced.13335] [Medline: 29265426]
26. Li W, Ma JE, Chan AA, Lee DJ, Smogorzewski J. Hidradenitis suppurativa through the lens of YouTube: a cross-sectional analysis [online ahead of print]. J Am Acad Dermatol 2020 Jun 06. [doi: 10.1016/j.jaad.2020.05.148] [Medline: 32522514]
27. St Claire KM, Rietcheck H, Patel R, Dunnick C, Dellavalle R. Dermatology on YouTube - an update and analysis of new trends. Dermatol Online J 2018 Dec 15;24(12):13030 [FREE Full text] [Medline: 30677792]
28. Mandal A. Rosacea and cosmetics (make-up). News Medical and Life Sciences. 2019. URL: https://www.news-medical.net/health/Rosacea-and-Cosmetics-(Make-Up).aspx#:~:text=Rosacea%20sufferers%20tend%20to%20have,and%20stinging%20of%20the%20face [accessed 2020-09-21]
29. Jappe U, Schnuch A, Uter W. Rosacea and contact allergy to cosmetics and topical medicaments--retrospective analysis of multicentre surveillance data 1995-2002. Contact Dermatitis 2005 Feb;52(2):96-101. [doi: 10.1111/j.0105-1873.2005.00514.x] [Medline: 15725288]
30. Diepgen T, Weisshaar E. Contact dermatitis: epidemiology and frequent sensitizers to cosmetics. J Eur Acad Dermatol Venereol 2007 Sep;21(Suppl 2):9-13. [doi: 10.1111/j.1468-3083.2007.02381.x] [Medline: 17716286]
31. Clay D, Vignoles VL, Dittmar H. Body Image and Self-Esteem Among Adolescent Girls: Testing the Influence of Sociocultural Factors. J Res Adolescence 2005 Nov;15(4):451-477. [doi: 10.1111/j.1532-7795.2005.00107.x]
32. Stapleton P, Crighton GJ, Carter B, Pidgeon A. Self-esteem and body image in females: The mediating role of self-compassion and appearance contingent self-worth. Humanistic Psychol 2017 Sep;45(3):238-257. [doi: 10.1037/hum0000059]
33. Huynh TT. Burden of Disease: The Psychosocial Impact of Rosacea on a Patient's Quality of Life. Am Health Drug Benefits 2013 Jul;6(6):348-354 [FREE Full text] [Medline: 24991368]
34. Riddoch LH. It takes one to know one: exploring patient dialogue on rosacea web-based platforms and their potential for significant harm. J Dermatolog Treat 2019 Feb;30(1):52-62. [doi: 10.1080/09546634.2018.1468067] [Medline: 29676186]

12

Skin of Color Representation on Wikipedia

William Kim[1], MA, BSc; Sophia M Wolfe[1], BSc; Caterina Zagona-Prizio[1], BSc; Robert P Dellavalle[1,2,3], MD, PhD, MSPH

[1]University of Colorado School of Medicine, Aurora, CO, United States

[2]Dermatology Service, Rocky Mountain Regional VA Medical Center, Eastern Colorado Health Care System, Aurora, CO, United States

[3]Colorado School of Public Health, Aurora, CO, United States

Corresponding Author:
William Kim, MA, BSc
University of Colorado School of Medicine
13001 E 17th Pl
Aurora, CO, 80045
United States

Email: william.kim@cuanschutz.edu

Abstract

Background: Wikipedia is one of the most popular websites and may be a go-to source of health and dermatology education for the general population. Prior research indicates poor skin of color (SOC) photo representation in printed dermatology textbooks and online medical websites, but there has been no such assessment performed to determine whether this discrepancy also exists for Wikipedia.

Objective: The aim of this study was to investigate the number and quality of SOC photos included in Wikipedia's skin disease pages and to explore the possible ramifications of these findings.

Methods: Photos of skin diseases from Wikipedia's "List of Skin Conditions" were assigned by three independent raters as SOC or non-SOC according to the Fitzpatrick system, and were given a quality rating (1-3) based on sharpness, size/resolution, and lighting/exposure.

Results: We identified 421 skin disease Wikipedia pages and 949 images that met our inclusion criteria. Within these pages, 20.7% of images of skin diseases (196 of 949 images) were SOC and 79.3% (753 of 949 images) were non-SOC ($P<.001$). There was no difference in the average quality for SOC (2.05) and non-SOC (2.03) images ($P=.81$). However, the photo quality criteria utilized (sharpness, size/resolution, and lighting/exposure) did not capture all aspects of photo quality. Another limitation of this analysis is that the Fitzpatrick skin typing system is prone to subjectivity and was not originally intended to be utilized as a non-self SOC metric.

Conclusions: There is SOC underrepresentation in the gross number of SOC images for dermatologic conditions on Wikipedia. Wikipedia pages should be updated to include more SOC photos to mend this divide to ameliorate access to accurate dermatology information for the general public and improve health equity within dermatology.

KEYWORDS

skin of color; Wikipedia; dermatology; skin photographs; skin color; dermatology; eHealth; representation; SOC; skin conditions; photos; images; medical images

Introduction

Wikipedia provides a broad range of information for the general public as the 8th most visited website in the United States and the 13th most visited website in the world [1]. Wikipedia may also be a go-to source of health education for the general population, including for information about dermatologic conditions. For example, the Wikipedia pages for psoriasis and leprosy have over 1 million views each, and one project to improve dermatologic Wikipedia pages found that 40 of these pages had over 10 million views combined [2]. Most of the pages dedicated to skin diseases have accompanying pictures to highlight these common skin pathologies, and the Cochrane Skin Wikipedia Initiative, supported by a board-certified dermatologist, has recently updated 80 dermatologic Wikipedia pages with information and photographs from Cochrane reviews [3]. However, many of the skin disease Wikipedia pages often do not offer adequate photo representation of skin of color (SOC) individuals. As more research on dermatologic conditions for SOC individuals emerges, it is clear that certain conditions such as melanoma, plaque-type psoriasis, and acne can present visually differently in people with darker skin compared to people with lighter skin [4]. These variable presentations can also alter treatment; for example, acne treatment may be based on expected hyperpigmentation levels [4].

Given these visual variations in skin disease presentations based on an individual's skin color, adequate SOC photo representation on Wikipedia is important for the information to be applicable to and usable by people of all skin colors. Ensuring accurate skin disease photo representation contributes to health equity by allowing individuals of all skin colors to access relevant information. Therefore, the aim of this study was to investigate the number and quality of SOC photos included in Wikipedia's skin disease pages and explore the possible ramifications of these findings.

Methods

Skin diseases from Wikipedia's "List of Skin Conditions" page (that either specified dermatology as a specialty in the article or were discussed in a separate dermatology textbook) were included in this study [5]. We followed the categorization system from Wikipedia's "List of Skin Conditions" for the major categories listed in Table 1 and Table 2 [6]. Each category of skin condition contained multiple individual skin pages. For example, under the category acneiform eruptions, there were pages on neonatal acne and acne vulgaris, among others. Each page had varying amounts of information on the skin pathology, with some more extensive pages including signs and symptoms, causes, pathophysiology, diagnoses, management, prognosis, and epidemiology, in addition to photographs displaying the associated skin findings. In our review, we categorized these photographs into Fitzpatrick skin types, with Fitzpatrick scores of 1-3 deemed as non-SOC and Fitzpatrick skin types 4-6 deemed as SOC [7,8].

Three raters independently counted the images on each skin page, assigned the Fitzpatrick type, and scored the photo quality [7,8]. The raters were third-year medical students at the University of Colorado School of Medicine who were interested in dermatology, with all raters having a bachelor's degree and one having a master's degree. The photos were rated on a scale of 1-3, with 1 being poor quality, 2 being average quality, and 3 being excellent quality. Each photo was assessed for sharpness, size/resolution, and lighting/exposure. A photo received a score of 1 if it failed all three of these criteria, 2 if it had 2/3 criteria, and 3 if it met all three criteria. Any discrepancies in photo quality among the raters were discussed until a consensus was reached.

Our photo quality criteria were chosen as dermatology is an exceedingly visual specialty that requires clear images to accurately identify and interpret skin pathology. Black and white images, paintings and drawings, or images with ambiguous Fitzpatrick type were excluded, as were images unrelated to the skin disease. Some images appeared in more than one article, and these were counted more than once, as they were important in the context of each individual article. The quality and quantity of images were then compared between the SOC and non-SOC groups using the Student t test.

Table 1. Percentage of skin of color (SOC) to non-SOC photos on the Wikipedia list of skin conditions.

Skin condition	Non-SOC photos, n (%)	SOC photos, n (%)	Total number of photos
Acneiform eruptions	13 (81)	3 (19)	16
Autoinflammatory syndromes	3 (60)	2 (40)	5
Chronic blistering	11 (92)	1 (8)	12
Conditions of the mucous membranes	30 (91)	3 (9)	33
Conditions of the skin appendages	43 (78)	12 (22)	55
Conditions of the subcutaneous fat	8 (89)	1 (11)	9
Congenital anomalies	9 (82)	2 (9)	11
Connective tissue diseases	48 (92)	4 (8)	52
Dermal and subdermal growths	45 (66)	23 (34)	68
Dermatitis	32 (84)	6 (16)	38
Disturbances of pigmentation	12 (71)	5 (29)	17
Drug eruptions	11 (79)	3 (21)	14
Endocrine-related	7 (50)	7 (50)	14
Eosinophilic	2 (100)	0 (0)	2
Epidermal nevi, neoplasms, and cysts	45 (88)	6 (12)	51
Erythemas	11 (92)	1 (8)	12
Genodermatoses	31 (74)	11 (26)	42
Infection-related	146 (67)	71 (33)	217
Lichenoid eruptions	2 (40)	3 (60)	5
Lymphoid-related	11 (92)	1 (8)	12
Melanocytic nevi and neoplasms	36 (92)	3 (8)	39
Monocyte- and macrophage-related	3 (75)	1 (25)	4
Mucinoses	3 (75)	1 (25)	4
Neurocutaneous	11 (79)	3 (21)	14
Noninfectious immunodeficiency-related	2 (100)	0 (0)	2
Nutrition-related	0 (0)	4 (100)	4
Papulosquamous hyperkeratotic	12 (100)	0 (0)	12
Pregnancy-related	6 (86)	1 (14)	7
Pruritic	8 (67)	4 (33)	12
Psoriasis	15 (100)	0 (0)	15
Reactive neutrophilic	8 (100)	0 (0)	8
Recalcitrant palmoplantar eruptions	2 (100)	0 (0)	2
Resulting from errors in metabolism	10 (100)	0 (0)	10
Resulting from physical factors	65 (88)	9 (12)	74
Urticaria and angioedema	7 (100)	0 (0)	7
Vascular-related	45 (90)	5 (10)	50

Table 2. Average quality rating of skin of color (SOC) and non-SOC photos.

Categories	Average quality of non-SOC photos	Average quality of SOC photos
Acneiform eruptions	1.69	2.33
Autoinflammatory syndromes	1.67	2.5
Chronic blistering	2.27	2.0
Conditions of the mucous membranes	2.07	1.67
Conditions of the skin appendages	1.74	1.75
Conditions of the subcutaneous fat	2.0	2.0
Congenital anomalies	2.33	2.0
Connective tissue diseases	1.92	1.75
Dermal and subdermal growths	2.24	2.65
Dermatitis	1.78	1.5
Disturbances of pigmentation	1.5	2.6
Drug eruptions	2.36	2.67
Endocrine-related	2.43	2.67
Eosinophilic	1.5	N/A[a]
Epidermal nevi, neoplasms, and cysts	2.31	2.17
Erythemas	2.36	2.0
Genodermatoses	1.77	2.09
Infection-related	2.08	1.89
Lichenoid eruptions	1.5	1.33
Lymphoid-related	1.55	3.0
Melanocytic nevi and neoplasms	1.64	2.0
Monocyte- and macrophage-related	2.0	2.0
Mucinoses	1.67	2.0
Neurocutaneous	1.64	2.0
Noninfectious immunodeficiency-related	1.5	N/A
Nutrition-related	N/A	1.75
Papulosquamous hyperkeratotic	1.75	N/A
Pregnancy-related	2.0	1.0
Pruritic	1.38	3.0
Psoriasis	2.27	N/A
Reactive neutrophilic	2.25	N/A
Recalcitrant palmoplantar eruptions	2.0	N/A
Resulting from errors in metabolism	2.5	N/A
Resulting from physical factors	2.29	2.0
Urticaria and angioedema	2.43	N/A
Vascular-related	2.18	2.0

[a]N/A: not applicable.

Results

We identified 421 skin disease Wikipedia pages and 949 images that met our inclusion criteria. Within these pages, 20.7% of images of skin diseases (196 of 949 images; s=1.52 cm) were SOC (Table 1) and 79.3% (753 of 949 images; s=2.02 cm) were non-SOC, representing a significant difference (*P*<.001); the s values are the standard deviations of the *t* tests. Lichenoid eruptions had the highest percentage of SOC photos (60%) with 3 out of 5 images being SOC images. Categories with no SOC representation included eosinophilic, noninfectious immunodeficiency-related, papulosquamous hyperkeratotic, psoriasis, reactive neutrophilic, recalcitrant palmoplantar eruptions, resulting from errors of metabolism, and urticaria and angioedema. The average quality for SOC images was 2.05 (s=0.79 cm) compared to 2.03 (s=0.75 cm) in non-SOC images (P=.81) (Table 2).

Discussion

Principal Findings

This study found significantly fewer SOC images compared to non-SOC images in the dermatology-related Wikipedia skin pages. There was no significant difference in photo quality between SOC and non-SOC photos.

Limitations

This study highlights the discrepancies in the total number of SOC photos represented on Wikipedia's list of skin conditions. However, our findings did not show a significant difference in the quality of SOC vs non-SOC photos. This may have been influenced by the small range of the rating scale (1-3) or the photo quality criteria utilized (sharpness, size/resolution, and lighting/exposure). If the rating scale was more granular, it may have allowed for more nuanced differences in photo quality to emerge between the SOC and non-SOC mean photo qualities. Additionally, other aspects of photo quality, including noise amount, noise pattern, and compression quality, may have led to differences in photo quality between SOC and non-SOC photographs. The study was also limited by the nature of the Fitzpatrick skin typing system, which was not originally intended to be utilized as a non-self SOC metric [9]. Therefore, some SOC individuals fell into our grouping of non-SOC (Fitzpatrick skin types 1-3), which may have influenced our results.

Recommendations

Regardless of the quality of the photographs, there is underrepresentation in the total number of images for SOC dermatologic conditions on Wikipedia. Previous research has shown SOC photo underrepresentation in a wide range of resources, including printed dermatology textbooks [7], online websites such as VisualDx and Dermnet [7], and USMLE preparatory materials [8]. Alvarado et al [7] assessed the percentages of dark-skin (Fitzpatrick types 5 and 6) images across a variety of dermatologic resources [7]. DermNet NZ had 2.8% dark skin images, whereas VisualDx had 28.5% dark skin images [7]. In comparison, our study found 20.7% SOC images on Wikipedia (Fitzpatrick types 4-6).

Compared to websites such as VisualDx (ranked in position 113,182) and Dermnet (ranked in position 26,412), Wikipedia (ranked in position 8) has substantially more US internet traffic and engagement as evidenced by the listed rankings on the Alexa website [1]. Although VisualDx and Dermnet are well-known sources of dermatology information for the medical community, they may not be as well utilized by the general public. Wikipedia is arguably one of the main sources of dermatology information for the general public, and the discrepancies in SOC representation have a larger influence on the public's perception of dermatologic disease and care compared to other dermatology resources previously reported in the literature. Possible ramifications of this discrepancy include decreased access to accurate information for SOC patients, skewed societal perceptions of how dermatologic conditions manifest in SOC individuals, inadequate treatment, and potentially poorer outcomes.

Specific dermatology-related Wikipedia pages that need updating with more SOC photographs to reflect the higher rates in individuals with SOC include hyperpigmentation, acral lentiginous melanoma, melasma, pityriasis alba, acne, and atopic dermatitis [4,10,11]. Wikipedia's "melasma" skin page has only one photograph highlighting skin pathology, and it is of an ambiguous Fitzpatrick skin type. Similarly, Wikipedia's atopic dermatitis page has only one picture, and it is of a non-SOC individual. Potentially lethal skin diseases should also have their pages updated. For example, acral lentiginous melanoma is a dangerous skin pathology that disproportionately affects SOC individuals but has no SOC skin photographs on Wikipedia [4].

One skin page that did have a significant number of SOC photographs was "keloid" (under the dermal and subcutaneous growth category) with 20 of 26 photographs being SOC photos, which is more aligned with the higher rates seen in black patients [12]. The other Wikipedia skin pages should be updated similarly to more closely match population statistics in order to improve access to accurate information and potentially improve safety.

Conclusion

Wikipedia pages should be updated to include more SOC photos. Given that Wikipedia is open to editing, more teams dedicated to updating the material information on SOC dermatology findings and presentations, particularly those supported by board-certified dermatologists, can help bolster the information available. Doing so will help mend the divide between SOC and non-SOC photos on Wikipedia's dermatology pages and improve access to accurate dermatology information for the general public, thereby improving health equity within dermatology.

References

1. Alexa. URL: https://www.alexa.com/siteinfo [accessed 2021-05-31]
2. Hutton MO, Dawson JE, Lee KC, Shumaker PR, Doney E, Dellavalle RP. Improving Wikipedia skin disease content. J Am Acad Dermatol 2019 Nov;81(5):1193-1195. [doi: 10.1016/j.jaad.2019.03.063] [Medline: 30928466]
3. Cochrane Skin Wikipedia Initiative. Cochrane Skin. URL: https://skin.cochrane.org/our-evidence/cochrane-skin-wikipedia-initiative [accessed 2021-05-17]

4. Jothishankar B, Stein SL. Impact of skin color and ethnicity. Clin Dermatol 2019;37(5):418-429. [doi: 10.1016/j.clindermatol.2019.07.009] [Medline: 31896399]
5. Bolognia JL, Jorizzo JJ, Schaffer JV, Callen JP, Cerroni L, Heymann WR, et al. Dermatology, 3rd edition. London: Elsevier; 2012.
6. List of skin conditions. Wikipedia. URL: https://en.wikipedia.org/wiki/List_of_skin_conditions [accessed 2021-05-14]
7. Alvarado SM, Feng H. Representation of dark skin images of common dermatologic conditions in educational resources: A cross-sectional analysis. J Am Acad Dermatol 2021 May;84(5):1427-1431. [doi: 10.1016/j.jaad.2020.06.041] [Medline: 32565205]
8. Jones VA, Clark KA, Shobajo MT, Cordova A, Tsoukas MM. Skin of color representation in medical education: an analysis of popular preparatory materials used for United States medical licensing examinations. J Am Acad Dermatol 2020 Aug 01:online ahead of print. [doi: 10.1016/j.jaad.2020.07.112] [Medline: 32750385]
9. Ware OR, Dawson JE, Shinohara MM, Taylor SC. Racial limitations of fitzpatrick skin type. Cutis 2020 Feb;105(2):77-80. [Medline: 32186531]
10. Davis SA, Narahari S, Feldman SR, Huang W, Pichardo-Geisinger RO, McMichael AJ. Top dermatologic conditions in patients of color: an analysis of nationally representative data. J Drugs Dermatol 2012 Apr;11(4):466-473. [Medline: 22453583]
11. Kim Y, Blomberg M, Rifas-Shiman SL, Camargo CA, Gold DR, Thyssen JP, et al. Racial/ethnic differences in incidence and persistence of childhood atopic dermatitis. J Invest Dermatol 2019 Apr;139(4):827-834 [FREE Full text] [doi: 10.1016/j.jid.2018.10.029] [Medline: 30414911]
12. McGinty S, Siddiqui WJ. Keloid. StatPearls. 2020 Aug 16. URL: https://www.ncbi.nlm.nih.gov/books/NBK507899/ [accessed 2021-06-26]

Abbreviations

SOC: skin of color

13

Google Trends in Dermatology: Scoping Review of the Literature

Torunn Elise Sivesind[1], MD; Mindy D Szeto[1], MS; William Kim[2], MA; Robert Paul Dellavalle[1,3], MD, MSPH, PhD

[1]Department of Dermatology, University of Colorado School of Medicine, Aurora, CO, United States

[2]University of Colorado School of Medicine, Aurora, CO, United States

[3]Dermatology Service, Rocky Mountain Regional VA Medical Center, Aurora, CO, United States

Corresponding Author:
Robert Paul Dellavalle, MD, MSPH, PhD
Department of Dermatology
University of Colorado School of Medicine
1665 Aurora Ct
Aurora, CO, 80045
United States

Email: robert.dellavalle@cuanschutz.edu

Abstract

Background: Google Trends is a powerful online database and analytics tool of popular Google search queries over time and has the potential to inform medical practice and priorities.

Objective: This review aimed to survey Google Trends literature in dermatology and elucidate its current roles and relationships with the field.

Methods: A literature search was performed using PubMed to access and review relevant dermatology-related Google Trends studies published within the last 5 years.

Results: Current research utilizing Google Trends data provides insight related to skin cancer, pruritus, cosmetic procedures, and COVID-19. We also found that dermatology is presently the highest-searched medical specialty—among 15 medical and surgical specialties as well as general practitioners. Google searches related to dermatology demonstrate a seasonal nature for various skin conditions and sun-related topics, depending on a region's inherent climate and hemi-sphere. In addition, celebrity social media and other viral posts have been found to potentiate Google searches about dermatology and drive public interest.

Conclusions: A limited number of relevant studies may have been omitted by the simplified search strategy of this study, as well as by restriction to English language articles and articles indexed in the PubMed database. This could be expanded upon in a secondary systematic review. Future re-search is warranted to better understand how Google Trends can be utilized to improve the quality of clinic visits, drive public health campaigns, and detect disease clusters in real time.

KEYWORDS

Google Trends; search trends; internet; infodemiology; infoveillance; search terms; dermatology; skin cancer; databases

Introduction

Google Trends is an online database and analytics tool provided by Google (Google LLC, Mountain View, CA) that reports the relative popularity of a particular search term on Google compared to the peak number of Google searches related to that term over a certain period of time [1,2]. A search volume index (SVI) between 0 to 100 is then generated [2,3], reflecting trends and peak popularity for the term over a given timespan. Data are normalized by Google Trends such that ratios are created, which relate the search volume of an individual search term to the aggregate search volume for all queries, for a given geographic location and time range. These ratios are then proportionally transformed to a scale of 0 to 100 based on a search term's relative magnitude compared to all searches [2,4].

It is also possible to find the true search volume (rather than relative volume) by using the Google Keyword Planner [4], which allows one to assess a particular term for its total number of Google searches over a specified timeframe in a specific location. Patterns and changes in topic popularity may be examined via investigating different time periods or different locations after separately downloading each result and then comparing these side-by-side. In a similar manner, it is also possible to compare the relative popularity of topics by conducting separate searches utilizing different search terms.

Recently, many medical specialties, including dermatology, have started using Google Trends data to better understand population interest in various topics, such as sunscreen, sunburn, skin cancer, and melanoma [1]. Knowledge gained from Google Trends has the potential to guide public health interventions, improve patient education, and tailor health care to patient concerns. Google Trends data are of particular interest to the field of dermatology; in a 2018 study, Ransohoff and Sarin [5] found that, among medical specialists and general practitioners, the most frequently searched physicians were dermatologists.

This study was undertaken to provide a scoping [6] preliminary review of literature in the field of dermatology that highlights the use of Google Trends, to elucidate the current relationship between dermatology and Google Trends, describe limitations of its use, and guide future directions for research and application to patient care.

Methods

A literature review was performed using the PubMed database to tabulate the total number of Google Trends studies from 2016 to 2020. To isolate the relevant dermatology-related publications, the following search string was utilized on August 4, 2020, resulting in 53 articles for initial screening: ((((“Dermatology”[Mesh]) OR “Skin Diseases”[Mesh]) OR “Cosmetic Techniques”[Mesh]) OR “Cosmeceuticals”[Mesh]) AND (google trends AND (y_5[Filter])). The search term “y_5” was included to filter articles published within the last 5 years (2016-2020). Screening of title and abstract for these articles was performed independently by 2 authors with education and experience in dermatology (TS, WK), and of these, 26 were ultimately chosen for inclusion in this review after determination of relevance.

Results

The total number of Google Trends publications over the last 5 years, along with the dermatology-related subset of 26 articles screened is displayed and tabulated by year in Multimedia Appendix 1.

Summary information for the 26 dermatology-specific articles included in this review is captured in Table 1.

Table 1. Summary of dermatology-related Google Trends publications (2016-2020) included in the review.

Topic and article citation	Google Trends location(s) analyzed	Key findings
Skin-related topics of public interest		
Ransohoff JD, Sarin KY. Referred by Google: mining Google Trends data to identify patterns in and correlates to searches for dermatological concerns and providers. Br J Dermatol; 2018 [5]	US, UK, South Africa, Singapore, worldwide	During the study window (September 2011-September 2016), searches originating in the United States revealed that dermatology is the most frequently searched medical specialty, followed by psychiatry and ophthalmology. This correlates with the proportion of self-referred patients, not with overall volume of visits. Countries in the southern hemisphere, such as South Africa, demonstrate a reversed seasonal search trend for dermatologists compared to countries in the northern hemisphere. Countries without distinct seasons, such as Singapore, had no seasonal variation in searches.
Hopkins ZH, Secrest AM. An international comparison of Google searches for sunscreen, sunburn, skin cancer, and melanoma: Current trends and public health implications. Photodermatol Photoimmunol Photomed; 2019 [1]	US, UK, Canada, Australia, New Zealand	From January 1, 2004 to December 31, 2017, sunscreen and sunburn had the highest intraterm correlation, with both searches rising. Searches for skin cancer and melanoma decreased during the study window for all countries except New Zealand and the United Kingdom. Countries with rising rates of melanoma displayed higher searches for all terms. Recommended online skin cancer prevention campaigns use the search terms "sunburn" and "sunscreen."
Seidl S, Schuster B, Rüth M, Biedermann T, Zink A. What do Germans want to know about skin cancer? A nationwide Google search analysis from 2013 to 2017. J Med Internet Res; 2018 [7]	Germany	From November 2013 to October 2017, the highest volume search terms related to nonmelanoma skin cancer and melanoma included "skin cancer," "white skin cancer," "basalioma," and "melanoma." The most-searched anatomic area of nonmelanoma skin cancer was ""nose" and for melanoma, "nails." This suggested that this information can be utilized to focus educational campaigns.
Callaghan DJ. Use of Google Trends to examine interest in Mohs micrographic surgery: 2004 to 2016. Dermatol Surg; 2018 [8]	US	During the study window (2004-2016), there was a rise in searches for "Mohs surgery," positively correlated with a rise in the SVI[a] for "basal cell carcinoma" and "squamous cell carcinoma," but without a similar correlation for "melanoma" or "skin cancer."
Huang X, Baade P, Youlden DR, Youl PH, Hu W, Kimlin MG. Google as a cancer control tool in Queensland. BMC Cancer; 2017 [9]	Australia	Increases in the monthly ASR[b] for breast cancer, melanoma, and prostate cancer were significantly correlated with increases in monthly SVIs. Colorectal cancer did not show this significant correlation. However, the predictive powder of SVIs to account for ASR variances was different for each cancer type, suggesting that more research is needed for internet search–based cancer surveillance.
Zink A, Schuster B, Rüth M, Pereira MP, Philipp-Dormston WG, Biedermann T, Ständer S. Medical needs and major complaints related to pruritus in Germany: a 4-year retrospective analysis using Google AdWords Keyword Planner. J Eur Acad Dermatol Venereol; 2019 [10]	Germany	During the study window (June 2013-April 2017), the most searched German language Google terms on the topic of pruritus included "atopic eczema," the lay term for psoriasis; "Schuppenflechte"; and "psoriasis." A seasonal trend was noted, with the lowest searches for pruritus occurring in the summer.
Motosko C, Zakhem G, Ho R, Saadeh P, Hazen A. Using Google to trend patient interest in botulinum toxin and hyaluronic acid fillers. J Drugs Dermatol; 2018 [11]	US	Search volume for queries related to neuromodulators and hyaluronic acid–based fillers was positively correlated with the number of procedures performed in the same year and year prior.
Wang S, Manudhane A, Ezaldein HH, Scott JF. A review of the FDA's 510(k) approvals process for electromagnetic devices used in body contouring. J Dermatolog Treat; 2019 [12]	US	Google Trends SVI for the term "Emsculpt" grew during 2018, reaching a peak in July.
Seth D, Wang S, Ezaldein HH, Merati M, Scott JF. Over-the-counter light therapy for acne: a cross-sectional retrospective analysis. Dermatol Online J; 2019 [13]	US	During the study window (2010-2018), SVI for "acne light therapy mask" peaked in 2016.

Topic and article citation	Google Trends location(s) analyzed	Key findings
Dey M, Zhao SS. COVID-19 and Kawasaki disease: an analysis using Google Trends. Clin Rheumatol; 2020 [14]	Worldwide	Searches for "Kawasaki disease" rose sharply in April 2020; "Kawasaki disease" SVI was highest in Europe, possibly reflecting pediatric manifestation of COVID-19 in European populations. This suggests the use of Google Trends to detect disease clusters in real time.
Seasonality of searches		
Kardeş S. Seasonal variation in the internet searches for psoriasis. Arch Dermatol Res; 2019 [15]	US, UK, Canada, Ireland, Australia, New Zealand	Public interest in psoriasis-related information shows seasonal variability, with interest peaking in late winter and early spring.
Zink A, Schuster B, Rüth M, Pereira MP, Philipp-Dormston WG, Biedermann T, Ständer S. Medical needs and major complaints related to pruritus in Germany: a 4-year retrospective analysis using Google AdWords Keyword Planner. J Eur Acad Dermatol Venereol; 2019 [10]	Germany	During the study window (June 2013-April 2017), the most searched German language Google terms on the topic of pruritus included "atopic eczema," the lay term for psoriasis" "Schuppenflechte"; and "psoriasis." A seasonal trend was noted, with the lowest searches for pruritus occurring in the summer.
Tizek L, Schielein M, Rüth M, Ständer S, Pereira MP, Eberlein B, Biedermann T, Zink A. Influence of Climate on Google Internet Searches for Pruritus Across 16 German Cities: Retrospective Analysis. J Med Internet Res; 2019 [16]	Germany	Between August 2014 and July 2018, "pruritis" and "anal pruritis" were the most searched terms for the topic of pruritis, with more searches related to chronic than to acute pruritis. Temperature had a larger effect on searches than particle matter, humidity, and sunshine duration, with a peak in searches during winter.
Kirchberger MC, Kirchberger LF, Eigentler TK, Reinhard R, Berking C, Schuler G, Heinzerling L, Heppt MV. Interest in tanning beds and sunscreen in German-speaking countries. J Dtsch Dermatol Ges; 2017 [17]	Germany, Austria, Switzerland	During the study window (2004-2016), worldwide searches for sunscreen increased, while tanning bed searches decreased. Conversely, for German-speaking countries, there were more searches for tanning beds than for sunscreen. More education regarding prevention of UV[c] damage is needed for those residing in German-speaking countries.
Toosi B, Kalia S. Seasonal and geographic patterns in tanning using real-time data from Google Trends. JAMA Dermatol; 2016 [18]	Canada, US, Australia	Public interest in tanning salons and tanning beds has been declining since 2010 in Canada and since 2012 in the United States and Australia. Interest in tanning is seasonal — highest in March in the northern hemisphere, highest in September in the southern hemisphere.
Ransohoff JD, Sarin KY. Referred by Google: mining Google Trends data to identify patterns in and correlates to searches for dermatological concerns and providers. Br J Dermatol; 2018 [5]	US, UK, South Africa, Singapore, worldwide	During the study window (September 2011-September 2016), searches originating in the United States revealed that dermatology is the most frequently searched medical specialty, followed by psychiatry and ophthalmology. This correlates with the proportion of self-referred patients, not with overall volume of visits. Countries in the southern hemisphere, such as South Africa, demonstrate a reversed seasonal search trend for dermatologists compared to countries in the northern hemisphere. Countries without distinct seasons, such as Singapore, were found to have no seasonal variation in searches.
Kluger N. Insights into worldwide interest in tattoos using Google Trends. Dermatology; 2019 [19]	Worldwide	Public interest in tattoos increased steadily during the study window (January 2004-December 2018). Interest in tattoos demonstrates a seasonal pattern, peaking in the summer months.
Celaj S, Deng J, Murphy BL, Kundu RV. Analysis of population inquiry on practices for ultraviolet radiation protection. Dermatol Online J; 2017 [20]	US	During the study window (2004-2015), "broad spectrum sunscreen" SVI was highest in June and lowest in winter. After an FDA[d] announcement in 2011 regarding broad spectrum sunscreen labeling, the SVI for "broad spectrum sunscreen" increased. The "sunblock" and "sunscreen" SVIs were highest in June and lowest in December but were not affected by the FDA 2011 announcement. This suggests that Google Trends can be utilized to monitor campaigns or public health policy changes similar to the 2011 FDA announcement.

Topic and article citation	Google Trends location(s) analyzed	Key findings
Kluger N, Bouchard LJ. A comparative study of Google Search trends for melanoma, breast cancer and prostate cancer in Finland. Dermatology; 2019 [21]	Finland-based; included data from Belgium, Italy, Portugal, and Sweden	Compared public interest in melanoma to breast and prostate cancer, using Google Trends (January 1, 2010-January 1, 2019). The "melanoma" SVI was maximal in early summer. SVI peaks for the terms related to breast and prostate cancer were positively correlated with awareness campaigns for those diseases. This suggests a second public health campaign for melanoma awareness should be timed during winter (lowest public interest period).
Xu S, Thyssen JP, Paller AS, Silverberg JI. Eczema, atopic dermatitis, or atopic eczema: analysis of global search engine trends. Dermatitis; 2017 [22]	English, Russian, Japanese, Turkish, German (specified languages searched)	From 2014 to 2016, searches for eczema increased, while "atopic dermatitis" and "atopic eczema" searches remained stable. Authors recommended the universal use of "atopic dermatitis" rather than "eczema" due to the term's ambiguous nature. Seasonal climate changes were associated with flares of severity for atopic dermatitis and corresponded with search trends.
Hsiang EY, Semenov YR, Aguh C, Kwatra SG. Seasonality of hair loss: a time series analysis of Google Trends data 2004-2016. Br J Dermatol; 2018 [3]	8 English-speaking countries (did not specify)	SVI for terms related to hair loss demonstrated seasonality, with peaks in summer and autumn. This suggests symptoms of hair loss are greatest in summer and autumn.
Social media's impact on searches		
Ward B, Ward M, Paskhover B. Google Trends as a resource for informing plastic surgery marketing decisions. Aesthetic Plast Surg; 2018 [23]	US	Highly publicized plastic surgery events and celebrity social media posts have a significant impact on search volume for related topics.
Noar SM, Leas E, Althouse BM, Dredze M, Kelley D, Ayers JW. Can a selfie promote public engagement with skin cancer? Prev Med; 2018 [24]	US	Searches related to skin cancer, skin cancer prevention, and tanning increased during the period May 13-17, 2005, after a cancer selfie Facebook post went viral. This suggests that public health practitioners can utilize Google Trends to build on viral posts in real time to potentiate positive health benefits.
Limitations and strengths of Google Trends		
Martinez-Lopez A, Ruiz-Villaverde R, Molina-Leyva A. Google search trends in psoriasis: a pilot evaluation of global population interests. J Eur Acad Dermatol Venereol; 2018 [25]	Worldwide	This was a pilot study to assess primary topics of interest to those with psoriasis. The search term with the most growth during the period 2004-2016 was "kim kardashian psoriasis."
Kluger N. Tattoo side effects worldwide: a Google Trends-based time series analysis. Acta Dermatovenerol Alp Pannonica Adriat; 2019 [26]	Worldwide	SVI for tattoo-related symptoms increased during the study window (January 1, 2004-December 31, 2018).
Corazza M, Amendolagine G, Musmeci D, Forconi R, Borghi A. Sometimes even Dr Google is wrong: An unusual contact dermatitis caused by benzoyl peroxide. Contact Dermatitis; 2018 [27]	Italy	The study compared SVI for 3 chronic diseases to searches for "dermatitis," noting that only "diabetes" was searched more frequently than "dermatitis." This demonstrates likelihood of self-diagnosis of dermatitis via the internet. Search volume for the medication Benzac peaked in autumn and winter, aligning with seasonal acne flares.
Hessam S, Salem J, Bechara FG, Haferkamp A, Heidenreich A, Paffenholz P, Sand M, Tsaur I, Borgmann H. Hidradenitis suppurativa gains increasing interest on World Wide Web: a source for patient information? Int J Dermatol; 2017 [28]	Worldwide	Search queries related to HS[e] have risen over the last decade. HS-related website analysis demonstrates a need for improvement in quality and readability to raise disease awareness and allow earlier patient presentation for undiagnosed patients.
Lospinoso DJ, Lospinoso JA, Miletta NR. The impact of ultraviolet radiation on sunburn-related search activity. Dermatol Online J; 2017 [29]	US	A strong positive association between the UV index and SVI for sunburn-related terms was demonstrated. This suggests tracking search terms for sun protective measures as an indication of public awareness and efficacy of public health programs.

[a]SVI: search volume index.

[b]ASR: age-standardized incidence rate.

[c]UV: ultraviolet.

[d]FDA: Food and Drug Administration.

[e]HS: hidradenitis suppurativa.

Discussion

Skin-Related Topics of Public Interest

Notably, dermatology was reported by Ransohoff and Sarin [5] to be the most searched medical specialty in a comparative study of 15 medical specialties. To compare relative specialist popularity using Google Trends data, the study [5] used the search term "physician," to enable all specialist search terms to be normalized to the SVI of this term (the most popular term) and thus enabled an accurate comparison across all 15 physician specialties. However, the study by Ransohoff and Sarin [5] also found that, despite being the most searched specialty, dermatology ranked sixth in number of clinic visits per specialty and revealed that dermatologists had one of the highest percentages of self-referred patients. The authors concluded that the high rate of dermatology Google searches correlates with the proportion of self-referred patients rather than the number of clinic visits, and therefore, changes in online search volume may better reflect how patients initiate care with dermatologists rather than demonstrate real-time vacillations in clinic volume [5].

Several papers also describe the use of Google Trends to gather information about user searches related to skin cancer and skin cancer prevention. Google Trends searches for "sunscreen" and "sunburn" are growing in the United States, United Kingdom, Canada, Australia, and New Zealand [1]. Conversely, searches for "skin cancer" and "melanoma" are declining for one or both terms in the United States, Canada, and Australia [1].

In Germany, the most searched term in the skin cancer–related category was "forms of skin cancer," followed by "skin alterations" [7]. Seidl et al [7] also noted that the most searched anatomic locations of melanoma were "nails" and "eyes," while for nonmelanoma skin cancer, the most searched locations were "nose" and "face." A 2018 study [8] of US-based Google searches discovered that the search terms "Mohs surgery," "basal cell carcinoma," and "squamous cell carcinoma" rose during the years 2004 to 2016. This finding aligns with a rise in the use of Mohs micrographic surgery during this time, according to reports from Medicare and the National Ambulatory Medical Survey [8].

A study by Huang et al [9] using data from the Queensland Cancer Registry from January 2006 to December 2012 reported that increases in the monthly age-standardized incidence rates (ASR) for melanoma correlated with increases in the monthly SVI for search terms "skin cancer" and "melanoma." Additionally, through use of a multiple linear regression model, Huang et al [9] reported that the predictive power of the "skin cancer" SVI to explain variance in melanoma ASR was 17.9%, noting that the search term "skin cancer" includes both melanoma and keratinocyte carcinomas and thus may better predict rates of melanoma than the specific search term "melanoma," since online users may not be able to distinguish different skin cancer types when performing Google searches.

Google Trends has also been utilized to study pruritus. According to a 2019 study conducted in Germany by Zink et al [10] that utilized the Google Keywords Planner to determine search volume, it was discovered that for German language Google searches regarding pruritus, the most searched terms included "atopic eczema" (24.3%), the common term for psoriasis, "Schuppenflechte" (17.8%), "psoriasis" (13.4%), and the German word for pruritus, "Juckreiz" (2.9%).

Gauging public interest in certain cosmetic procedures and treatments is another application of Google Trends data. A 2018 study by Motosko et al [11] found that the number of procedures employing botulinum toxin and/or hyaluronic acid–derived fillers correlated significantly with the search volume for related search terms over the period spanning 2005 to 2016, while Wang et al [12] noted search volume expansion for "Emsculpt," a body contouring technique, during 2018. Similarly, a study by Seth et al [13] reported an increase in the search term "acne light therapy mask" in 2016, reflecting a parallel increase in public interest in light-emitting diode therapy for inflammatory acne.

Of particular interest given the currently evolving pandemic, a 2020 study by Dey and Zhao [14] examined the relationship between COVID-19 and Kawasaki disease using Google Trends data. The study found that the search frequencies of Kawasaki disease in 2019 and 2020 were similar until April 2020, when reports of a Kawasaki-like disease in children with COVID-19 emerged. From February to May 2019, searches for Kawasaki disease were highest in Indonesia, the Philippines, and Malaysia — regions where the disease is more commonly found. However, from February to May 2020, searches for Kawasaki disease were highest in France, Switzerland, and Italy, a finding that reflects our current knowledge of the multisystem inflammatory syndrome in children (MIS-C), associated with COVID-19 and aligning with MIS-C clusters in Europe during this time [22,30]. While popularity of search terms may be confounded by news or social media–driven popularity, Dey and Zhao [14] noted that the association revealed through Google Trends data could highlight its potential future utility in identifying real-time disease clusters.

Seasonality of Searches

Google searches related to dermatology demonstrate a seasonal nature for several skin diseases. A 2019 study by Kardeş [15] found that searches for "psoriasis" were elevated in the late winter and early spring and were lower in the late summer and early fall, with statistically significant results from the United Kingdom, Canada, Ireland, Australia, and New Zealand and noted a trend toward seasonal variation in US-based searches.

In Germany, Google searches for "pruritus" were lowest in the summer [10] and highest in the winter [16]. Additionally, "tanning bed" was searched most in March and May, while "sunscreen" search volume was highest in June [17]. Toosi and Kalia [18] reported that public interest in tanning for Canada and the United States was highest in March and for Australia, was highest in September. Countries in the southern hemisphere, such as South Africa, demonstrate a reversed seasonal search trend compared to countries in the northern hemisphere; countries without distinct seasons, such as Singapore, were found to have no seasonal variation in searches [5]. According to Kluger [19], the term "tattoo" was searched most during the summer and least during winter: Searches for the term "tattoo" are highest from July to August in the northern hemisphere and reach a peak in January for regions in the southern hemisphere. Interestingly, Kluger [26] found that searches for symptoms of tattoo-related complications, such as pruritus and induration, rose during the period 2004 through 2018 inclusive — however, interpretation of these results is difficult, as the search volume increase could reflect either a real increase in tattoo side effects or be secondary to rising popularity of tattoos [26].

Search patterns for sunscreen in the United States have shown similar seasonal trends [20]. A US-based study found the search terms "skin cancer" and "tanning" were highest in the early summer months, while "sunburn" was highest in the late summer; the monthly timing of these trends was noted to be reversed in countries of the southern hemisphere, such as South Africa [5]. "Melanoma" was found to have the highest searches in the early summer months of either hemisphere [5,21].

In a study of worldwide Google Trends data spanning 5 languages, 4 of these demonstrated peaks in SVI for the term "eczema" in line with seasonal climate changes that are associated with flares of severity for atopic dermatitis, speaking to both the seasonality of searches and to the widespread usage of "eczema" as a synonym for atopic dermatitis [31]. Hsiang et al [3] studied "hair loss" search volume, with data from the top 4 most populous countries of both hemispheres and observed the highest SVI occurred in the summer and autumn, with the lowest search volume corresponding to the spring. The authors noted these results suggest a correlative relationship between hair loss and seasonality and that hair loss is greatest in the summer and autumn. This is in line with other studies that have noted the percentage of telogen phase hairs peaks in the late summer, with a smaller peak in the spring, and therefore, maximal hair loss occurs at the end of summer and during the fall [32].

Social Media's Impact on Searches

Social media has been found to influence dermatology-related search volume on Google. A 2018 study by Ward et al [23] found that the average interest level of fillers increased by 30.31 points (relative to a maximum SVI of 100) in the time period after Kylie Jenner stated that she underwent lip augmentation with Juvederm in April 2015, compared to searches conducted in the period prior (January 2004 through March 2015). Additionally, a study by Noar et al [24] noted that after a highly graphic skin cancer selfie went viral on Facebook, all search queries for skin cancer, skin cancer prevention, and tanning significantly increased, with May 13, 14, and 15 of 2017 being the 6th, 8th, and 40th most searched days for skin cancer since the inception of Google Trends on January 1, 2004.

Limitations and Strengths of Google Trends

The main limitation of utilizing Google Trends to accurately assess public interest in a certain dermatologic topic is that it relies on the ability to access the internet, which is variable [25,26]. Individuals who are of lower socioeconomic status and educational background may not have access to a computer or smart device through which they can use Google. Additionally, individuals who are of older age may choose not to use a computer and thus would not use Google. As a result, certain groups of individuals who may be at higher risk for particular dermatologic conditions may not use Google and are omitted from Google Trends. This would imply that the dermatologic interests of people in older age groups or lower socioeconomic status may not be accurately or fully represented in Google Trends data, which could bias the information it presents and limits extrapolation to the broader population.

Thus, while Google Trends is a powerful tool for assessing the public's dermatologic interest, it is important to consider which populations are unequally represented with this instrument and find other tools to fill these gaps. While Google accounts for approximately 91% of the market share of online searches worldwide (according to available data from January 2021), it is vital to note that search engines other than Google may be utilized, along with specific health information websites; therefore, analysis of a variety of search engines could potentially capture a more complete picture of current trends in skin-related topics of public interest.

Nevertheless, Google Trends may be a useful tool for dermatologists to gauge areas of skin concern and topics of interest, as patients may perform searches on Google for questions they are not comfortable asking their dermatologists in a clinic visit [11]. Additionally, the increasing use of Google to search skin diseases may highlight the increased prevalence of self-diagnosis and self-treatment [27,28]. Therefore, it could be useful for professional medical organizations to take note of which skin diseases and dermatology-related terms are most often searched and to notify individual dermatologists, who could then dedicate additional time to patient education, reaffirm facts, and dispel misconceptions and misinformation.

One potential public health benefit of Google Trends would be to focus on highly searched terms in order to guide and drive health campaigns. For example, in 2019, Hopkins and Secrest [1] recommended online skin cancer prevention campaigns to focus on the search terms "sunburn" and "sunscreen" as these 2 terms have demonstrated increasing search frequency from 2004 to 2016. These public health campaigns can be specifically tailored to complement and make the most of current public interest [7]. Frequency of searched terms can serve as a proxy for public awareness and speak to the efficacy of public health programs [29].

Another possible use of Google Trends is for dermatologists to quickly detect the presence of viral social media content related to dermatology, such as the skin cancer selfie that went viral on Facebook in 2017, and to then engage with the online public and utilize this viral content to strengthen public health campaigns [24]. Lastly, as the study by Dey and Zhao [14] of COVID-10 and Kawasaki-like disease illustrates, Google Trends has the potential to be utilized in identifying disease clusters in real time, meriting further research to better understand how dermatology may leverage this tool in early identification of public health concerns in the future.

Limitations of This Scoping Review

Limitations of this review article include its simplified search strategy, which included only English language publications, restriction to the PubMed database, and lack of previous studies examining Google Trends and dermatology. Google Trends is a relatively new tool (2006 conception), and therefore, not many dermatology publications highlight the use of Google Trends in dermatology. For example, in 2020, there was only 1 dermatology Google Trends publication out of 174 total publications discussing Google Trends, as illustrated in Multimedia Appendix 1. This highlights the gap in prior literature on the intersection of these 2 topics, which weakens the conclusions we can generate from existing research. While we lay the groundwork with this survey and scoping review of related literature [6], in order to better assess the utility of Google Trends in dermatology, further research in this area is required.

Summary

Review of the literature illustrates that assessment of Google Trends data related to dermatology has been studied, with topics including skin cancer, pruritus, cosmetic procedures, social media, clinic visits, and the associated Kawasaki-like disease of COVID-19 (MIS-C). Additionally, a seasonal nature of search terms has been widely reported in the literature, varying according to hemisphere. The main limitation of Google Trends as a research tool is access to and use of the internet. Further research is needed to better understand how this search tool can be utilized to improve the quality of clinic visits, drive public health campaigns, and detect disease clusters in real time.

References

1. Hopkins ZH, Secrest AM. An international comparison of Google searches for sunscreen, sunburn, skin cancer, and melanoma: Current trends and public health implications. Photodermatol Photoimmunol Photomed 2019 Mar;35(2):87-92. [doi: 10.1111/phpp.12425] [Medline: 30198586]
2. Google L. FAQ about Google Trends data: how is google trends data normalized? Trends Help. URL: https://support.google.com/trends/answer/4365533?hl=en&ref_topic=6248052 [accessed 2021-05-08] [WebCite Cache ID 73eSYBJXk]
3. Hsiang EY, Semenov YR, Aguh C, Kwatra SG. Seasonality of hair loss: a time series analysis of Google Trends data 2004-2016. Br J Dermatol 2018 Apr;178(4):978-979. [doi: 10.1111/bjd.16075] [Medline: 29048738]
4. Churick N. How to Use Google Trends for Keyword Research: 7 Effective Ways. ahrefs blog. 2019 Dec 30. URL: https://ahrefs.com/blog/how-to-use-google-trends-for-keyword-research/ [accessed 2021-05-08]
5. Ransohoff JD, Sarin KY. Referred by Google: mining Google Trends data to identify patterns in and correlates to searches for dermatological concerns and providers. Br J Dermatol 2018 Mar;178(3):794-795. [doi: 10.1111/bjd.15491] [Medline: 28338220]
6. Munn Z, Peters MDJ, Stern C, Tufanaru C, McArthur A, Aromataris E. Systematic review or scoping review? Guidance for authors when choosing between a systematic or scoping review approach. BMC Med Res Methodol 2018 Nov 19;18(1):143 [FREE Full text] [doi: 10.1186/s12874-018-0611-x] [Medline: 30453902]
7. Seidl S, Schuster B, Rüth M, Biedermann T, Zink A. What Do Germans Want to Know About Skin Cancer? A Nationwide Google Search Analysis From 2013 to 2017. J Med Internet Res 2018 May 02;20(5):e10327 [FREE Full text] [doi: 10.2196/10327] [Medline: 29698213]
8. Callaghan DJ. Use of Google Trends to Examine Interest in Mohs Micrographic Surgery: 2004 to 2016. Dermatol Surg 2018 Feb;44(2):186-192. [doi: 10.1097/DSS.0000000000001270] [Medline: 28930787]
9. Huang X, Baade P, Youlden DR, Youl PH, Hu W, Kimlin MG. Google as a cancer control tool in Queensland. BMC Cancer 2017 Dec 04;17(1):816 [FREE Full text] [doi: 10.1186/s12885-017-3828-x] [Medline: 29202718]
10. Zink A, Schuster B, Rüth M, Pereira MP, Philipp-Dormston WG, Biedermann T, et al. Medical needs and major complaints related to pruritus in Germany: a 4-year retrospective analysis using Google AdWords Keyword Planner. J Eur Acad Dermatol Venereol 2019 Jan;33(1):151-156. [doi: 10.1111/jdv.15200] [Medline: 30067284]
11. Motosko C, Zakhem G, Ho R, Saadeh P, Hazen A. Using Google to Trend Patient Interest in Botulinum Toxin and Hyaluronic Acid Fillers. J Drugs Dermatol 2018 Nov 01;17(11):1245-1246. [Medline: 30500150]
12. Wang S, Manudhane A, Ezaldein HH, Scott JF. A review of the FDA's 510(k) approvals process for electromagnetic devices used in body contouring. J Dermatolog Treat 2019 Nov;30(7):727-729. [doi: 10.1080/09546634.2019.1566589] [Medline: 30614316]
13. Seth D, Wang S, Ezaldein HH, Merati M, Scott JF. Over-the-counter light therapy for acne: a cross-sectional retrospective analysis. Dermatol Online J 2019 Jan 15;25(1):13030. [Medline: 30710908]
14. Dey M, Zhao SS. COVID-19 and Kawasaki disease: an analysis using Google Trends. Clin Rheumatol 2020 Aug;39(8):2483-2484 [FREE Full text] [doi: 10.1007/s10067-020-05231-z] [Medline: 32557254]
15. Kardeş S. Seasonal variation in the internet searches for psoriasis. Arch Dermatol Res 2019 Aug;311(6):461-467. [doi: 10.1007/s00403-019-01921-0] [Medline: 31025101]
16. Tizek L, Schielein M, Rüth M, Ständer S, Pereira MP, Eberlein B, et al. Influence of Climate on Google Internet Searches for Pruritus Across 16 German Cities: Retrospective Analysis. J Med Internet Res 2019 Jul 12;21(7):e13739 [FREE Full text] [doi: 10.2196/13739] [Medline: 31301128]
17. Kirchberger MC, Kirchberger LF, Eigentler TK, Reinhard R, Berking C, Schuler G, et al. Interest in tanning beds and sunscreen in German-speaking countries. J Dtsch Dermatol Ges 2017 Dec;15(12):1192-1198. [doi: 10.1111/ddg.13380] [Medline: 29148618]
18. Toosi B, Kalia S. Seasonal and Geographic Patterns in Tanning Using Real-Time Data From Google Trends. JAMA Dermatol 2016 Feb;152(2):215-217. [doi: 10.1001/jamadermatol.2015.3008] [Medline: 26719968]

19. Kluger N. Insights into Worldwide Interest in Tattoos Using Google Trends. Dermatology 2019;235(3):240-242 [FREE Full text] [doi: 10.1159/000496986] [Medline: 30826808]
20. Celaj S, Deng J, Murphy BL, Kundu RV. Analysis of population inquiry on practices for ultraviolet radiation protection. Dermatol Online J 2017 Oct 15;23(10):13030 [FREE Full text] [Medline: 29469800]
21. Kluger N, Bouchard LJ. A Comparative Study of Google Search Trends for Melanoma, Breast Cancer and Prostate Cancer in Finland. Dermatology 2019;235(4):346-347 [FREE Full text] [doi: 10.1159/000498987] [Medline: 30999301]
22. Toubiana J, Poirault C, Corsia A, Bajolle F, Fourgeaud J, Angoulvant F, et al. Kawasaki-like multisystem inflammatory syndrome in children during the covid-19 pandemic in Paris, France: prospective observational study. BMJ 2020 Jun 03;369:m2094 [FREE Full text] [doi: 10.1136/bmj.m2094] [Medline: 32493739]
23. Ward B, Ward M, Paskhover B. Google Trends as a Resource for Informing Plastic Surgery Marketing Decisions. Aesthetic Plast Surg 2018 Apr;42(2):598-602. [doi: 10.1007/s00266-017-1019-4] [Medline: 29218476]
24. Noar SM, Leas E, Althouse BM, Dredze M, Kelley D, Ayers JW. Can a selfie promote public engagement with skin cancer? Prev Med 2018 Jun;111:280-283. [doi: 10.1016/j.ypmed.2017.10.038] [Medline: 29109014]
25. Martinez-Lopez A, Ruiz-Villaverde R, Molina-Leyva A. Google search trends in psoriasis: a pilot evaluation of global population interests. J Eur Acad Dermatol Venereol 2018 Oct;32(10):e370-e372. [doi: 10.1111/jdv.14944] [Medline: 29573479]
26. Kluger N. Tattoo side effects worldwide: a Google Trends-based time series analysis. Acta Dermatovenerol Alp Pannonica Adriat 2019 Sep;28(3):125-127 [FREE Full text] [Medline: 31545390]
27. Corazza M, Amendolagine G, Musmeci D, Forconi R, Borghi A. Sometimes even Dr Google is wrong: An unusual contact dermatitis caused by benzoyl peroxide. Contact Dermatitis 2018 Dec;79(6):380-381. [doi: 10.1111/cod.13086] [Medline: 30079477]
28. Hessam S, Salem J, Bechara FG, Haferkamp A, Heidenreich A, Paffenholz P, et al. Hidradenitis suppurativa gains increasing interest on World Wide Web: a source for patient information? Int J Dermatol 2017 Jul;56(7):726-732. [doi: 10.1111/ijd.13601] [Medline: 28321845]
29. Lospinoso DJ, Lospinoso JA, Miletta NR. The impact of ultraviolet radiation on sunburn-related search activity. Dermatol Online J 2017 Aug 15;23(8):13030 [FREE Full text] [Medline: 29469736]
30. Bautista-Rodriguez C, Sanchez-de-Toledo J, Clark BC, Herberg J, Bajolle F, Randanne PC, et al. Multisystem Inflammatory Syndrome in Children: An International Survey. Pediatrics 2021 Feb;147(2):e2020024554. [doi: 10.1542/peds.2020-024554] [Medline: 33234669]
31. Xu S, Thyssen JP, Paller AS, Silverberg JI. Eczema, Atopic Dermatitis, or Atopic Eczema: Analysis of Global Search Engine Trends. Dermatitis 2017;28(4):276-279. [doi: 10.1097/DER.0000000000000273] [Medline: 28722692]
32. Kunz M, Seifert B, Trüeb RM. Seasonality of hair shedding in healthy women complaining of hair loss. Dermatology 2009;219(2):105-110. [doi: 10.1159/000216832] [Medline: 19407435]

Abbreviations

ASR: age-standardized incidence rate
MIS-C: multisystem inflammatory syndrome in children
SVI: search volume index

14

Identifying and Responding to Health Misinformation on Reddit Dermatology Forums with Artificially Intelligent Bots Using Natural Language Processing: Design and Evaluation Study

Monique A Sager[1], BA; Aditya M Kashyap[2], PhD; Mila Tamminga[1], BS; Sadhana Ravoori[2], BE; Christopher Callison-Burch[2], PhD; Jules B Lipoff[3], MD

[1]Perelman School of Medicine, University of Pennsylvania, Philadelphia, PA, United States
[2]Department of Computer Science, University of Pennsylvania, Philadelphia, PA, United States
[3]Department of Dermatology, University of Pennsylvania, Philadelphia, PA, United States

Corresponding Author:
Jules B Lipoff, MD
Department of Dermatology
University of Pennsylvania
3737 Market Street, Suite 1100
Penn Medicine University City
Philadelphia, PA, 19104
United States

Email: jules.lipoff@pennmedicine.upenn.edu

Abstract

Background: Reddit, the fifth most popular website in the United States, boasts a large and engaged user base on its dermatology forums where users crowdsource free medical opinions. Unfortunately, much of the advice provided is unvalidated and could lead to the provision of inappropriate care. Initial testing has revealed that artificially intelligent bots can detect misinformation regarding tanning and essential oils on Reddit dermatology forums and may be able to produce responses to posts containing misinformation.

Objective: To analyze the ability of bots to find and respond to tanning and essential oil–related health misinformation on Reddit's dermatology forums in a controlled test environment.

Methods: Using natural language processing techniques, we trained bots to target misinformation, using relevant keywords and to post prefabricated responses. By evaluating different model architectures across a held-out test set, we compared performances.

Results: Our models yielded data test accuracies ranging 95%-100%, with a Bidirectional Encoder Representations from Transformers (BERT) fine-tuned model resulting in the highest level of test accuracy. Bots were then able to post corrective prefabricated responses to misinformation in a test environment.

Conclusions: Using a limited data set, bots accurately detected examples of health misinformation within Reddit dermatology forums. Given that these bots can then post prefabricated responses, this technique may allow for interception of misinformation. Providing correct information does not mean that users will be receptive or find such interventions persuasive. Further studies should investigate this strategy's effectiveness to inform future deployment of bots as a technique in combating health misinformation.

KEYWORDS

bots; natural language processing; artificial intelligence; Reddit, medical misinformation; health misinformation; detecting misinformation; dermatology; misinformation

Introduction

Background

Health misinformation—defined as information that is incorrect, and possibly intended to deceive [1]—is rampant on the internet. Well-intentioned social media users often advise each other regarding health care treatments and home remedies. Prior studies have assessed health misinformation on Facebook and Twitter, yet one of the most active communities in health care discussions remains less investigated: the social media forums of Reddit [2]. As a social media and commentary platform with 330 million users, Reddit is the fifth most popular site in the United States [3]. The forums, known as subreddits, also cover nearly every medical specialty; for example, dermatology (known as "r/Dermatology"), cardiology, and others.

One of the most active medical forums on Reddit is r/Dermatology, with users seeking to crowdsource for free medical opinions. Indeed, posts often begin with variations of "I cannot afford a dermatologist." The advice ranges from homeopathic remedies suggested by uncredentialled users to evidence-based medical treatments offered by dermatologists volunteering their time on the forum. A significant portion of medical advice from nonphysicians promotes non–evidence-based homeopathic treatments over scientifically validated medical treatments. For example, a user posting a photograph of a suspicious mole may be falsely reassured by other posters that in-person evaluation is unnecessary or that it can be resolved with the application of essential oils. Given that Reddit posts are anonymous, people may be empowered to reveal their medical concerns more candidly. In contrast, the public nature of a forum such as Facebook may discourage candid sharing [4]. Thus, the design of Reddit makes it a uniquely promising target for studying this crowdsourcing and potential health misinformation.

The audience for Reddit dermatology forums is large and highly engaged; over 55,000 users follow r/Dermatology, over 1.3 million users follow r/SkincareAddiction, and over 19,000 follow r/essentialoils [5]. These users (known as Redditors), log in globally, though a majority are from the United States (58%) [6]. While the majority of Redditors are young men, the skin care forums are largely female-dominated. Subreddit r/SkincareAddiction is one of the largest dermatology-related forums with 87% of female users, of whom 70% are between 19 and 29 years old [7].

Prior Work

Our previous work has used the artificial intelligence subfield of natural language processing techniques to analyze Reddit dermatology forums' content [8]. Our data suggest that these forums are a rich source of patient engagement, presenting an untapped opportunity for expert involvement. Our study aimed to investigate the feasibility of engaging in these forums using bots, with the goal of intercepting health misinformation.

Preliminary analysis of Reddit dermatology forums identified a potential target: rampant confusion and misinformation regarding sun exposure. For instance, many users had questions about the dangers of sun exposure, questioning if these supposed dangers are a scam perpetuated by sunscreen companies. Further, tanning beds were often touted as a cure for acne and other skin conditions. Sun exposure–related misinformation was identified as a good target for intervention because of the clear consensus on guidance from the medical establishment. Indoor tanning devices are classified as the highest class of carcinogens by the World Health Organization, and it is well established that tanning bed use is a risk factor for developing melanoma, with multiple tanning bed sessions increasing the risk of melanoma [9-11]. Melanoma leads to an estimated 7000 deaths per year in the United States [12].

Essential oil (EO) use and safety was selected as a second target of misinformation. Users discussed EOs as a remedy for many health conditions, though no such efficacy has been established in the medical literature, and EO use is not without risk. For instance, 1 user solicited information on using EOs to treat Sjogren syndrome and was told to seek out a local herbalist.

In this context, we aimed to develop artificially intelligent bots for Reddit forums as a means to intercept and correct health misinformation.

Methods

Methods Overview

To develop bots to intercept health misinformation, we developed 2 sets of machine learning models: 1 targeting posts that discussed sun exposure or tanning, and the second for posts that discussed EOs. We used Google's BigQuery application programming interface (API) to query publicly available Reddit data [13], pulling from the forums r/Dermatology, r/essentialoils, and r/tanning from January 2018 to August 2019. Google BigQuery API analyses 100% of full-text posts. We used the API to extract Reddit posts and comments that belonged to the subreddits we targeted and then locally ran our scripts over the entirety of the text posts. Using the data from BigQuery, we filtered by subreddit and searched for keywords (Textbox 1) [14].

Textbox 1. Keywords used.

Essential oil–related keywords

- essential oils
- Bay
- cinnamon bark
- clove
- frankincense
- citronella
- cumin
- lemongrass
- lemon verbena
- oregano
- thyme
- lavender
- nutmeg
- peppermint
- tea tree
- cinnamon leaf
- camphor oil
- oil of wintergreen
- jasmine
- ylang-ylang
- sandalwood oil

Tanning-related keywords

- sun exposure
- tanning
- tanning bed
- base tan

For the sun exposure/tanning data set, we included all posts from the r/tanning subreddit as positive training instances in addition to posts from r/Dermatology, which contained tanning-related keywords. The remaining posts from r/Dermatology were taken as negative training instances. Similarly, for the essential oils data set, all posts from the r/essentialoils subreddit were considered positive training instances in addition to posts from r/Dermatology that contained EO-related keywords. Positive training instances meant that the targeted content was identified, while negative training instances indicated that no such content was identified within the post. Next, we removed the search keywords from the positive comments to ensure that the classification task was nontrivial.

Two medical student annotators read through over 350 posts on the aforementioned forums and annotated posts as containing misinformation or not. This analysis was performed to determine that a sufficient number of posts contained misinformation in r/essentialoils and r/tanning to establish those forums as misinformation in our data set. To annotate the posts, the annotators used UpToDate and PubMed. UpToDate is the most frequently utilized clinical decision database for physicians, and all information included is evidence-based and peer reviewed [15]. PubMed (the database of science journals for the National Library of Medicine of the National Institutes of Health) supplemented with additional journal articles when needed.

As mentioned, during bot development, we trained the bot to treat all comments related to "tanning" or "essential oils" as positive for misinformation. As a result, we did not exclude posts with phrases such as "avoid tanning," despite the risk of causing the bot to respond to posts containing accurate information. This workflow was chosen because we felt that false positives were acceptable, but false negatives (where misinformation is present and we failed to reply to it) could be harmful. After the bot had been trained to identify "misinformation" versus "valid posts," our human annotators reviewed posts to ascertain the number of false positives vs false negatives, using the aforementioned annotation. In our training data set, the percentage of false positives for EOs and tanning was 2% and 5% respectively.

Once the quality of these data sets was verified, we were then able to posit an "accuracy" score for each model to determine how much true misinformation they could assimilate. These scores were calculated by evaluating the trained models on a held-out test set.

Given a smaller proportion of positive training instances (21% and 5% for EOs and tanning, respectively), we created a balanced data set by undersampling the negative examples. We performed a train-test split on this balanced data set (details about their sizes are shown in Table 1).

Table 1. Number of instances in the data set.

	Essential oils	Tanning
Training instances, n	1971	586
Test instances, n	221	66

In this study, we aimed to examine the theoretical ability of bots to detect and respond to misinformation. In developing our methods, we found that by using natural language processing techniques, bots can learn differentiating terms such as "tanning," "essential oils," or "sun exposure." These bots have the ability to post prefabricated responses to comments related to a variety of skin conditions. These responses were developed and condensed from the American Academy of Dermatology (AAD) into user-friendly lengths and include a link for viewers to directly access the AAD website.

When these terms are identified, bots can reflexively provide condensed AAD recommendations in a comment. For example, with a mention of sun exposure, the bot can post a brief response detailing risk factors such as blistering sunburns, rates of skin cancer in the United States, and recommendations on sunscreen use. For EOs, the bot can return guidance on safe usage and potential adverse reactions. To be clear, these responses have not been posted in any live forums on Reddit, but the design was aimed at a live endpoint in the future.

Model Creation

We compared the test accuracy for 3 different models. The first model included a baseline logistic regression model, which used a simple bag-of-words representation considering unigram, bigram, and trigram features. A vocabulary consisting of the 20,000 most frequent ngrams was chosen after converting the text to lowercase.

The second model involved fine-tuning a pretrained Bidirectional Encoder Representations from Transformers (BERT) model [16] with a fully connected feed forward classification layer on top. The posts in the training data were first tokenized using a word piece tokenizer, following which [CLS] and [SEP] tokens were appended to the beginning and end of the sequences, respectively. Adam optimizer with a learning rate of 2e-5 and Binary Cross Entropy Loss was used to finetune this model over 4 epochs.

For the third model, we developed a fine-tuned XLNet model [17] with a single feed forward layer on top for classification. The optimizer, loss, and model hyperparameters were similar to those selected for the BERT model. The held-out test data set was used to evaluate each model's performance and estimate the prediction error.

Results

Test accuracies by model are shown in Table 2. We compared the results against a random baseline (where there is an equal probability for each label to be picked for a test instance). Our preliminary results show that all 3 models had high test accuracies for both EOs and tanning. The baseline logistic regression model performed well with an accuracy of over 95%. The top positive features of the logistic regression model included words such as "diffuser" and "blends" for essential oils, "bronzer" and "St. Tropez" for tanning, and top negative features included words such as "rash" and "acne." The XLNet fine-tuned model was also effective, with a test accuracy over 98%, while the BERT fine-tuned model had the highest test accuracy of 100%.

Table 2. Validation accuracy of the models.

Model	Test accuracy for "essential oils," %	Test accuracy for "tanning," %
Random predictor	50.00	50.00
Logistic regression model	97.29	95.65
BERT[a] fine-tuned	99.56	100
XLNet fine-tuned	98.70	98.61

[a]BERT: Bidirectional Encoder Representations from Transformers.

Discussion

Principal Findings

Our study demonstrates, in a test environment, the ability for artificially intelligent bots to identify health misinformation related to tanning and EOs on Reddit forums, which have the ability to subsequently post corrective prefabricated responses. These results raise the question of whether benevolent bots should play a role in identifying and intercepting health misinformation on live forums. To date, social media bots have largely failed to promote credible sources. An analysis of 14 million Twitter messages by Shao et al [18] in 2017 revealed that social media bots overwhelmingly spread information from low-credibility sources. They reported that bots can "tailor misinformation" to "target those who are most likely to believe it." The public's vulnerability to misinformation is further enhanced by inundation of such untruths from multiple sources. For instance, similar tweets, news stories, and Facebook articles popping up on social media feeds, even if all incorrect, may appear to falsely validate each other [19]. By automatically targeting inaccuracies with accurate medical information, we can potentially interrupt this inundation of untruths.

Beyond the issue of noncredible bots, media coverage related to bots has focused on their potential negative impact on society. These concerns mainly revolve around the use of malicious bots to alter outcomes of elections, seed political and social turmoil, or even endanger lives via public health propaganda. One recent study showed, for example, that bots and Russian trolls on Twitter post more content about vaccination than the average user [20]. However, we would argue that the potential upside makes benevolent bots, at the very least, worthy of further study, with any potential impacts carefully studied before transitioning from proof of concept to real-world application.

Specifically, while bots have been used to spread misinformation, they can also be harnessed proactively to disseminate information from high-credibility sources, such as the National Institutes of Health and various academies of medicine. Indeed, some nonmedical projects have already attempted to harness the power of benevolent bots. For example, the United States Geological Service uses @earthquakeBot, a bot that detects earthquakes of 5.0 magnitude and automatically alerts the public. In 2017, the World Economic Forum experimented with an official Twitter bot, @forumfactbot, to combat misinformation about its funding sources, targeting World Economic Forum–related misinformation in tweets and automatically linking to accurate stories [21]. These examples show how transparent, fact-based bots have previously been harnessed to combat misinformation on social media. The creators of any benevolent bot must preemptively consider all ethical and practical issues prior to and during implementation.

Though concerns about bots are justified, our study builds on a growing body of work arguing that bots can—and should—be studied as forces for public health benefits. Many believe that a critical part of combating misinformation is the strong assertion of the truth, with many effective (though nonbot) examples such as Politifact, Factcheck.org, and Snopes [19]. Others have suggested that the public health community should "go on the offense with our messages," and perhaps benevolent bots could be 1 avenue to deliver such messages [22]. This reveals the possibility that those with malicious intent could use bots to further their own interests or stymie healthy discussions of differing viewpoints.

Strengths and Limitations

Our approach has several limitations. Methodologically, we chose to have the bot treat all posts on the r/essentialoils and r/tanning subreddit forums as misinformation. The basis for this assumption came from having annotators read through over 350 posts on r/tanning and r/essentialoils and determine that a sufficient number of posts contained misinformation, which we would be able to consider it misinformation in our data set. Of note, an additional limitation is that while the annotators used evidence-based sources and support from a senior physician to annotate the posts for misinformation, there was no formal training prior to the annotation process. Thus, no standards were developed from which a formal training process could be created.

Many posts simply promoted the practice of tanning, which is undoubtedly misinformation given consensus among experts regarding the risk of melanoma with tanning. Similarly, many posts promoted EO use instead of evidence-based medical treatments. For r/Dermatology, more information was deemed accurate and thus required a different strategy. We considered only posts containing those keywords included in this study on r/Dermatology as misinformation.

Given that bots consider entire forums as misinformation, they are highly sensitive but fairly nonspecific. We run the risk of automatically posting replies to posts containing phrases such as "avoid tanning." This reflexivity could prompt users to consider the bots as unreliable and thus begin to ignore the responses. In future iterations, we intend to refine this approach to increase the specificity of posts captured.

The bots currently only search for a limited set of keywords, as shown in Multimedia Appendix 1 [23-26]. Given that these keywords do not encompass all the words that users describe when discussing tanning or essential oils, we are inevitably missing posts containing misinformation. We hope to increase the effectiveness of the bots by including a wider set of keywords in future searches, such as commonly used words for tanning in countries outside of the United States.

Furthermore, to be an effective public health intervention, we must assume that users will read both the post containing the misinformation and any corrective responses. However, the massive amount of content on these forums makes it impossible for a casual browser to read everything. Many posts on Reddit are either unread or only have 1 or 2 comments in response to them. The forums are constantly refreshed as new content is generated, meaning that our responses to a post could be buried under a new post within a few hours. One safeguard against this is the "search" function that exists within the forums; if a user is searching for advice on a topic such as "tanning," Reddit returns results spanning back to the creation of the forum, which could be years prior. The user can then see all posts about the topic, including those that have our responses attached to them.

Another factor complicating Reddit visibility of posts is the order in which posts are displayed. Responses to Reddit posts are displayed in order of how often they are "upvoted," which is essentially the same function as a "like" on Facebook. Thus, a highly upvoted but inaccurate opinion could become the top comment users see, lending it more visibility than our post. Future research could benefit from addressing how to boost the visibility of validated information, such as running advertisements or "featured spots" on social media sites.

A final limitation is that even if users see factual evidence opposing misinformation, they may disregard corrective responses. Politics and sociology have repeatedly demonstrated that when facts are incongruent with a person's opinion, a person may in fact disregard the facts presented to them and cling to the misinformation, a phenomenon called "cognitive consistency" [27,28]. Ideological beliefs, or simply rumors heard enough to have reached a "social consensus," can impair one's ability to assess the validity of a statement and lead readers to process incongruent information less fluently [27,28]. Further, users may not be receptive to corrective information provided by nonhuman users; indeed, the presence of bots could potentially interrupt a tacit community standard and violate users' trust, even if bots were completely transparent in their roles to correct health misinformation.

Conclusions

In our study, our bot models all had high test accuracies, which suggests that artificially intelligent bots may accurately target Reddit posts containing commonly misunderstood health content. The ability to consistently detect comments at risk of misinformation is merely the first step toward using benevolent bots to disseminate high-quality scientific information to the public. Our ultimate goal is to test a novel method of addressing dermatology misinformation on Reddit by posting active replies with bots to posts deemed misinformation. Our results suggest that using artificial intelligence is a potentially beneficial and valid method of targeting misinformation on the internet. Having now established feasibility of both detecting misinformation and reflexively responding to it in test environments, subsequent steps include testing the bots on Reddit and other social media forums, with user satisfaction surveys and links to track user engagement with bot-delivered posts. While this initial work has focused on a subset of dermatology misinformation, it demonstrates proof of concept of the potential for using bots to promote fact-based discussions on any medical topic or public health conversation. Thus, we anticipate continued and necessary work to explore and validate the potential for benevolent bots in the health misinformation space.

References

1. Misinformation. Cambridge Dictionary. URL: https://dictionary.cambridge.org/us/dictionary/english/misinformation [accessed 2021-07-28]
2. De Choudhury M, De S. Mental Health Discourse on reddit: Self-Disclosure, Social Support, and Anonymity. 2014 Presented at: Eighth International AAAI Conference on Weblogs and Social Media (ICWSM-14); June 1-4, 2014; Ann Arbor, MI URL: https://ojs.aaai.org/index.php/ICWSM/article/view/14526
3. Hutchinson A. Reddit now has as many users as twitter, and far higher engagement rates. Social Media Today. 2018. URL: https://www.socialmediatoday.com/news/reddit-now-has-as-many-users-as-twitter-and-far-higher-engagement-rates/521789/ [accessed 2019-11-06]
4. Newman M, Lauterbach D, Munson S, Resnick P, Morris M. It's not that i don't have problems, i'm just not putting them on facebook: challenges and opportunities in using online social networks for health. 2011 Presented at: CSCW '11: Computer Supported Cooperative Work; March 19-23, 2011; Hangzhou. [doi: 10.1145/1958824.1958876]
5. Subreddit Stats: Statistics for every subreddit. URL: https://subredditstats.com/ [accessed 2021-03-29]
6. Sattelberg W. The Demographics Of Reddit: Who Uses The Site? ALPHR. 2021. URL: https://www.techjunkie.com/demographics-reddit/ [accessed 2019-11-05]
7. [Meta] They're finally here: the ScA Survey results!. Reddit. URL: https://www.reddit.com/r/SkincareAddiction/comments/6nagon/meta_theyre_finally_here_the_sca_survey_results/ [accessed 2019-11-05]
8. Okon E, Rachakonda V, Hong HJ, Callison-Burch C, Lipoff JB. Natural language processing of Reddit data to evaluate dermatology patient experiences and therapeutics. J Am Acad Dermatol 2020 Sep;83(3):803-808. [doi: 10.1016/j.jaad.2019.07.014] [Medline: 31306722]
9. Indoor Tanning: The Risks of Ultraviolet Rays. US Food and Drug Administration. 2015. URL: https://www.fda.gov/consumers/consumer-updates/indoor-tanning-risks-ultraviolet-rays [accessed 2021-08-23]
10. Mogensen M, Jemec GB. The potential carcinogenic risk of tanning beds: clinical guidelines and patient safety advice. Cancer Manag Res 2010 Oct 28;2:277-282 [FREE Full text] [doi: 10.2147/CMR.S7403] [Medline: 21188119]
11. Ting W, Schultz K, Cac NN, Peterson M, Walling HW. Tanning bed exposure increases the risk of malignant melanoma. Int J Dermatol 2007 Dec;46(12):1253-1257. [doi: 10.1111/j.1365-4632.2007.03408.x] [Medline: 18173518]
12. American Cancer Society. 2019. URL: https://www.cancer.org/content/dam/cancer-org/research/cancer-facts-and-statistics/annual-cancer-facts-and-figures/2019/cancer-facts-and-figures-2019.pdf [accessed 2021-08-23]
13. Using BigQuery with Reddit Data. Pushshift. URL: https://pushshift.io/using-bigquery-with-reddit-data/ [accessed 2021-03-20]

14. Google Cloud Platform, SQL Workspace: Reddit Comments 2018_01. URL: https://console.cloud.google.com/bigquery?project=fh-bigquery&page=table&t=2018_01&d=reddit_comments&p=fh-bigquery&redirect_from_classic=true&ws=!1m5!1m4!4m3!1sfh-bigquery!2sreddit_comments!3s2018_01 [accessed 2021-03-20]
15. About UpToDate. Wolters Kluwer. URL: https://www.wolterskluwer.com/en/solutions/uptodate/about [accessed 2021-06-20]
16. Devlin J, Chang MW, Lee K, Toutanova K. BERT: Pre-training of Deep Bidirectional Transformers for Language Understanding. arXiv Preprint posted online May 24, 2019. [FREE Full text]
17. Yang Z, Dai Z, Yang Y, Carbonell J, Salakhutdinov R, Le QV. XLNet: Generalized Autoregressive Pretraining for Language Understanding. arXiv Preprint posted online January 2, 2020. [FREE Full text]
18. Shao C, Ciampaglia GL, Varol O, Yang K, Flammini A, Menczer F. The spread of low-credibility content by social bots. Nat Commun 2018 Nov 20;9(1):4787 [FREE Full text] [doi: 10.1038/s41467-018-06930-7] [Medline: 30459415]
19. West DM. How to combat fake news and disinformation. Brookings. 2017. URL: https://www.brookings.edu/research/how-to-combat-fake-news-and-disinformation/ [accessed 2019-11-23]
20. Broniatowski DA, Jamison AM, Qi S, AlKulaib L, Chen T, Benton A, et al. Weaponized health communication: Twitter bots and Russian trolls amplify the vaccine debate. Am J Public Health 2018 Oct;108(10):1378-1384. [doi: 10.2105/AJPH.2018.304567] [Medline: 30138075]
21. Stroppa A, Hanley M. How can we defeat fake news? World Economic Forum. 2017. URL: https://www.weforum.org/agenda/2017/02/how-can-we-defeat-fake-news-automate-the-right-to-reply/ [accessed 2019-12-02]
22. Lowry M, Fouse D. Communicating research in an era of misinformation. Am J Public Health 2019 May;109(5):645. [doi: 10.2105/AJPH.2019.305048] [Medline: 30969830]
23. Ismail F, Nixon R. Allergic contact dermatitis to essential oils. DermNet NZ. 2020. URL: https://www.dermnetnz.org/topics/allergic-contact-dermatitis-to-essential-oils/ [accessed 2021-07-28]
24. Henley DV, Lipson N, Korach KS, Bloch CA. Prepubertal gynecomastia linked to lavender and tea tree oils. N Engl J Med 2007 Feb 01;356(5):479-485. [doi: 10.1056/NEJMoa064725] [Medline: 17267908]
25. Morris MC, Donoghue A, Markowitz JA, Osterhoudt KC. Ingestion of tea tree oil (Melaleuca oil) by a 4-year-old boy. Pediatr Emerg Care 2003 Jun;19(3):169-171. [doi: 10.1097/01.pec.0000081241.98249.7b] [Medline: 12813303]
26. Del Beccaro MA. Melaleuca oil poisoning in a 17-month-old. Vet Hum Toxicol 1995 Dec;37(6):557-558. [Medline: 8588296]
27. Lewandowsky S, Ecker UKH, Seifert CM, Schwarz N, Cook J. Misinformation and its correction: continued influence and successful debiasing. Psychol Sci Public Interest 2012 Dec;13(3):106-131. [doi: 10.1177/1529100612451018] [Medline: 26173286]
28. Winkielman P, Huber DE, Kavanagh L, Schwarz N. Fluency of consistency: When thoughts fit nicely and flow smoothly. In: Gawronski B, Strack F, editors. Cognitive consistency: A Fundamental Principle in Social Cognition. New York, NY: Guilford Press; 2012:89-111.

Abbreviations

AAD: American Academy of Dermatology
API: application programming interface
BERT: Bidirectional Encoder Representations from Transformers
EO: essential oil

15

Instagram Content Addressing Pruritic Urticarial Papules and Plaques of Pregnancy

Ashley Payton[1,2*], BS, MS; Benjamin K P Woo[1*], MD

[1]Department of Psychiatry, Olive View Medical Center, University of California Los Angeles Medical Center, Sylmar, CA, United States

[2]College of Osteopathic Medicine of the Pacific, Western University of Health Sciences, Pomona, CA, United States

[*]all authors contributed equally

Corresponding Author:
Ashley Payton, BS, MS
Department of Psychiatry
Olive View Medical Center
University of California Los Angeles Medical Center
14445 Olive View Drive
Cottage H1
Sylmar, CA, 91342
United States

Email: aapayton16@gmail.com

Abstract

Background: Pruritic urticarial papules and plaques of pregnancy (PUPPP) is the most commonly diagnosed pregnancy-specific dermatosis. It presents with intense pruritus and can be difficult to manage, which encourages mothers to look to social media for camaraderie and advice.

Objective: This study aimed to characterize the sources and thematic content of Instagram posts in order to define influential groups of users. Our goal was to determine the status of online discourse surrounding PUPPP and elucidate any potential space for health care provider intervention via creation of Instagram accounts dedicated to information dissemination for patient populations.

Methods: Three hashtag categories were selected (#PUPPP, #PUPPPs, and #PUPPPrash), and the top public posts from each were analyzed and organized by source and by thematic content. The numbers of likes and comments were also recorded.

Results: Among the top 150 posts in each hashtag category, only 428 posts in total were eligible for this analysis. Majority (316/428, 73.8%) of posts were created by mothers who experienced PUPPP. These posts were testimonial accounts in nature. A small fraction of posts (14/428, 3.3%) were generated by physician accounts. Posts from blogs with extensive followings garnered the most attention in the form of likes and comments.

Conclusions: Mothers experiencing PUPPP comprised the majority of accounts posting under the hashtags selected. The most common themes included pictures of the rash and personal testimonies. Posts under blog posts received the most likes and comments on average. There is space for physician and health care specialists to improve their social media presence when it comes to discourse surrounding PUPPP. Patients are seeking out communities on social media, like Instagram, in order to have questions answered and obtain advice on management. Accounts with large followings tend to have more likes and more comments, which encourages information dissemination and awareness. Thus, we suggest that physicians create content and potentially partner with blog-type accounts to improve outreach.

KEYWORDS

pruritic urticarial papules and plaques of pregnancy; dermatology; rash; pregnancy; obstetrics; dermatosis; Instagram; social media; patient education

Introduction

Pruritic urticarial papules and plaques of pregnancy (PUPPP) is the most common pregnancy-specific dermatosis affecting about 1 in 200 pregnancies [1]. It is also known as polymorphic eruption of pregnancy. PUPPP is more common in primiparous women and is characterized by erythematous papular lesions that classically arise within the confines of striae distensae on the gravid abdomen [1,2].

Typically, the eruptions begin on the abdomen and can spread to the thighs, arms, and buttocks, with onset occurring typically in the third trimester [3,4]. Symptoms tend to resolve 7 to 10 days postpartum [4]. However, this rash can be very pruritic, extensive, and difficult to manage for patients, especially in multiple gestation cases [4]. Many mothers try antipruritus creams and medications, with little or short-lasting relief. This could be one factor driving mothers with PUPPP to seek support in various outlets, including social media.

Social media has taken the spotlight in recent years as a tool for human interaction, which has changed how we learn from and engage with peers. Particularly within younger generations that grew up with internet access, it is increasingly common to find that people turn to social media for information and advice. A recent survey found that 72% of people reported turning to the internet to look up health information within the last year [5]. The convenience of the internet at the tips of our fingers has made it a preferred source for many Americans searching for answers.

Social media has become a way for patients with various unique conditions to post and find camaraderie with others who have similar afflictions, including during pregnancy [6]. We must be cognizant of the power that social media has to influence our decision-making ability in this regard [7,8]. Endorsements on social media sites, such as Instagram, have been shown to activate reward centers of the brain, making social media a powerful tool for peer influence [8]. According to Instagram's webpage, it boasts of having over 1 billion users worldwide. The Pew Research Center generated an estimate that roughly 72% of American adults have at least one social media account and that 37% have an Instagram account as of 2019 [9]. Creating posts for Instagram is free, and posts can be made available to the public. This makes the app a cost-effective and efficient way for health care specialists to widely distribute quick medical information to the public at large. In light of this, it is important to analyze how patient populations interact with content on social media so that we can determine whether there is space for health care professionals to provide evidence-based medical information and quell patient skepticism about information they are finding online.

PUPPP is a lesser publicized affliction, and thus, its discussion is not common in the public arena despite its relatively high prevalence in pregnant and postpartum mothers [1]. The rash can dramatically impact mothers during pregnancy and alter their experience. We hope to be able to shed some light on what information is being distributed on popular social media sites. In this study, we seek to characterize posts regarding PUPPP circulated on Instagram from the public. It is our goal to determine what discourse is generated by and for these pregnant mothers in order to define a potential space for increased physician and health care provider intervention, education, and advocacy.

Methods

Data Collection

Using the Instagram app, hashtag-based key terms were searched and identified (n=3; #PUPPP, #PUPPPs, and #PUPPPrash). Note that capitalization does not make a difference on the app hashtag search function; thus, "#PUPPP" yields the same result as "#puppp."

The top 150 posts from each tag were selected for analysis from all public posts. To be included in the study, the picture's caption had to include information or opinions regarding PUPPP. We excluded posts that were considered private because they would not be readily accessible to the public when using Instagram's search function. We excluded posts that had irrelevant material (ie, posts about puppies that were tagged within the #puppp thread and posts that did not include content regarding PUPPP) or were repeat tags (ie, posts tagged in the #puppp and #puppps categories). With these criteria, two of the tag categories yielded fewer than 150 posts that qualified for the study.

Data Analysis

Each post was assigned exclusively to a category based on source. The categories included the following: (1) mother, (2) physician/health care provider, (3) health care organization, (4) company/product, and (5) blog/blogger (Table 1). For further clarification, the category for physician/health care provider was scrutinized even further to determine if posts were from physicians or other providers such as midwives and doulas. In order for a post to be determined to be from a mother, caption information was taken into account and designation was granted if first person language was used. Many of these posts were accompanied by "selfies" that contributed to the decision of assigning a post to the mother category.

Characterization of the thematic content of each post was then determined by the team. Thematic content was categorized nonexclusively, meaning that each post could be assigned to more than one category based on image content as well as accompanying caption content. These categories included the following: (1) testimony, (2) educational information, (3) picture of PUPPP rash, (4) therapy advice & guidance, (5) blog post, and (6) product promotion (Table 1).

Table 1. Stratification methodology of Instagram posts that met the inclusion criteria.

Post source categories (exclusive assignment)[a]	Thematic content categories (nonexclusive assignment)[a]
1. Mother	1. Testimony
2. Physician/health care provider	2. Educational information
3. Health care organization	3. Picture of PUPPP[b] rash
4. Company/product	4. Therapy advice & guidance
5. Blog/blogger	5. Blog post
	6. Production promotion

[a]Individual posts could be placed exclusively in one category based on their source but were nonexclusively categorized by content of the post.
[b]PUPPP: pruritic urticarial papules and plaques of pregnancy.

The numbers of comments and endorsements or "likes" were recorded for each post after the characterization process. The average numbers of likes and comments were then calculated within each tag category.

Results

Tags

As of November 23, 2020, there were 2100 posts tagged with #PUPPP, 599 posts tagged with #PUPPPs, and 189 posts tagged with #PUPPPrash, which were publicly available on Instagram (totaling 2888 posts).

After determining which posts were eligible for study, 150 were included under #PUPPP, 141 were included under #PUPPPs, and 137 were included under #PUPPPrash (totaling 428 posts).

Source Categorization

Posts in all three tags were placed into one of five designated categories for characterization of the source. Overall, we found that the majority of posts available were created and shared by those who identified themselves as mothers (316/428, 73.8%), followed by blogs (58/428, 13.6%), companies (28/428, 6.5%), physicians or health care providers (14/428, 3.3%), and health care organizations (12/428, 2.8%) (Table 2).

Table 2. Post source categorization.

Tag category	Post source, n (%)				
	Mothers	Health care organizations	Physicians and health care providers	Companies	Blogs
#PUPPP (N=150)	134 (89.3%)	9 (6.0%)	7 (4.7%)	0 (0%)	0 (0%)
#PUPPPs (N=141)	132 (93.6%)	1 (0.7%)	0 (0%)	8 (5.7%)	0 (0%)
#PUPPPrash (N=137)	50 (36.5%)	2 (1.5%)	7 (5.1%)	20 (14.6%)	58 (42.3%)
Overall (N=428)	316 (73.8%)	12 (2.8%)	14 (3.3%)	28 (6.5%)	58 (13.6%)

In all categories, except for #PUPPPrash, mothers themselves were the predominant posters of content regarding PUPPP. In #PUPPPrash, the largest portion of content and discussion involved blogs (58/137, 42.3%), most of which were identified as "maternity lifestyle blogs" where women share experiences, advice, and information regarding pregnancy and motherhood to their followers (Table 2).

Only 14 posts came from health care providers overall, seven of which were from physicians licensed with an MD (Doctorate in Medicine) or DO (Doctorate in Osteopathic Medicine) medical degree (Table 2). The other seven advertised themselves as mid-level providers, such as nurse practitioners, lactation consultants or midwives, and doulas. This content made up 3.3% (14/428) of the overall number of posts.

#PUPPP had the majority of posts from accounts deemed as "health care organizations," such as a public account, @skincancerderminstitute, a dermatology clinic. Nine of the 12 posts coming from health care organizations were in this tag group. Other organizations represented were centered on pregnancy and women's health.

The "companies" category, which we defined as any account tied to a business that advertised a product or service that they themselves sell and/or provide for financial gain, was most prominent in the #PUPPPrash category, comprising 14.6% (20/137) of all posts analyzed (Table 2). Of the 28 posts from companies, 20 were found under #PUPPPrash.

Thematic Content Analysis

All posts were categorized nonexclusively into six categories based on the content in the image or the caption associated with the image.

By and large, the category "testimony" comprised a majority of the posts across all three tag groups. Out of all 428 posts, 309 (72.2%) were classified as a "testimony" based on the content within the caption provided by the poster. This meant that 72.2% of all posts contained personal accounts and anecdotes from mothers who had experienced PUPPP during one or more of their pregnancies (Table 3). Most of these testimonies were mothers describing their journeys, expressing frustration with the pruritic rash, and providing encouragement to their followers who may be experiencing the same affliction.

Table 3. Analysis of thematic content of posts in each tag category and overall (N=428).

Theme[a]	Tag category			
	#PUPPP, n	#PUPPPs, n	#PUPPPrash, n	Across all tags, n (%)
Testimony	91	94	124	309 (72.2%)
Education	20	8	1	29 (6.8%)
Therapy advice	10	14	5	29 (6.8%)
Blog post	0	11	89	100 (23.4%)
Production promotion	15	23	5	43 (10.0%)
Picture of rash	58	55	115	228 (53.3%)

[a]Posts were nonexclusively categorized, that is, each post could be tallied in more than one of the six themes represented.

Posts were given a designation under the category "education" if they provided objective and factual medical information about PUPPP. Posts in this category, for example, included infographics, diagrams, and other texts that would provide information to moms about what PUPPP is, what the symptoms are, and what standard treatment includes, and/or provide epidemiological information. A popular fact included frequently in educational posts was that about 1 in 150 to 200 women will be affected by PUPPP [1,3].

Overall, 228 (53.3%) posts contained a picture of a rash directly. Pictures of a rash included an exposed abdomen with signs of PUPPP. Within the PUPPPrash tag, one picture of one blogger's rash was reposted 78 times with a copied caption. In the PUPPP and PUPPPs groups, pictures were all personal, meaning they were of the user's own rash.

Another important finding was that 100 of the 428 (23.4%) posts were from an account that advertised being a blog (Table 3). Blog posts either came from blog accounts, such as accounts that advertised being a "personal" or "maternity" blog, or from mothers who were self-promoting their own personal blogs. Of these 100 posts, 89 were found under the PUPPPrash tag.

Therapy advice included posts in which accounts offered advice on which over-the-counter products or home remedies worked best for the poster's PUPPP. These posts only comprised 6.8% (n=29) of all posts.

Lastly, product promotion included posts in which a specific product or service was advertised for financial gain by the poster. These posts included products, such as herbal soap bars, creams, and essential oils, designed to help with the symptoms of PUPPP. These posts could have links to the vendor's Instagram page or website for consumers to purchase products directly. Product promotion posts comprised 10.0% (43/428) of all posts and were more represented in the PUPPPs group followed by the PUPPP group (Table 3).

Endorsement and Follower Interaction

The number of likes was recorded for each post during analysis, and the average was calculated for each subsection. The highest average number of likes was found in the PUPPPrash tag with 2371.52. The same category also resulted in the highest average number of comments of 34.34 (Table 4).

Table 4. Likes and comments broken down by tag category.

Tag category	Mean number of endorsements	Range for the number of likes	Mean number of comments	Range for the number of comments
#PUPPP	50.53	0-458	10.46	0-65
#PUPPPs	67.39	1-1452	8.57	0-46
#PUPPPrash	2371.52	4-38,350	34.34	0-389

The PUPPPrash group had the highest average number of likes but also had the largest range of likes from 4 to 38,350. This category had 10 posts with more than 10,000 likes and 32 posts with between 1000 and 9999 likes. No other category had a post with more than 10,000 likes. PUPPPrash also had the largest average number of comments per post with a range of 0 to 389 (Table 4).

Of note, the PUPPPrash category also had the highest concentration of blog accounts (Table 3). These accounts tended to have more followers, which may have accounted for the higher number of likes and comments per post.

Discussion

Principal Findings

The presence of PUPPP on the social media app Instagram is significant yet small in comparison to the estimated number of pregnancies affected each year. With a little under 3000 posts available to the public on the popular app and around 3.7 million births in the United States annually, there appears to be a gap in discourse surrounding this common dermatosis [10]. A search on the Instagram interface reveals that other sequelae of pregnancy, such as hyperemesis gravidarum, have more dedicated posts. For example, searching #hyperemesisgravidarum on Instagram returned approximately 49,200 posts as of November 30, 2020. Despite the low census of posts for PUPPP, the posts included in this analysis represented a diverse pool of sources as well as themes.

Interestingly, the overwhelming majority of posts came from mothers who were affected by the rash. These posts tended to contain testimonial captions and frequently included pictures of the mother's own rash. Based on caption analysis, most of these testimonial posts were intended to bring awareness to a condition that is considered "embarrassing" by many moms. Posts would include candid accounts of the mothers' experiences with combating PUPPP. Posts like this help to normalize the discourse and make others feel more comfortable discussing their rash with their followers. Some moms even included pictures of their exposed rash. These vulnerable pictures could put others at ease if the rash looks similar to their own. Overall, these testimonial posts really highlight the community's honesty with PUPPP and willingness to share their experiences for the benefit of others.

The amount of posts coming from health care professionals made up a small fraction of the sample (14/428, 3.3%). As a potential space for physicians to impact the public beyond their clinical domain, this analysis has made it apparent that there is room for improvement on the part of physicians to guide online discussion. Only 14 of all 428 posts were from professional health care providers, and only seven of those were from physicians (Table 2). A post that is created by a trained medical professional might be viewed as more credible by the public than a post from a layperson, meaning these posts could be more influential. The posts that did come from these accounts tended to be educational in nature with the goal of teaching followers about PUPPP. Again, only a small percentage of posts offered educational material signaling a place for growth for specialists who see and treat patients with PUPPP.

The posts that this study found to garner the most attention, in the form of likes and comments, were blog posts, although they made up only 23.4% (100/428) of the posts across all three investigated tags. Some of these posts gained tens of thousands of likes and hundreds of comments. The blog accounts that many of these "high-earning" posts came from boasted large followings, which may have been a contributing factor for the greater interaction of these posts than posts from any one mother. This makes sense given that Instagram's algorithm puts pictures from accounts you follow into one's home feed. Therefore, the more followers an account has, the more interaction its posts will receive. Many of the blogs that earned the most likes were advertised as maternity blogs, and the posts dealt with topics and issues for expecting mothers as well as new mothers. It is possible that mothers who have experienced complications during their pregnancy seek out and follow pregnancy-specific blogs on Instagram in the hope of finding camaraderie and reassurance in their peers and influential users.

Limitations and Future Directions

Several limitations became apparent during our analysis. First, Instagram has introduced a new policy that does not allow the general public to view all available posts. Currently, there is a disclaimer when one searches any given hashtag that states not all of the most recent posts will show up on the content feed. This is part of a new initiative by social media companies to stop the spread of misinformation.

On Instagram, we are not able to definitively determine the age or gender of the person posting the content as this information is not distributed by each user's account. This limited our analysis particularly when looking at the posts coming from mothers affected by PUPPP. Access to the demographic information of the mothers would have given us a better idea of what audience characteristics are better represented on Instagram.

There is future potential for a similar study to analyze the content of the comment sections. Previous studies have demonstrated that examining user comments on social media can provide an in-depth view of questions and concerns brought up by patients [11,12]. Characterization of the comments from followers in order to discover the nature of supportive or inquisitive feedback under each post could strengthen the argument that patients are seeking quality medical information on Instagram. A dive into the nuances of conversation between followers and posters could further elucidate the exact needs and curiosities of patients opting to research conditions on social media.

Other studies could be designed with this paradigm in order to examine other lesser known medical conditions in all specialties. It could be interesting to investigate some more "taboo" conditions as well in order to see how willing online users would be to ask about them behind the comfort and convenience of the keyboard rather than in person to their physician.

Clinical Applications and Conclusions

This study demonstrated that there is a considerable presence on Instagram of the most common dermatosis specific to pregnancy, PUPPP. We were able to examine this common skin condition of pregnancy through the unique lens of publicly available Instagram content. Through the use of hashtags on the popular social media app, we found that mothers with PUPPP readily expressed their experiences, asked questions, and shared advice with their followers. At times, these moms would even share their opinions on various treatments and therapies as well and generate dialogue among one another.

Importantly, there are very few physicians actively posting clinically valid information about the rash, which could address many of the questions and concerns that these mothers pose online. Health care professionals, such as dermatologists and obstetricians, should be aware of this social media presence and consider increasing their influence on applications since a high number of patients turn to internet communities for support.

One suggestion we propose is for physicians to increase their social media presence by creating public professional accounts that display their credentials [13]. In this way, physicians can advertise their professional accounts to the existing clientele and reach patient populations beyond those that they personally serve. Once an account is established, posts can be made that combine informative graphics with educational text. Therefore, if physicians generate more content and use hashtags so that their posts are searchable, they could reach a larger audience interested in the topic. It might also behoove the physician to partner with bloggers, such as maternity bloggers in our case, in order to quickly gain visibility and reach a larger audience already seeking information and support [13].

The spread of misinformation has also become a topic of discussion in recent years as social media has become a dominant forum for peer conversation [13]. With the rise of social media as an arena for sharing, it has become apparent that perpetuation of incorrect medical statements may create mistrust and fear among patients [14]. Serious false information has been disseminated, such as the belief that vaccines cause autism, because physicians abuse the trust built. It is the duty of physicians, including physicians participating in online discourse, to ensure that facts are checked. Physicians are in a particularly unique position to create posts containing evidence-based information while also being key opinion leaders.

In a time where we have immediate access to any information through the internet, misinformation is rampant and physicians work hard to dispel concerns that patients bring in with them to the examination room. We suggest that clinicians build up their social media presence to offer legitimate responses and medical information to patients looking for quick answers before their next doctor's appointment.

References

1. Lehrhoff S, Pomeranz MK. Specific dermatoses of pregnancy and their treatment. Dermatol Ther 2013;26(4):274-284. [doi: 10.1111/dth.12078] [Medline: 23914884]
2. Zhu P, Fung A, Woo BKP. Consumer Preference of Products for the Prevention and Treatment of Stretch Marks: Systematic Product Search. JMIR Dermatol 2020 Jun 4;3(1):e18295. [doi: 10.2196/18295]
3. Aronson IK, Bond S, Fiedler VC, Vomvouras S, Gruber D, Ruiz C. Pruritic urticarial papules and plaques of pregnancy: Clinical and immunopathologic observations in 57 patients. Journal of the American Academy of Dermatology 1998 Dec;39(6):933-939. [doi: 10.1016/s0190-9622(98)70265-8] [Medline: 9843004]
4. Matz H, Orion E, Wolf R. Pruritic urticarial papules and plaques of pregnancy: polymorphic eruption of pregnancy (PUPPP). Clin Dermatol 2006;24(2):105-108 [FREE Full text] [doi: 10.1016/j.clindermatol.2005.10.010] [Medline: 16487883]
5. Zhao Y, Zhang J. Consumer health information seeking in social media: a literature review. Health Info Libr J 2017 Dec;34(4):268-283 [FREE Full text] [doi: 10.1111/hir.12192] [Medline: 29045011]
6. Baker B, Yang I. Social media as social support in pregnancy and the postpartum. Sex Reprod Healthc 2018 Oct;17:31-34. [doi: 10.1016/j.srhc.2018.05.003] [Medline: 30193717]
7. Lam NH, Woo BK. Efficacy of Instagram in Promoting Psychoeducation in the Chinese-Speaking Population. Health Equity 2020 Apr 01;4(1):114-116 [FREE Full text] [doi: 10.1089/heq.2019.0078] [Medline: 32258963]
8. Sherman LE, Payton AA, Hernandez LM, Greenfield PM, Dapretto M. The Power of the Like in Adolescence: Effects of Peer Influence on Neural and Behavioral Responses to Social Media. Psychol Sci 2016 Jul;27(7):1027-1035 [FREE Full text] [doi: 10.1177/0956797616645673] [Medline: 27247125]
9. Social Media Fact Sheet. Pew Research Center for Internet and Technology. 2019. URL: http://www.pewinternet.org/fact-sheet/social-media/ [accessed 2020-12-01]
10. Martin JA, Hamilton BE, Osterman MJK, Driscoll AK. Births: Final Data for 2018. Natl Vital Stat Rep 2019 Nov;68(13):1-47 [FREE Full text] [Medline: 32501202]
11. Chong KPL, Guo JZ, Deng X, Woo BKP. Consumer Perceptions of Wearable Technology Devices: Retrospective Review and Analysis. JMIR Mhealth Uhealth 2020 Apr 20;8(4):e17544 [FREE Full text] [doi: 10.2196/17544] [Medline: 32310148]
12. Chung S, Woo BK. Using Consumer Perceptions of a Voice-Activated Speaker Device as an Educational Tool. JMIR Med Educ 2020 Apr 24;6(1):e17336 [FREE Full text] [doi: 10.2196/17336] [Medline: 32329740]
13. Trethewey SP. Strategies to combat medical misinformation on social media. Postgrad Med J 2020 Jan 15;96(1131):4-6. [doi: 10.1136/postgradmedj-2019-137201] [Medline: 31732511]
14. Larson HJ. The biggest pandemic risk? Viral misinformation. Nature 2018 Oct 16;562(7727):309-309. [doi: 10.1038/d41586-018-07034-4] [Medline: 30327527]

Abbreviations

PUPPP: pruritic urticarial papules and plaques of pregnancy

16

Risks and Benefits of Using Social Media in Dermatology

Moshe Y Bressler[1,2], BS; Eugene Grudnikoff[3], MD; Yaakov Bressler[2], BA; Rebecca Tamez[2], MD; John G Zampella[4], MD

[1]New York Institute of Technology College of Osteopathic Medicine, Old Westbury, NY, United States

[2]Department of Dermatology, Jamaica Hospital Medical Center, Richmond Hill, NY, United States

[3]Department of Psychiatry, South Oaks Hospital, Amityville, NY, United States

[4]Ronald O Perelman Department of Dermatology, New York University, New York, NY, United States

Corresponding Author:
John G Zampella, MD
Ronald O Perelman Department of Dermatology
New York University
555 Madison Ave, 4th Floor
New York, NY, 10022
United States

Email: John.zampella@nyulangone.org

Abstract

Background: Dermatological information on social media is often presented by nondermatologists. Increasing the online engagement of trained dermatologists may improve information quality, patient education, and care.

Objective: Our study assesses dermatologists' perceptions of social media and patterns of use to identify barriers limiting engagement.

Methods: In our cohort study, a 36-item online survey was distributed to dermatologists in the United States; responses were captured on a 1-100 sliding scale.

Results: Of 166 initiated surveys, 128 valid responses were submitted. Dermatologists showed greater concern for social media risk-related issues (mean 77.9, SD 15.1) than potential benefits (mean 61.8, SD 16.4; *P*<.001). Leading concerns were poor patient care, nonevidence-based information, and breaching patient privacy. Benefits included interphysician collaboration, patient education, and public health awareness. The most avid and enthusiastic social media users were millennials (mean total optimism score 67.5, SD 14.9) and baby boomers (mean total optimism score 63.1, SD 11.2) compared with Generation X dermatologists (mean total optimism score 52.2, SD 16.3, *P*<.001). Of 128 dermatologists, 103 (82.4%) plan on increasing their social media use (*P*=.003). Predictors showing an intent to increase future social media use were younger age, integration into professional use, and an optimistic view (r2=.39; *P*<.001).

Conclusions: Dermatologists perceive the risk of social media to be considerable but still intend to increase its use, likely recognizing the value and importance of social media to the field.

KEYWORDS

social media; dermatologist; generational differences; Instagram; Facebook; information quality; patient education; online content; risk; benefit; dermatology; cross-sectional; survey; online health information

Introduction

Americans spend an average of 142 minutes per day on social media, and this number is expected to rise [1]. It is no surprise that patients have turned to social media for information regarding health care, with reports of more than 125 million Americans using social media to search for health-related information [2]. The use of social media as a health care resource has documented benefits. Studies point to improved patient well-being and empowerment through the use of social media, especially among those with new medical diagnoses [3].

Patient use of social media also has its downfalls, with little quality control or regulation of the information posted to social media platforms. Patients often encounter misinformation with potentially harmful outcomes [4,5]. Campaigns such as the #VerifyHealthcare movement encourages physicians on social media to validate their credentials to help identify posts with reliable medical information; however, the extent to which such interventions alter health literacy has not been evaluated [6].

Indeed, false information tends to spread 6 times faster on social media than factual information [7,8], and re-educating patients to correct false information can be challenging [9]. For health-related content, a physician's engagement on social media is effective in spreading quality information and has the potential to reach millions of people [10]. The barriers preventing practitioners and experts from participating are likely multifactorial but may involve concerns over privacy violations [11], fear of litigation [12], and uncertainty surrounding patient-physician boundaries on social media [13].

Dermatologists were early adopters of social media, and many continue to make educational and relevant content for consumers. A recent study showed that "top influencer" dermatologists have large social media audiences and provide a valuable educational service to patients [14]. However, these influencers may not be sufficient to combat the gaps in public health education, as other studies show that as little as 4%-5% of dermatology-related content on Instagram is posted by board-certified dermatologists [2,15].

To increase dermatologist engagement and the positive outcomes associated with a strong physician presence on social media, we aim to understand the perceptions and behaviors of dermatologists in the United States using social media. With this understanding, we can appropriately guide policies to promote safe and effective participation on social media while mitigating risks.

Methods

Study Design

Using the SurveyMonkey tool (SVMK Inc), we created and distributed an anonymous, open, online survey of 36 questions (Multimedia Appendix 1) to board-certified dermatologists and dermatology residents enrolled in an Accreditation Council for Graduate Medical Education (ACGME)–accredited program in accordance with the Checklist for Reporting Results of Internet eSurveys (CHERRIES) [16]. Participants disclosing non-US–based practices were screened. Multiple entries were prevented by limiting duplicate IP address entries. The survey design was created using prior models [17] and piloted by 6 dermatologists and 2 dermatology residents.

The survey was distributed using an academic listserv (Association of Professors in Dermatology [APD]), which was distributed to 486 members and the private Facebook group "Board Certified Dermatologists," with more than 4500 board-certified dermatologists. Survey questions used a 0-100 sliding scale, where 100 represented maximal agreement. Information collected included demographic data, social media usage patterns and preferences, and perceptions of social media, including positive and negative effects of social media and its effect on relationships. Upon completion, users were able to share the survey with their peers using our web landing page.

Data Analysis

Data were stratified for credentials, degree, employment type, years of experience, years on social media, geographical region, favorite social media platform, and generational differences. We compared millennials (ages 23-38 years in 2019), Generation X (ages 39-54 years), and baby boomers (ages 55-73 years) using definitions outlined by Pew Research [18]. Chi-square and ANOVA tests were used for the analysis of categorical and continuous variables, respectively. When an omnibus ANOVA F-test revealed significant differences between multiple groups, we performed group-to-group post hoc analyses; the Fisher exact test was used due to low *n* in some cells. A *t* test was used for group comparisons with unequal variances. Variables associated at $P<.1$ with a response of "yes" or "maybe" regarding the intention to increase social media use were entered in a backward elimination multiple linear logistic regression model to identify variables independently associated with intent to increase social media use. All analyses were 2-sided with alpha set at .05, and they were conducted using JMP statistical software (version 9.0; SAS Institute Inc).

We created a scoring system to evaluate positive and negative perceptions of social media by calculating the net sum-average of all the responses in each category. Potential benefits yielded a total optimism score, risks and concerns yielded a total pessimism score (wherein a higher value indicates greater pessimism), and a positive or negative effect on relationships generated the total relationship scores (wherein a higher value indicates a positive effect on relationships).

Results

Respondent Demographics

Of 166 initiated surveys, 128 were valid—38 entries were disqualified from the analysis due to a location outside of the United States, or a nonphysician or nondermatologist status.

Of the 128 valid entries, 48 (37%) respondents were male and 80 (63%) were female, with an average age of 38.7 (SD 9.7) years and an average time in clinical practice of 9.3 (SD 9.2) years. Of the 128 respondents, 36 were residents (28%) and 93 (72%) were board-certified dermatologists; 117 (91%) had Doctor of Medicine (MD) degrees and 11 (9%) had Doctor of Osteopathic Medicine (DO) degrees; 71 (57%) were millennials, 42 (34%) were Generation X, and 12 (10%) were baby boomers.

The respondents were evenly distributed by sex (*P*=.72) and geographical region (*P*=.34). Our sample was representative of the US dermatological workforce. Additional demographic, experience, and employment characteristics are reported in Table 1.

Table 1. Demographic characteristics of survey responders (n=128).

Variable	Total (n=128)	Millennial (n=71, 56.8%)	Generation X (n=42, 33.6%)	Baby boomer (n=12, 9.6%)	*P* value
Age in years, mean (SD)	38.7 (9.7)	31.9 (3.0)	44.1 (4.4)	59.6 (6.6)	<.001[a]
Gender, n (%)					.72
Female	80 (62.5)	47 (66.2)	26 (61.9)	6 (54.6)	
Male	48 (37.5)	24 (33.8)	16 (38.1)	5 (45.5)	
Region, n (%)					.34
Midwest	17 (13.3)	9 (12.7)	6 (14.3)	2 (16.7)	
Northeast	54 (42.2)	34 (47.9)	14 (33.3)	3 (25.0)	
South	40 (31.3)	20 (28.2)	16 (38.1)	3 (25.0)	
West	18 (14.1)	8 (11.3)	6 (14.3)	4 (33.3)	
Clinical experience in years, mean (SD)	9.3 (9.2)	3.5 (3.3)	7.3 (10.1)	29.4 (9.9)	<.001[b]
Employment, n (%)					.016[c]
Academic institution	79 (61.7)	40 (58.0)	28 (66.7)	8 (66.7)	
Equity owner of a group practice	4 (3.1)	0 (0.0)	3 (7.1)	1 (8.3)	
Owner of a solo practice	12 (9.4)	5 (7.3)	4 (9.5)	3 (25.0)	
Group practice, hospital or health care system	32 (25.0)	24 (34.8)	7 (16.7)	0 (0.0)	

[a]Age: all post hoc comparisons significant at *P*<.001.

[b]Years of clinical experience: all post hoc comparisons significant at *P*<.001.

[c]Employment: millennials are less likely to be employed as equity owners of a group practice vs. nonmillennials (*P*=.035) and more likely to be employed at a group practice or hospital (*P*=.007; baby boomers are less likely to be employed at a group practice or hospital (*P*=.036).

Social Media Practices

Among the 128 respondents, 120 (93.8%) reported using social media across a variety of platforms, including Facebook (109/128, 85.2%), Instagram (85/128, 66%), and LinkedIn (51/128, 40%; Table 2), for an average of 45.9 (SD 35.2) minutes/day. Millennials had used social media for an average of 11.8 (SD 3.0) years, significantly longer than either GenX (mean 9.4, SD 3.6 years) or baby boomers (mean 6.2, SD 3.4 years; *P*<.001). The overall time spent on social media for professional use was 16.9 (SD 24.3) minutes/day and 31.1 (SD 22.0) minutes/day for personal use; millennials spent more total time on social media compared to baby boomers and GenX respondents. Unexpectedly, baby boomers' time spent on social media for professional use (mean 17.3, SD 18.9 minutes/day) was comparable to that of millennials (mean 21.6, SD 28.6 minutes/day; *P*=.67).

Owners of private practices and solo practitioners spent more time on social media for professional use compared to all other respondents (mean 41.7, SD 41.5 minutes/day vs. mean 13.9, SD 20.2 minutes/day; *P*<.001), while physicians working at academic institutions spent less time on social media (mean 11.6, SD 18.6 minutes/day vs. mean 24.8, SD 29.9 minutes/day; *P*=.003). Overall, 44% (53/128) of physicians found Instagram to be the most valuable platform, followed by Facebook (49/128, 40.7%), and preferences varied by generation. Social media usage patterns and preferences are reported in Table 2.

Table 2. Social media patterns and preferences observed from the survey responses (n=128).

Variable	Total (n=128)	Millennial (n=71, 56.8%)	Generation X (n=42, 33.6%)	Baby boomer (n=12, 9.6%)	*P* value
Years of social media use, mean (SD)	10.6 (3.7)	11.8 (3.0)	9.4 (3.6)	6.2 (3.4)	<.001[a]
Personal time spent on social media, min/day, mean (SD)	31.1(22.0)	38.5(20.2)	22.7(21.9)	15.0 (12.8)	<.001[b]
Professional time spent on social media, min/day, mean (SD)	16.9 (24.3)	21.6 (28.6)	8.5 (13.1)	17.3 (18.9)	.021[b]
Total time spent on social media, min/day, mean (SD)	45.9 (35.2)	59.6 (34.7)	30.5 (29.2)	29.6 (25.5)	<.001[c]
Plan to increase social media use, n (%)	103 (82.4)	67 (94.4)	28 (66.7)	8 (66.7)	.001[d]
Platforms with an active account, n (%)					
Facebook	109 (85.2)	62 (87.3)	36 (85.7)	8 (66.7)	.18
Instagram	85 (66.4)	58 (81.7)	21 (50.0)	4 (33.3)	<.001[e]
LinkedIn	51 (39.8)	25 (35.2)	19 (45.2)	5 (41.7)	.56
Reddit	16 (12.5)	8 (11.3)	5 (11.9)	2 (16.7)	.87
Snapchat	33 (25.8)	30 (42.3)	2 (4.8)	0 (0.0)	<.001[f]
Twitter	29 (22.7)	14 (19.7)	11 (26.2)	3 (25.0)	.71
WhatsApp	49 (38.3)	32 (45.1)	15 (35.7)	2 (16.7)	.15
YouTube	35 (27.3)	18 (25.4)	12 (28.6)	3 (25.0)	.93
Most valuable platform, n (%)	Instagram, 53 (44.4)	Instagram, 42 (60.0)	Facebook, 22 (59.5)	Facebook, 6 (50.0)	.004[g]
Location where social media is accessed, n (%)					
Home	114 (89.1)	66 (93.0)	35 (83.3)	10 (83.3)	.24
Work	54 (42.2)	38 (53.5)	11 (26.2)	4 (7.6)	.014[h]
During commute	32 (25.0)	24 (33.8)	5 (11.9)	2 (16.7)	.027[i]

[a]Years on social media: all post hoc comparisons significant at *P*<.033.

[b]Time spent on social media: all post hoc comparisons significant at *P*<.031.

[c]Time on social media above average: millennial>GenX, *P*<.001; millennial>baby boomer, *P*<.001.

[d]Plan to increase social media use: millennial>GenX, *P*<.001; millennial>baby boomer, *P*=.013.

[e]Active Instagram account: all post hoc comparisons significant at *P*<.02.

[f]Active Snapchat account: all post hoc comparisons significant at *P*<.036.

[g]Most valuable platform: Facebook, GenX>millennials, *P*<.001; Instagram, millennial>GenX, *P*<.001 , millennial>baby boomers, *P*<.001.

[h]Social media use at work: GenX>millennials, *P*<.001.

[i]Social media use during commute: millennial>GenX, *P*=0.014.

Perceptions

Overall, dermatologists perceived that social media has many benefits and uses (total optimism score 61.8, SD 16.4). There was strong agreement that social media use increases patient education (69.4, SD 20.6), while less agreement concerning access to care or strengthening the doctor-patient relationship (50.3, SD 21.8, and 46.1, SD 24.7, respectively). Millennials (67.5, SD 14.9) and baby boomers (63.1, SD 11.2) were more optimistic about the benefits of social media than the GenX physicians (52.2, SD 16.3; *P*<.001 and *P*=.030, respectively). Attitudes and perceptions regarding social media are reported in Table 3 and Figure 1.

Dermatologists showed greater concern for risk-related issues on social media compared to potential benefits (mean score 77.9, SD 15.1 vs. mean score 61.8, SD 16.4, paired *t* test; *P*<.001). The greatest concerns were that social media use contributes to the substitution of proper dermatological care with unqualified providers (88.5, SD18.0), promotion of nonevidence-based products (82.1, SD 20.6), and the threat of breaching patients' privacy (78.9, SD 19.9); however, this varied by generation, with millennials being less pessimistic than GenX dermatologists (*P*=.018).

Most dermatologists believed that social media use improves relationships with friends (65.3, SD 21.0) and professional colleagues (61.4, SD 22.3) but were more neutral about social media's effect on relationships with patients (50.3, SD 21.2).

Table 3. Future users versus nonusers of social media (n=128).

Survey question	Response score by generation, mean (SD)				P value[a,b]
	Total (n=128)	Millennial (n=71, 56.8%)	Generation X (n=42, 33.6%)	Baby boomer (n=12, 9.6%)	
Perceived benefits related to social media					
Help deliver health care	61.9 (24.2)	67.3 (24.7)	52.3 (22.3)	65.8 (19.5)	.005
Improve clinical knowledge	68.2 (24.6)	74.7 (20.5)	59.2 (27.9)	63.6 (22.9)	.003
Increase interphysician collaboration	75.3 (21.2)	81.3 (19.0)	67.6 (23.4)	73.3 (17.3)	.005
Help recruit patients	65.7 (22.1)	71.9 (21.2)	55.9 (23.3)	63.1 (11.8)	<.001
Strengthen doctor-patient relationship	46.1 (24.7)	54.4 (23.9)	32.7 (23.2)	43.0 (16.1)	<.001
Increase patient education	69.4 (20.6)	74.0 (22.6)	61.6 (16.4)	70.8 (15.6)	.008
Increase access to care	50.3 (21.8)	56.5 (19.5)	38.5 (22.4)	55.3 (20.6)	<.001[b]
Good tool for public awareness	68.8 (22.6)	73.8 (20.7)	59.5 (24.9)	73.9 (18.4)	.004[b]
Good tool for patient compliance	51.5 (22.2)	54.1 (23.1)	44.5 (21.0)	59.0 (17.9)	.040[b]
Total optimism score	61.8 (16.4)	67.5 (14.9)	52.2 (16.3)	63.1 (11.2)	<.001[b]
Perceived risks related to social media					
Could damage professional reputation	74.9 (21.4)	72.5 (23.3)	80.9 (15.8)	72.4 (22.5)	.11
Breach patient privacy	78.9 (19.9)	75.0 (21.4)	84.1 (16.3)	82.8 (17.1)	.044
Untruthfulness	70.1 (26.3)	65.9 (25.8)	79.5 (25.1)	69.4 (19.9)	.024
Emphasis on superficial values	72.9 (24.0)	70.6 (25.0)	78.2 (22.1)	73.3 (24.0)	.27
Boosts nonevidence-based products	82.1 (20.6)	80.5 (20.2)	85.2 (21.9)	86.6 (12.4)	.38
Allows for unqualified substitution of care	88.5 (18.0)	88.7 (18.0)	86.5 (20.1)	91.7 (9.3)	.66
Total pessimism score	77.9 (15.1)	75.5 (14.8)	82.4 (15.0)	79.4 (12.7)	.058
Perceived social media effect on relationships					
Affects relationships with family	54.1 (22.5)	60.3 (20.7)	41.9 (22.7)	57.8 (19.9)	.002[b]
Affects relationships with friends	65.4 (21.1)	70.7 (20.3)	55.4 (20.8)	64.4 (18.5)	.006
Affects professional relationships	61.3 (22.3)	68.0 (21.5)	51.4 (23.2)	59.9 (15.9)	.011
Affects relationships with patients	50.2 (21.2)	51.6 (26.0)	47.0 (18.5)	53.6 (7.9)	.68
Average effect on relationships	60.2 (19.1)	60.3 (20.7)	41.9 (22.7)	57.8 (19.9)	.002[b]

[a]All significant *P* values ≤.05 for millennials vs. GenX.

[b]*P*≤.05 for GenX vs. baby boomer; there were no significant differences between millennials and baby boomers.

Figure 1. Generational differences of social media use and perceptions. Survey questions were answered on a 0-100 agreement scale. The radar chart demonstrates the average for each question grouped by generation. Questions calculated toward the total optimism score are highlighted teal, pessimistic questions are highlighted pink, and questions affecting relationships are highlighted yellow. (*) denotes statistically significant different answers by generation using a Fisher test, P≤.05. min/d: minutes per day; SM: social media.

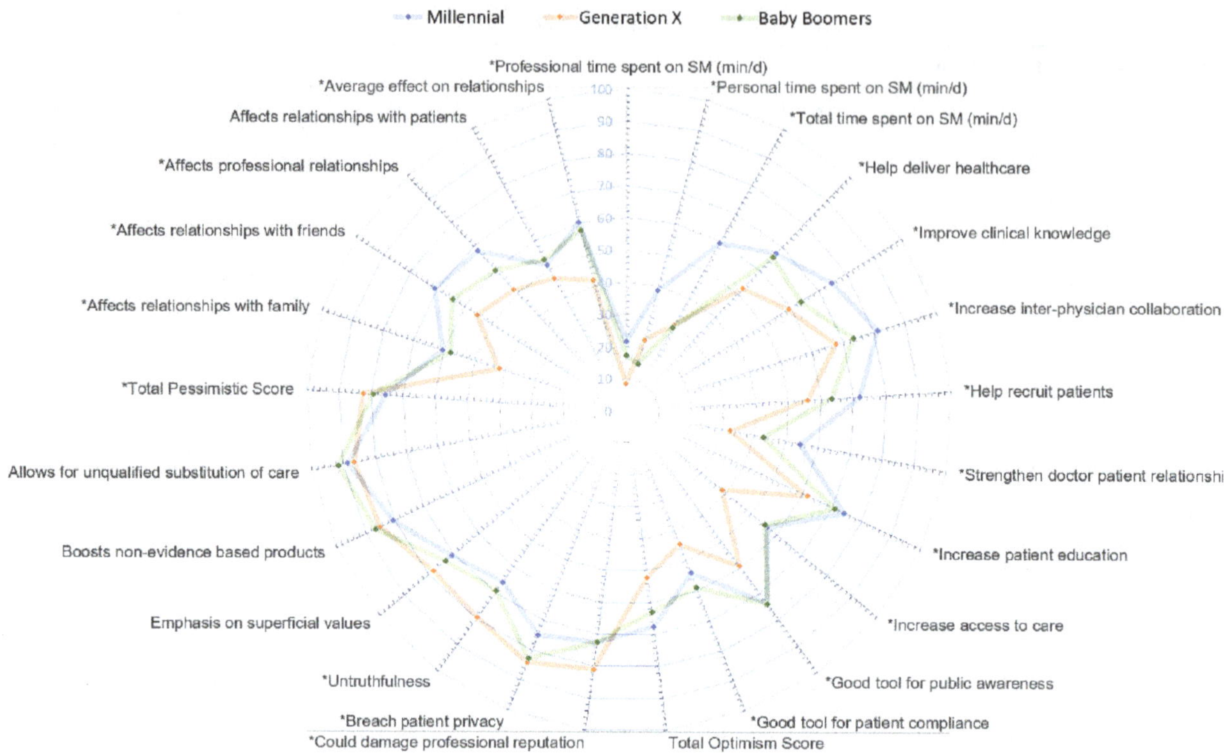

Future Users vs. Nonusers

Of the 128 dermatologists surveyed, 103 (82.4%) are actively or considering increasing their social media usage. The variables independently associated with a plan to use more social media in the future were younger age (*P*=.023), use at work (*P*=.028), and average optimism (*P*<.001) in the logistic regression model using backward elimination. In contrast, other variables (eg, average pessimism, employment type, favorite social media platform) were codependent or not significant (final model r^2=.390, *P*<.001).

Discussion

Principal Findings

Our survey of US dermatologists demonstrates that there are many perceived risks and benefits of social media. These views vary significantly across generations, yet our data suggest the perceived benefits outweigh the associated risks. Our study provides insight into physicians' perceptions of social media; the results may serve as a guide to promoting dermatologist engagement on social media.

The total pessimism score revealed a general negativity surrounding social media use among dermatologists. Pessimism was driven by perceived risks of poor patient care, misinformation, damage to professional reputation, and privacy breaches, consistent with prior reports of social media risks [2,11–13] (Figure 1). Mitigating these risks will be essential for increasing the engagement of dermatologists on social media.

Indeed, the risks associated with physicians sharing information online have been identified as a key area for social media research [13], with little data currently reported. Patient privacy violations resulting from posting and sharing patient photographs are common among some specialties [19] and represent real concern, as images can be downloaded and reshared, increasing patient exposure to privacy breaches. The lack of clear guidelines for sharing photos of patients online may cause physicians to avoid creating patient-centered content altogether [20].

Alternatively, there is promising optimism for social media use among dermatologists. The total optimism score calculated from our survey reflects the perceived benefits of social media, which include increased health care access, improved education, and improved public health (Figure 1). Despite a more prominent, uniform, overall pessimism score acknowledging inherent risks, a preponderance of those surveyed (103/128, 82.4%) plan to increase social media usage. Using a linear regression model, we found that optimism predicts an increase in future social media usage, while the pessimism score has no predictive value. This implies that perceived benefits outweigh the risks.

Additional predictors of increasing social media use are younger age and use at work. Dermatologists may be moving to social media for economic reasons, and younger physicians may consider a social media presence necessary to compete in a modern medical marketplace. This is likely a self-reinforcing process where physicians that use social media to recruit more patients will benefit most and feel more positively about it. Alternatively, physicians who are currently not using social media are not exposed to its benefits and therefore view social media as nonadvantageous. Studies suggest that 32% of people have made health decisions using social media [21] and may explain that one of the perceived benefits of social media discovered in our survey was the ability to recruit patients. A recent study by Murphy et al [22] found that 43% of all patients consider social media to be moderately to extremely important in choosing a dermatologist, particularly for patients seeking cosmetic procedures [23-25].

Perception of benefits and risks of social media varied by generation. Unexpectedly, millennials (ages 23-38 years in 2019) and baby boomers (ages 55-73 years) shared similar views of social media, while GenX (ages 39-54 years) tended to be the least optimistic. Prior studies show that older internet users are less optimistic about social media [26]; however, the common notion that older practitioners are less likely to adapt to emerging technologies may not be true [27]. The discovery that millennials have more optimism regarding social media may not be surprising; however, the shift in demographics is important, as millennials are now the largest proportion of the adult US population [28]. It is likely that millennial and Generation Z (ages 7-23 years) patients will drive an increased need for quality dermatologic information on social media. This underscores the importance of mitigating risks to encourage dermatologists of all generations to engage on social media.

Finally, our survey found that educational and collaborative capabilities were cited among the key advantages of using social media. The rapid dissemination and easy accessibility of new treatments, interesting cases, and continuing medical education through social media highlight this benefit. The perceived benefit of educational opportunities stands in contrast to the lower utilization of social media by academic dermatologists uncovered in our survey. A list of the top influencers in dermatology was recently published [14]; however, less than half (14/30) were faculty at academic institutions, highlighting an opportunity for academic dermatologists to engage on social media.

Limitations

Our study was limited by a small sample size. Our sample population demonstrates similar demographics to other studies [29]; however, few responses from baby boomers require caution in the interpretation of our generational results. Similarly, bias toward positive social media perceptions may have been introduced by delivering our survey using a social media platform. The APD listserv was utilized to mitigate this bias and increase the practice diversity of our cohort.

Our survey's completion rate was 77.7% (128/166); however, a response rate could not be calculated since our survey was posted online and was shareable. We mitigated this by tracking clicks on our survey, which produced 166 respondents.

Conclusion

Our survey identified risks that act as barriers and perceived benefits driving increased social media usage. Views varied significantly among generations, with millennial and baby boomer dermatologists expressing more optimistic outlooks than Generation X. Our research can be used to develop best practices to mitigate risks of privacy violation, litigation, and poor patient care, while promoting education and collaboration can help shape the presence of dermatology on social media.

References

1. Salim S. How much time do you spend on social media? Research says 142 minutes per day. Digital Information World. URL: https://www.digitalinformationworld.com/2019/01/how-much-time-do-people-spend-social-media-infographic.html [accessed 2020-05-12]
2. Park JH, Christman MP, Linos E, Rieder EA. Dermatology on Instagram: An Analysis of Hashtags. J Drugs Dermatol 2018 Apr 01;17(4):482-484 [FREE Full text] [Medline: 29601627]
3. Smailhodzic E, Hooijsma W, Boonstra A, Langley D. Social media use in healthcare: A systematic review of effects on patients and on their relationship with healthcare professionals. BMC Health Serv Res 2016 Aug 26;16:442 [FREE Full text] [doi: 10.1186/s12913-016-1691-0] [Medline: 27562728]
4. Tan A, Gutierrez D, Milam EC, Neimann AL, Zampella J. Patient health-seeking behavior on WeChat: Social media and dermatology. JAAD Case Reports 2020 Feb;6(2):136-138. [doi: 10.1016/j.jdcr.2019.11.015]
5. Julian AK, Welch J, Bean MM, Shahid S, Perna FM. Information About Sunscreen on YouTube and Considerations for Sun Safety Promotion: Content Analysis. JMIR Dermatol 2020 Jun 2;3(1):e14411. [doi: 10.2196/14411]
6. Croley JAA. Emerging roles of social media in dermatology. Cutis 2019 Jan;103(1):E13-E14. [Medline: 30758345]
7. Vosoughi S, Roy D, Aral S. The spread of true and false news online. Science 2018 Dec 09;359(6380):1146-1151. [doi: 10.1126/science.aap9559] [Medline: 29590045]
8. Nsoesie EO, Cesare N, Müller M, Ozonoff A. COVID-19 Misinformation Spread in Eight Countries: Exponential Growth Modeling Study. J Med Internet Res 2020 Dec 15;22(12):e24425 [FREE Full text] [doi: 10.2196/24425] [Medline: 33264102]
9. Granter SR, Papke DJ. Opinion: Medical misinformation in the era of Google: Computational approaches to a pervasive problem. Proc Natl Acad Sci U S A 2018 Jun 19;115(25):6318-6321. [doi: 10.1073/pnas.1808264115] [Medline: 29921726]
10. Pulido CM, Ruiz-Eugenio L, Redondo-Sama G, Villarejo-Carballido B. A New Application of Social Impact in Social Media for Overcoming Fake News in Health. Int J Environ Res Public Health 2020 Apr 03;17(7) [FREE Full text] [doi: 10.3390/ijerph17072430] [Medline: 32260048]
11. Gómez-Zúñiga B, Fernandez-Luque L, Pousada M, Hernández-Encuentra E, Armayones M. ePatients on YouTube: Analysis of Four Experiences From the Patients' Perspective. Med 2.0 2012 Apr 25;1(1):e1. [doi: 10.2196/med20.2039]

12. George D, Rovniak L, Kraschnewski J. Dangers and opportunities for social media in medicine. Clin Obstet Gynecol 2013 Sep;56(3):453-462 [FREE Full text] [doi: 10.1097/GRF.0b013e318297dc38] [Medline: 23903375]
13. Campbell L, Evans Y, Pumper M, Moreno M. Social media use by physicians: A qualitative study of the new frontier of medicine. BMC Medical Informatics and Decision Making 2016 Jul 15;16(1):91 [FREE Full text] [doi: 10.1186/s12911-016-0327-y] [Medline: 27418201]
14. Sierro TJ, Young PM, Kassabian SK, Wu KK, Armstrong AW. Dermatologists in social media: A study on top influencers, posts, and user engagement. J Am Acad Dermatol 2020 Nov;83(5):1452-1455. [doi: 10.1016/j.jaad.2020.03.001] [Medline: 32151630]
15. Ranpariya V, Chu B, Fathy R, Lipoff JB. Dermatology without dermatologists? Analyzing Instagram influencers with dermatology-related hashtags. Journal of the American Academy of Dermatology 2020 Dec;83(6):1840-1842. [doi: 10.1016/j.jaad.2020.05.039]
16. Eysenbach G. Improving the quality of Web surveys: the Checklist for Reporting Results of Internet E-Surveys (CHERRIES). J Med Internet Res 2004 Sep 29;6(3):e34 [FREE Full text] [doi: 10.2196/jmir.6.3.e34] [Medline: 15471760]
17. Alsobayel H. Use of Social Media for Professional Development by Health Care Professionals: A Cross-Sectional Web-Based Survey. JMIR Med Educ 2016 Sep 12;2(2):e15. [doi: 10.2196/mededu.6232]
18. Dimock M. Where Millennials end and Generation Z begins. Pew Research Center. 2019. URL: https://www.pewresearch.org/fact-tank/2019/01/17/where-millennials-end-and-generation-z-begins/ [accessed 2019-01-17]
19. Fanti Silva DA, Colleoni R. Patient's Privacy Violation on Social Media in the Surgical Area. Am Surg 2018 Dec 01;84(12):1900-1905. [Medline: 30606346]
20. Nettrour J, Burch M, Bal B. Patients, pictures, and privacy: managing clinical photographs in the smartphone era. Arthroplast Today 2019 Mar;5(1):57-60 [FREE Full text] [doi: 10.1016/j.artd.2018.10.001] [Medline: 31020023]
21. Is Social Media Changing the Doctor-Patient Relationship? American Academy of Family Physicians. 2018 Jun 08. URL: https://www.aafp.org/news/practice-professional-issues/20180608commsurveys.html [accessed 2020-05-10]
22. Murphy E, Nelson K, Friedman A. The Influence of Dermatologists' Use of Social Media on Attracting Patients. J Drugs Dermatol 2020 May 01;19(5):532-538. [Medline: 32484619]
23. Maisel A, Waldman A, Furlan K, Weil A, Sacotte K, Lazaroff JM, et al. Self-reported Patient Motivations for Seeking Cosmetic Procedures. JAMA Dermatol 2018 Oct 01;154(10):1167-1174 [FREE Full text] [doi: 10.1001/jamadermatol.2018.2357] [Medline: 30140900]
24. Yoon S, Kim Y. Cosmetic Surgery and Self-esteem in South Korea: A Systematic Review and Meta-analysis. Aesthetic Plast Surg 2020 Feb;44(1):229-238 [FREE Full text] [doi: 10.1007/s00266-019-01515-1] [Medline: 31637500]
25. Nayyar A, Jadi J, Garimella R, Elkins-Williams S, Gallagher K, Kalliainen L, et al. Are You on the Right Platform? A Conjoint Analysis of Social Media Preferences in Aesthetic Surgery Patients. Aesthet Surg J 2019 Aug 22;39(9):1019-1032 [FREE Full text] [doi: 10.1093/asj/sjy238] [Medline: 30239573]
26. Older internet users less likely to view the internet as a positive for society. Pew Research Center. 2019. URL: https://www.pewresearch.org/fact-tank/2019/09/09/us-generations-technology-use/ft_19-09-06_internetgenerations_older-internet-users-less-likely-view-internet-positive-society/ [accessed 2020-04-27]
27. Yarbrough AK, Smith TB. Technology acceptance among physicians: a new take on TAM. Med Care Res Rev 2007 Dec;64(6):650-672. [doi: 10.1177/1077558707305942] [Medline: 17717378]
28. Fry R. Millennials outnumbered Boomers in 2019. Pew Research Center. URL: https://www.pewresearch.org/fact-tank/2020/04/28/millennials-overtake-baby-boomers-as-americas-largest-generation/ [accessed 2020-05-10]
29. DeWane ME, Grant-Kels JM. A commentary on gender bias in dermatology and its perceived impact on career development among women dermatologists. International Journal of Women's Dermatology 2020 Dec;6(5):440-444 [FREE Full text] [doi: 10.1016/j.ijwd.2020.07.010]

Abbreviations

APD: Association of Professors in Dermatology

17

Public Interest in a Potentially Harmful, Non–Evidence-Based "Wellness" Practice: Cross-Sectional Analysis of Perineum Sunning

Ryan Ottwell[1*], BS; Micah Hartwell[1*], PhD; Tracy Beswick[2*], MD, PhD; Taylor Calli Rogers[1*], BS; Heather Ivy[3*], DO; Marcus Goodman[4*], DO; Matt Vassar[1], PhD

[1]Oklahoma State University Center for Health Sciences, Tulsa, OK, United States

[2]Center for Dermatology, Tulsa, OK, United States

[3]Philadelphia College of Osteopathic Medicine, Roswell, GA, United States

[4]Goodman Dermatology, Roswell, GA, United States

[*]these authors contributed equally

Corresponding Author:
Ryan Ottwell, BS
Oklahoma State University Center for Health Sciences
1111 W 17th Street
Tulsa, OK, 74017
United States

Email: ryan.ottwell@okstate.edu

Abstract

Background: Perineum sunning/tanning is a potentially harmful yet popular new health trend cultivated by a viral social media post, famous public figures, and subsequent media coverage.

Objective: Our primary objective is to evaluate public interest in perineum sunning/tanning.

Methods: Using an observational study design, we extracted data from Google Trends for the terms "perineum sunning," "perineum tanning," "Metaphysical Meagan," and "Josh Brolin"; and Twitter (via SproutSocial) for "perineum sunning" and "perineum tanning" from November 1, 2019, to December 31, 2019. UberSuggest was used to investigate monthly search volumes and user engagement. We used data from Google Trends and Twitter to construct autoregressive integrated moving average (ARIMA) models to forecast public interest in perineum sunning and perineum tanning had the post on social media never occurred. Next, we performed an integral function to calculate the cumulative increase in "perineum tanning" from the day after the post occurred to the end of the year as the area between the forecasted values and the actual values. Using Welch *t* tests, we compared forecasted and actual values for "perineum sunning" and "perineum tanning" using Twitter and Google Trends data over 1-, 2-, and 4-week periods after the social media post to determine if the increased volumes were statistically significant over time. Lastly, we monitored Google Trends for "perineum sunning" and "perineum tanning" through September 30, 2020, to capture trends during the summer months.

Results: Before the Instagram post went viral, there was no search interest in perineum sunning. ARIMA modeling for perineum tanning forecasted no increase in searches (0.00) if the post had not gone viral, while actual interest conveyed a relative cumulative increase of 919.00% from the day the post went viral through December 31, 2020. The term "perineum sunning" was mentioned on average 804 (SD 766.1) times daily for this 7-day period, which was also significantly higher than predicted ($P \leq .03$), totaling 5628 tweets for these 7 days. The increased volume of tweets and relative search interest from Google Trends remained significantly higher for both terms over the 1-, 2-, and 4-week intervals. User engagement showed that nearly 50% of people who searched for "perineum sunning" were likely to click a returned link for more information. Continued observance of search interest in perineum sunning demonstrated interest spikes in the summer months, June and July 2020.

Conclusions: Google Trends and Twitter data demonstrated that one social media post claiming non–evidence-based health benefits of regular sun exposure—without the use of sunscreen—generated significant public interest. Medical journals, dermatologists, and other health care professionals are obligated to educate and correct public misperceptions about viral wellness trends such as perineum sunning.

KEYWORDS
general dermatology; perineum sunning; perineum tanning; skin neoplasm; public health; social media; infodemiology; public interest; Google Trends; Twitter

Introduction

Social media may positively affect health behaviors or propagate potentially harmful health information [1,2]. On October 21, 2019, posts on the social media platform Instagram boasted that perineum sunning would improve focus, augment hormonal regulation, increase libido, regulate circadian rhythm, and enhance health and longevity. These posts claimed that only 30 seconds of perineum sunning was equivalent to one day's worth of sun exposure while also recommending against sunscreen use when perineum sunning [3]. The original post went viral in late November via Twitter, and again in December after well-known actor Josh Brolin received media coverage for the severe sunburn to his anogenital area after attempting perineum sunning.

Given the high potential for sunburns and cutaneous cancers resulting from this practice, our primary objective was to investigate the effects of social media and news coverage of perineum sunning on public interest by examining internet search volume, trends, and engagement, using publicly available data. A more informed understanding of the influence of social media on public search interest in potentially harmful practices like perineum sunning may assist dermatologists and medical journals when developing social media strategies to directly combat medical misinformation.

Methods

Google Trends [4] was used to collect daily relative search interest from November 1, 2019, to December 31, 2019, for "perineum sunning," "perineum tanning," "Metaphysical Meagan" (the Instagram user who published the original post), and "Josh Brolin" (who appeared in news stories on December 3, 2019, after getting a severe sunburn while performing this practice). Search interest from Google Trends is provided as a relative measure of total searches from 0-100 estimated from the highest peak within a given time frame. To explore public interest beyond Google Trends, we performed keyword searches for "perineum sunning" and "perineum tanning" occurring on Twitter via SproutSocial [5], a social media analytics platform. We also used UberSuggest [6] to collect monthly internet search volumes and user engagement (defined as a person clicking on the links returned from the search) for the terms "perineum sunning" and "perineum tanning."

Using Google Trends and Twitter data, we constructed autoregressive integrated moving average (ARIMA) models to forecast predicted values of relative search interest and tweets for the terms "perineum sunning" and "perineum tanning" from November 25, 2019, to the end of the year if the post on social media had not occurred. Next, we calculated the average number of tweets and Google Trends relative search interest for the terms "perineum sunning" and "perineum tanning," and using Welch's *t* tests, compared them to their respective forecasted values over 1-, 2-, and 4-week periods after the social media post to assess if the increased volumes were statistically significant over time. Using an integral function, we calculated the cumulative area between the forecasted baseline and the actual relative search interest data to provide the relative increased search interest through December 31, 2019, for "perineum sunning" from Google Trends. Lastly, Google Trends was monitored for the terms "perineum sunning" and "perineum tanning" through September 30, 2020, to capture public interest trends during the summer months. All analyses were conducted in R, version 3.2.1 (The R Foundation).

Results

Relative search interest for the four search terms through the end of 2019 are compared in Figure 1.

Based on the first 24 days of November, the ARIMA model forecasted that no interest (0.0) would have arisen in "perineum sunning" for the rest of the year if the social media post had not happened.

Relative search interest for perineum sunning and perineum tanning peaked the day after the social media post went viral. Keyword usage on Twitter showed that tweets significantly increased the day following the post with an increase of 2064 (95% CI 2054-2074) tweets over the predicted value (1) for perineum sunning. For the first 7 days after the post went viral, actual search interest for perineum sunning and perineum tanning were on average 42% (SD 33.0) and 43.6% (SD 35.9) higher than predicted, respectively. Additionally, the term "perineum sunning" was mentioned on average 804 (SD 766.1) times daily for this 7-day period, which was also significantly higher than predicted ($P \leq .03$), totaling 5628 tweets for these 7 days. The increased volume of tweets and relative search interest from Google Trends remained significantly higher for both terms over the 1-, 2-, and 4-week intervals (Table 1).

Figure 1. Google Trends analysis of the terms "perineum sunning," "perineum tanning," "Metaphysical Meagan," and "Josh Brolin," from November 1 to December 31, 2019.

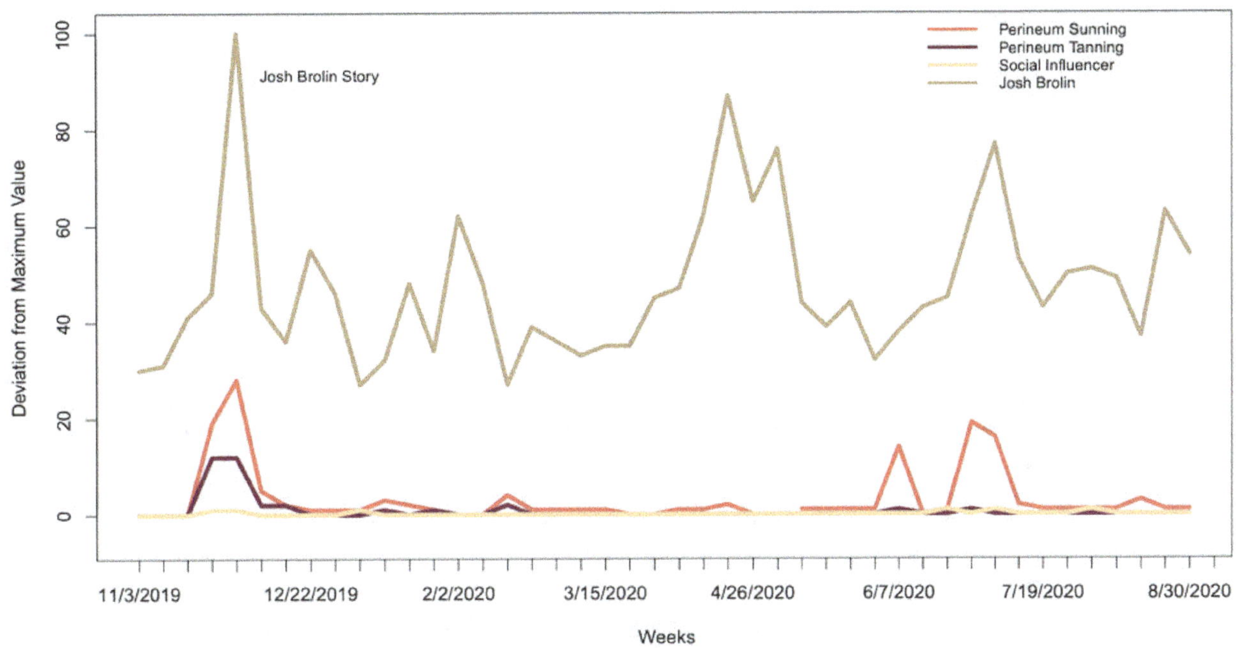

Table 1. Differences of means between actual and forecasted data from 1, 2, and 4 weeks after the social media post.

Search term	7 days			14 days			28 days		
	Forecast, mean (SD)	Actual, mean (SD)	*t* test (*df*=6); *P* value	Forecast, mean (SD)	Actual, mean (SD)	*t* test (*df*=13); *P* value	Forecast, mean (SD)	Actual, mean (SD)	*t* test (*df*=27); *P* value
Google Trends									
Perineum sunning[a] (%)	0 (0)	42.0 (33.0)	–4.2; .001	0 (0)	37.3 (32.4)	–4.3; <.001	0 (0)	21.2 (27.9)	–4.0; <.001
Perineum tanning[a] (%)	0 (0)	43.6 (35.9)	–3.2; .02	0 (0)	49.2 (31.3)	–5.9; <.001	0 (0)	30.6 (29.2)	–5.5; <.001
Twitter									
Perineum sunning[b]	2.8 (7.52)	804.1 (766.1)	–2.8; .03	1.4 (5.3)	573.4 (630.5)	–3.4; .004	0.7 (3.8)	299.2 (519.1)	–3.0; .005
Perineum tanning[b]	0.1 (0.0)	36.1 (37.4)	–2.5; .04	0.1 (0)	27.8 (28.4)	–3.6; .003	0.1(0)	15.0 (23.7)	–3.3; .002

[a]Data reflects average daily relative search interest (0%-100%).

[b]Data reflects average daily number of actual tweets.

The area under the curve (shaded in Figure 2) for "perineum tanning" indicated a cumulative increased interest of 919.00% from the day the post went viral to the end of the year.

Monthly search volumes from UberSuggest show no search interest in "perineum sunning" or "perineum tanning" before the post went viral on November 25, 2019. After the post, search volumes for the search terms "perineum sunning" and "perineum tanning" increased from 0 in October to a combined 52,599 searches for the remaining days in November and climbed to 67,598 searches in December. User engagement showed that nearly half of the individuals who searched for "perineum sunning" or "perineum tanning" were likely to click a returned link for more information. Search trends for perineum sunning showed additional spikes in the week of June 6 (29% of the original search interest peak), June 28 (60% of the original search interest peak), and July 5 (50% of the original search interest peak) (Figure 3).

Figure 2. ARIMA (autoregressive integrated moving average)-forecasted trend of "perineum tanning" from November 25 to December 31, 2019 (blue), and actual search trends (green) with the shaded area showing the cumulative area of increase.

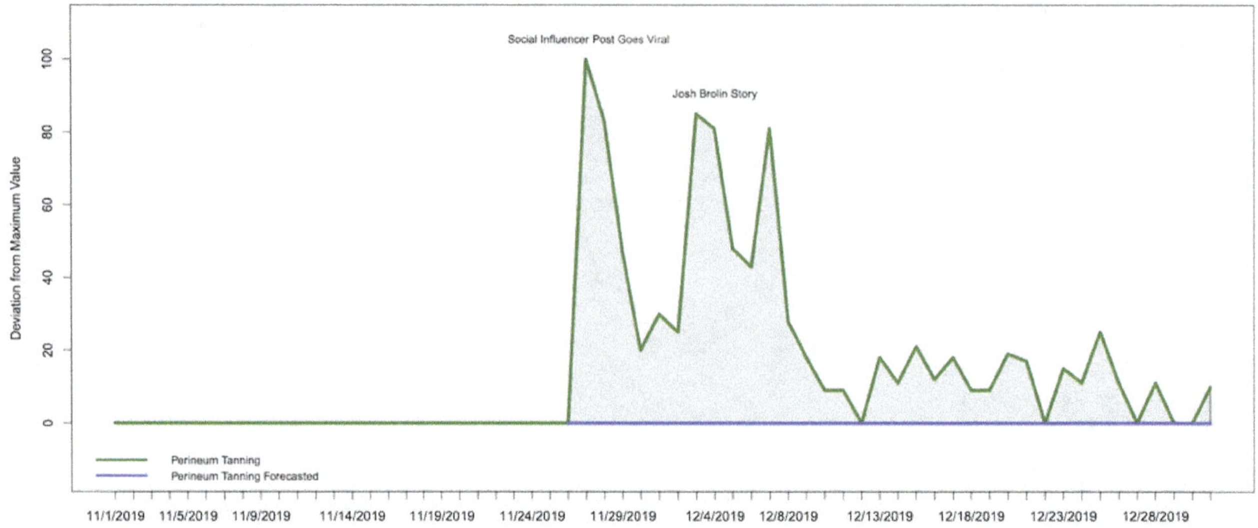

Figure 3. Google Trends analysis of the terms "perineum sunning" and "perineum tanning" from November 1 to September 30, 2020.

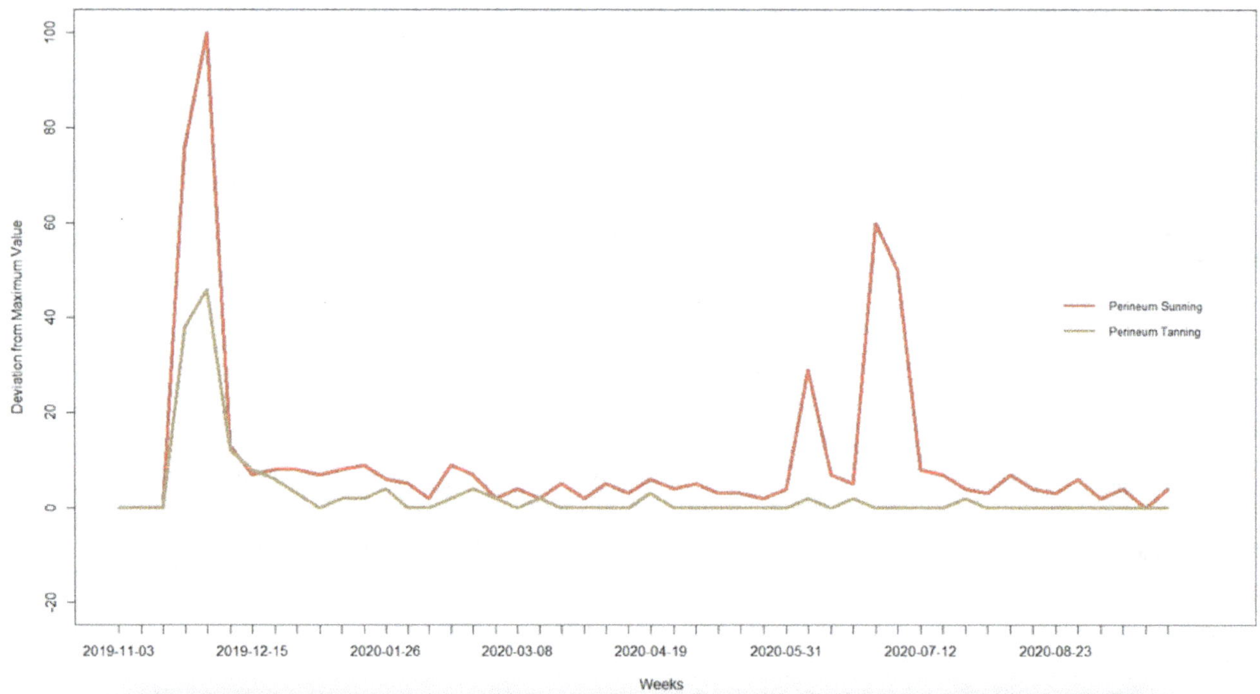

Discussion

Principal Findings

Our results show that one Instagram post, a subsequent viral tweet, and mainstream media coverage generated significant interest in perineum sunning. This new proposed health trend appeared in over 250 articles from numerous media outlets, which spurred others to engage in the behavior. For example, actor Josh Brolin attempted perineum sunning, which resulted in a severe sunburn to his anogenital area. Other iconic figures such as the famous American music producer Diplo, popular health author and entrepreneur Dave Aspery, and American actress Shailene Woodley have all shared their experience of perineum sunning through news media. Despite being deemed a "wellness" technique, the mainstream attention garnered by perineum sunning could lead to harmful health consequences.

Our trends analysis demonstrates continued public search interest in "perineum sunning" and "perineum tanning" for almost a year since the original post on October 21, 2019. Continued search interest in perineum sunning showed a resurgence during the summer months. This finding is concerning because UV exposure increases during the summer, and the solar radiation during these months has the greatest intensities of UV-B [7]. Additionally, Tripathi et al [8] found an increase in the prevalence and costs associated with sunburn-related emergency department visits, especially during the months of June, July, and August. While this study did not explore intent to act, if increased search interest during these summer months resulted in more people attempting this practice, they would be exposing themselves to more dangerous levels of UV radiation. While unsure why other spikes of public interest in perineum sunning occurred, we speculate that continued interest is being generated through social media platforms and ongoing news media coverage. Regardless of the reasons for the increased interest, our study suggests that people are continuing to search for perineum sunning, which may lead to higher rates of cutaneous malignancies and poorer health outcomes if more people attempt this unsafe wellness trend.

Exposure of skin to the UV rays present in sunlight has acute and chronic effects that can occur at doses of UV light that are nonerythemogenic. Short-term effects are sunburn (ranging from solar erythema to vesiculation/bullae formation) and tanning. Long-term effects include photoaging and UV-induced tumor formation [9,10]. It is well known that UV exposure is the most obvious risk factor for cutaneous malignancies such as melanoma, basal cell carcinoma, and squamous cell carcinoma [11]. To make matters worse, melanomas in less visible areas, such as the buttocks and perineum, have worse prognosis independent of tumor characteristics and visibility on self-skin examinations [10]. Furthermore, perineum skin is still vulnerable to risk of sunburn and, over time, cancer formation. To our knowledge, no study has shown perineal skin to have a special ability to generate more vitamin D production than other areas of the skin, nor is there any human evidence that sunning this specific area promotes positive changes in mood, increases libido, and improves regulation of hormones or circadian rhythm. Promotion of health misinformation, such as perineum sunning, via social media is quickly becoming a public health threat.

Non–evidence-based health trends and medical misinformation originating on social media are recognized challenges with serious public health implications (eg, antivaccination campaigns), which can place a significant burden on medical professionals and health care systems in one day, as our results show. Protecting the value of accurate medical information is of utmost importance as science and health information can be strategically manipulated by social media while perpetuating misinformation [12]. Strategies to combat the spread of misinformation require a collaborative approach involving medical journals, researchers, and physicians [13]. Doctors and health care professionals are encouraged to use social media platforms—the source of the majority of misinformation—as educational tools to promote accurate medical information and protect the integrity of online health information [14].

Along with health care professionals, journals must also be proactive in coordinating efforts to address public health misinformation that may harm the general public. We agree with Armstrong et al [15] and recommend journals publish articles with the intention of educating and redirecting public behavior at pertinent times when widespread dissemination of health misinformation has occurred. The *Journal of Medical Internet Research*, and its sister journal *JMIR Dermatology*, are two examples of journals that seem to be dedicated to publishing research focused on combating medical misinformation and raising awareness concerning the quality of health information on the internet [1,16-19]. For example, one study recently published by *JMIR Dermatology* evaluated the quality of sun-protection information by examining the most popular YouTube videos covering sunscreen [16]. Here the authors concluded that content about sunscreen use was often negative or failed to include important sunscreen use recommendations. Low-quality information surrounding sunscreen use, coupled with our study's results, further demonstrates the need for a collaborative approach to combat medical misinformation, especially in risky sun behaviors.

Limitations

Our study is limited by its cross-sectional design and should not be generalized. While Google Trends has been used to examine increased public interest and subsequent actions [20,21], our study did not determine intent. Therefore, future research in social media health trends may consider collecting participant surveys of *intent to act* after viewing the post. Lastly, by using Google Trends, we could only calculate relative search volumes.

Conclusion

Our findings suggest that it took only 24 hours for a potentially dangerous "health" trend to capture the spotlight of mainstream media outlets—an alarming exposé in the power of social media concerning perineum sunning. Additionally, continued observance of the search interest in perineum sunning showed a resurgence during the summer months. Exposure to sunlight is dangerous, and sensitive areas such as the perineum have worse prognosis even when detected during skin examinations. Dermatologists and physicians in other fields of medicine should be aware of perineum sunning and should consider that its popularity may warrant additional inquiry about sun exposure and tanning during patient encounters.

Acknowledgments

MV is funded through the US Department of Health and Human Services Office of Research Integrity and the Oklahoma Center for the Advancement of Science and Technology.

References

1. Park M, Sun Y, McLaughlin ML. Social Media Propagation of Content Promoting Risky Health Behavior. Cyberpsychol Behav Soc Netw 2017 May;20(5):278-285. [doi: 10.1089/cyber.2016.0698] [Medline: 28498046]
2. Smailhodzic E, Hooijsma W, Boonstra A, Langley DJ. Social media use in healthcare: A systematic review of effects on

patients and on their relationship with healthcare professionals. BMC Health Serv Res 2016 Aug 26;16(1):442 [FREE Full text] [doi: 10.1186/s12913-016-1691-0] [Medline: 27562728]
3. Groth L. So, Perineum Sunning is a Thing Now—Here's Why Doctors Definitely Don't Want You to Try It. Health. 2020 Feb 2. URL: https://www.health.com/mind-body/perineum-butt-sunning-wellness-trend [accessed 2020-02-09]
4. Google Trends. URL: https://trends.google.com/trends/?geo=US [accessed 2020-12-06]
5. Sprout Social. Social Media Management Solutions. URL: https://sproutsocial.com/?utm_source=google&utm_medium=cpc&utm_campaign=US_Brand_Sprout_Social_Phrase&utm_content=Brand_Sprout_Social_Brand_Name_Phrase&utm_term=sprout%20social&creative=436167110791&AdExtension=&Location=9026132&Matchtype=p&Device=c&gclid=Cj0KCQiA2af-BRDzARIsAIVQUOed2uHkbfe9oM6Uduxsl2WoLScsTHXwOJ6YBbnDOhIPqmelDYMZf7UaAm1nEALw_wcB&gclsrc=aw.ds [accessed 2020-12-04]
6. Ubersuggest. URL: https://app.neilpatel.com/en/ubersuggest [accessed 2020-12-06]
7. Scotto J, Nam J. Skin melanoma and seasonal patterns. Am J Epidemiol 1980 Mar;111(3):309-314. [doi: 10.1093/oxfordjournals.aje.a112902] [Medline: 7361755]
8. Tripathi R, Mazmudar RS, Knusel KD, Ezaldein HH, Bordeaux JS, Scott JF. Trends in emergency department visits due to sunburn and factors associated with severe sunburns in the United States. Arch Dermatol Res 2020 Apr 09. [doi: 10.1007/s00403-020-02073-2] [Medline: 32274574]
9. Howard MD, Wee E, Wolfe R, McLean CA, Kelly JW, Pan Y. Anatomic location of primary melanoma: Survival differences and sun exposure. J Am Acad Dermatol 2019 Aug;81(2):500-509. [doi: 10.1016/j.jaad.2019.04.034] [Medline: 31009667]
10. Gordon D, Hansson J, Eloranta S, Gordon M, Gillgren P, Smedby KE. Primary tumor sites in relation to ultraviolet radiation exposure and skin visibility correlate with survival in cutaneous melanoma. Int J Cancer 2017 Oct 01;141(7):1345-1354 [FREE Full text] [doi: 10.1002/ijc.30843] [Medline: 28635084]
11. Carcoforo P, Raiji M, Palini G, Pedriali M, Maestroni U, Soliani G, et al. Primary anorectal melanoma: an update. J Cancer 2012;3:449-453 [FREE Full text] [doi: 10.7150/jca.5187] [Medline: 23193431]
12. Merchant RM, Asch DA. Protecting the Value of Medical Science in the Age of Social Media and "Fake News". JAMA 2018 Dec 18;320(23):2415-2416. [doi: 10.1001/jama.2018.18416] [Medline: 30453315]
13. Trethewey SP. Strategies to combat medical misinformation on social media. Postgrad Med J 2020 Jan 15;96(1131):4-6. [doi: 10.1136/postgradmedj-2019-137201] [Medline: 31732511]
14. Rubin R. Getting Social: Physicians Can Counteract Misinformation With an Online Presence. JAMA 2019 Jul 31;322(7):598 [FREE Full text] [doi: 10.1001/jama.2019.10779] [Medline: 31365030]
15. Armstrong PW, Naylor CD. Counteracting Health Misinformation: A Role for Medical Journals? JAMA 2019 May 21;321(19):1863-1864. [doi: 10.1001/jama.2019.5168] [Medline: 31009036]
16. Julian AK, Welch J, Bean MM, Shahid S, Perna FM. Information About Sunscreen on YouTube and Considerations for Sun Safety Promotion: Content Analysis. JMIR Dermatol 2020 Jun 2;3(1):e14411. [doi: 10.2196/14411]
17. Mueller SM, Jungo P, Cajacob L, Schwegler S, Itin P, Brandt O. The Absence of Evidence is Evidence of Non-Sense: Cross-Sectional Study on the Quality of Psoriasis-Related Videos on YouTube and Their Reception by Health Seekers. J Med Internet Res 2019 Jan 16;21(1):e11935 [FREE Full text] [doi: 10.2196/11935] [Medline: 30664460]
18. Dunnsiri T, Kawashita T, Lee SC, Monga AK, Woo BKP. Assessing YouTube as an Educational Tool for Shingles: Cross-Sectional Study. JMIR Dermatol 2020 Sep 3;3(1):e20338 [FREE Full text] [doi: 10.2196/20338]
19. Park TH, Kim WI, Park S, Ahn J, Cho MK, Kim S. Public Interest in Acne on the Internet: Comparison of Search Information From Google Trends and Naver. J Med Internet Res 2020 Oct 26;22(10):e19427 [FREE Full text] [doi: 10.2196/19427] [Medline: 33104003]
20. Torgerson T, Khojasteh J, Vassar M. Public Awareness for a Sexual Assault Hotline Following a Grey's Anatomy Episode. JAMA Intern Med 2020 Mar 01;180(3):456-458 [FREE Full text] [doi: 10.1001/jamainternmed.2019.5280] [Medline: 31790540]
21. Ayers JW, Nobles AL, Dredze M. Media Trends for the Substance Abuse and Mental Health Services Administration 800-662-HELP Addiction Treatment Referral Services After a Celebrity Overdose. JAMA Intern Med 2019 Mar 01;179(3):441-442 [FREE Full text] [doi: 10.1001/jamainternmed.2018.6562] [Medline: 30640378]

Abbreviations

ARIMA: autoregressive integrated moving average

18

A Psychosocial Support Website from the British Association of Dermatologists for People Living with a Skin Condition: Mixed Methods Evaluation

Connor Heapy[1*], BSc, MSc, PhD; Kerry Montgomery[1*], BSc, MSc, PhD; Steven Ersser[2], BSc (Hons), RGN, PhD, PFHEA; Matt Gass[3], BA (Hons); Nina Goad[3], BA (Hons); Andrew R Thompson[4], BA (Hons), DClinPsy

[1]Department of Psychology, University of Sheffield, Sheffield, United Kingdom

[2]Department of Nursing, University of Bournemouth, Bournemouth, United Kingdom

[3]British Association of Dermatologists, London, United Kingdom

[4]Cardiff and Vale University Health Board / Cardiff University, South Wales Clinical Psychology Training, Cardiff, United Kingdom

[*]these authors contributed equally

Corresponding Author:
Andrew R Thompson, BA (Hons), DClinPsy
Cardiff and Vale University Health Board / Cardiff University
South Wales Clinical Psychology Training
11th Floor, Tower Building
70 Park Place
Cardiff, CF10 3AT
United Kingdom

Email: thompsona18@cardiff.ac.uk

Abstract

Background: There is a lack of psychological support for individuals with skin conditions, and few low-intensity self-help interventions are available.

Objective: This study aimed to test the acceptability and usability of a support website and its embedded self-help resources.

Methods: A mixed methods approach was utilized. A total of 583 participants (426 with a skin condition, 97 relatives and friends, and 60 dermatology professionals) viewed the British Association of Dermatologist's *SkinSupport* website and then completed a survey about their well-being and the usability of the website. A comparison group comprising 816 participants also completed the well-being measures. In total, 37 participants (19 living with a skin condition, and the relatives and friends of individuals with a skin condition, and 18 dermatology professionals) viewed the *SkinSupport* website and then took part in focus groups. Participants were recruited via social media, professional networks, and volunteer lists. Data from the survey were analyzed using descriptive and inferential statistics and qualitative content analysis.

Results: Both quantitative and qualitative responses suggest that the *SkinSupport* website was viewed positively by both patients and health professionals. Overall, 79.8% (417/523) of individuals with a skin condition, and the relatives and friends of individuals with a skin condition, said that they would use the website again; and 86.7% (52/60) of dermatology professionals said that they would recommend the site to somebody with a skin condition. Qualitative responses related to the website fell into 4 key themes: (1) appearance, (2) use and navigation, (3) information, and (4) areas for development.

Conclusions: The *SkinSupport* website was considered acceptable and usable. A range of areas requiring modification were identified. The website provides a useful resource that patients can access freely. Given the lack of services available to patients with skin conditions, health care professionals could routinely inform patients of this resource at assessment.

KEYWORDS

dermatology; psychology; surveys and questionnaires; interview; mobile phone

Introduction

Background

Skin conditions are common, affecting 54% of the UK population in any 12-month period [1]. Approximately 13 million people in England and Wales visit their general practitioner (GP) with a skin complaint each year, making it the most frequent reason for patients to visit their GP with a new problem [1,2]. Skin conditions may lead to difficulties in emotional, psychological, and social functioning [1,3]. Despite the potential negative impact that skin conditions can have on psychological well-being, access to psychological support for dermatology patients is acknowledged to be limited [1,4]. Although support websites and interventions exist for the group more broadly described as having a *visible difference*, many individuals with a skin condition will not identify themselves as having a visible difference and may, therefore, not find, or feel targeted by, such resources. In addition, there are many nonappearance-based issues associated with having a skin condition that do not apply to many other conditions that lead to a *visible difference*, such as pain and itch. As a result, the All Parliamentary Group on Skin has identified the provision of psychological services for people with skin conditions as a priority area for attention in 2019 [5].

Web-based self-help support has the potential to offer a cost-efficient method of addressing some of the gaps in the provision of psychosocial support for dermatology patients [5]. Such support can be considered as a *low-intensity* psychological intervention and is well-suited to individuals experiencing low-to-moderate levels of psychological distress [6]. Individuals could access such support in place of, or before, receiving more *intensive* forms of psychological therapy or support. Indeed, web-based self-help support has been found to improve individual well-being with a range of chronic health conditions [7]. However, there are few web-based self-help options available for people with skin conditions, and those that are available are condition-specific and not widely accessible (eg, cognitive-behavioral therapy–based web support for psoriasis [8]). Therefore, there is a need for a widely available self-help support tool for individuals with a range of skin conditions.

To address this need for psychological resources for individuals with a skin condition, the British Association of Dermatologists (BAD) launched a website, called *SkinSupport* [9], in July 2015. *Skin Support* was designed to support people living with a range of skin conditions and their relatives and friends, and as a signposting tool for professionals. The website was developed by a range of health care professionals and patient representatives. It includes access to downloadable self-help resources that have been subject to some evaluation. *SkinSupport* hosts a range of skin-specific psychosocial self-help information aimed at helping people to address common problems that are sometimes associated with skin conditions, such as how to regain confidence and improve low mood [10,11]. It also contains information and resources on different skin conditions, including treatment and causes.

Objectives

This study aimed to examine the acceptability and usability of the BAD *SkinSupport* website for people living with skin conditions and their relatives and friends. In addition, the acceptability and usability of the website as a signposting resource for professionals working with people living with skin conditions was examined. Evaluating this web-based resource is vital in ensuring that it serves its intended purpose of providing low-intensity psychosocial support for dermatology patients.

Methods

Design

A mixed methods approach was used to collect both qualitative and quantitative data using a web-based survey and focus group discussions. Qualitative methods using focus groups were adopted to capture novel, unanticipated responses that may be missed by a predetermined questionnaire [12]. Quantitative questionnaire survey methods were adopted to help summarize key acceptability and usability information across a large sample of individuals, allowing the generalizability of the findings to be examined. Using a single method approach to this question, therefore, would mean that crucial information on the acceptability and usability of the website would be missed. This pragmatic, mixed methods approach, therefore, allowed for a comprehensive assessment of the acceptability and usability of the *SkinSupport* website [13,14].

Participants

Both the questionnaire survey and the focus group were open to (1) individuals with a skin condition, (2) the relatives and friends of someone with a skin condition, and (3) dermatology professionals. To be involved in the study, participants were required to be able to speak fluent English and be aged ≥16 years. Any professional working with people with skin conditions was eligible to participate (eg, dermatologists, nurses, GPs, mental health workers and charities, etc).

Participants for the questionnaire survey (evaluation group) were recruited using a convenience sampling method. Participants for the focus groups were recruited via a purposive sampling method. For both parts of the study, participants living with a skin condition and their relatives and friends were recruited via a number of sources, including social media and volunteer lists (university and charity lists). Dermatology professionals were recruited via professional dermatology bodies, dermatology special interest groups, and staff working at a local National Health Service well-being service.

A comparison group of participants was also recruited for this study. These were individuals who had chosen to visit the *SkinSupport* website for purposes unrelated to the research project and then followed a link to a questionnaire on the website, inviting them to take part. This sample was recruited to check whether the participants who were involved in the website evaluation were typical of those who visited the *SkinSupport* website. Variables relevant to individuals with skin conditions were recorded and compared between the 2 samples.

Procedure

For the survey, participants in the evaluation group followed a web-based link to the questionnaire on the web-based survey platform Qualtrics. The survey first instructed participants to follow a link to the *SkinSupport* website before answering related questions. Participants in the comparison group were individuals who had visited the *SkinSupport* website before the current evaluation started. These participants were also asked to complete a series of established, validated questionnaires (patient health questionnaire 2 [PHQ-2], generalized anxiety disorder questionnaire 2 [GAD-2], and dermatology quality of life index [DLQI]).

In total, 3 focus groups were conducted for dermatology professionals and 3 focus groups for people living with skin conditions, and the relatives and friends of individuals with a skin condition. Participants were first sent a link to the website and asked to look at it. In addition, the website was displayed during the focus group discussion and participants were asked to comment on particular aspects. Focus groups were run by 2 authors of this paper, separately: CH and KM. Some focus group discussions took place in university settings and others in hotel conference room settings. A semistructured interview schedule was used to guide the focus groups, and the discussions were recorded using an encrypted digital recorder. The focus groups lasted approximately 60 min. Data were transcribed and uploaded into NVivo version 11 (QSR International) for thematic analysis. The qualitative data analysis was conducted by KM with supervision provided by AT.

Ethical approval was obtained from the Department of Psychology Ethics Committee, University of Sheffield.

Materials

The web-based survey assessed the acceptability and usability of the website as well as relevant demographic and clinical information. The acceptability and usability of the website were assessed by asking participants in the evaluation group for their opinions on a range of aspects of the website, including: (1) the appeal, (2) ease of use, (3) quality of information provided, (4) quality of self-help information, and (5) whether they would recommend the site.

The appeal of the website was assessed by asking participants to rate the home page and the rest of the website on a scale from *0* (not appealing) to *100* (very appealing). Participants were also asked to assess the balance of pictures and text on a 4-point Likert scale from *poor* to *excellent*. Ease of use was assessed by asking participants to rate on a 4-point Likert scale how easy they found the website to use, from *very easy to use* to *very difficult to use*. Quality of information provided was assessed by asking participants how helpful they found the information on the website from *0* (very unhelpful) to *100* (very helpful). Quality of self-help information provided was assessed by asking participants to rate on a 4-point Likert scale how easy the information was to understand, from *clear and easy to understand* to *very difficult to understand*. Participants were also asked to rate how helpful the self-help resource was from *0* (very unhelpful) to *100* (very helpful) and if they would use the techniques described in the self-help information from *0* (very unlikely) to *100* (very likely). Participants were also asked to rate on a 5-point Likert scale from *definitely* to *definitely not* whether they would use the website again, whether they would recommend the website to people living with a skin condition, and whether they would recommend the website to people supporting someone with a skin condition. Participants were also asked to provide any further comments on each of these areas in free-text response boxes.

The following demographic information was collected: age, gender, country of residence, ethnic group, and diagnosed skin condition (if relevant).

The DLQI is a 10-item measure of the impact of the skin condition on the patient's life in the last week. The DLQI has demonstrated good validity, reliability, and responsiveness to changes in a range of skin conditions [15,16].

PHQ-2 [17] is a 2-item measure of depression. PHQ-2 demonstrated good criterion and construct validity. PHQ-2 has a maximum score of 6, and a score of >3 is indicative of symptoms of major depression, with a sensitivity of 83% and specificity of 90% [17].

GAD-2 is a 2-item measure of the symptoms of GAD. GAD-2 has a maximum score of 6, and a score of >3 is indicative of clinically significant symptoms of GAD [18]. GAD-2 showed good sensitivity for GAD (88%), panic disorder (76%), and social anxiety disorder (70%) and good specificity (81%-83%) for all 3 disorders [17].

Website Development

The website development was guided from the outset by an expert advisory panel, comprising patients, psychiatrists, psychologists, dermatologists, and communications professionals. This panel was able to help guide the BAD through the many complexities involved in providing advice to potentially vulnerable service users or those in acute distress, and, crucially, to collate, evaluate, and commission the profusion of materials required. A large proportion of time and resources were allocated to the development and testing of the website, before a national rollout. This included beta testing of the site with medical professionals, the public, and patients. Patient information materials on the website were reviewed by a medical committee and seconded by experts every 3 years. This review date can be brought forward in response to known changes, such as withdrawal of a named drug or updates to guidelines.

Analysis

For the survey data, descriptive statistics were used to provide information on the demographics of participants in the evaluation group completing the survey. The current survey data for people living with skin conditions were compared with data collected by the BAD, before the launch of the survey (n=816), to examine any differences in anxiety, depression, and quality of life between website visitors and survey participants.

Qualitative free-text responses from the survey were analyzed using qualitative content analysis (QCA) [19]. QCA is a systematic text analysis technique that preserves the advantages of quantitative analysis, allowing frequencies of data to be reported while also providing a method to examine the experiences of participants using the *SkinSupport* website.

Qualitative data collected from the focus groups were analyzed using thematic analysis [20]. Thematic analysis is a method used to "identify, analyse and report patterns within data" to explain a particular phenomenon of interest [20]. Analysis of the focus group transcripts began by using line-by-line analysis, from which a list of key themes was generated from each group. These initial themes were then compared and contrasted to identify how the themes from each group fitted together. The aim was to preserve the integrity of the feedback gained from the individual groups within the final set of themes and to achieve internal saturation [21]. Detailed records of the analysis containing excerpts from the transcripts were maintained to enable checking.

Demographic data (age, gender, and ethnicity) of individuals in the evaluation group who would recommend the website to others were compared with those who would not recommend the website to others using a *t* test and chi-square test of homogeneity. Ethnicity was recoded into a dichotomous variable, to *white* and *nonwhite*, due to the relatively small number of participants with many of the *nonwhite* ethnic categories.

The qualitative results from the survey and focus groups were analyzed separately. These findings were then combined and summarized for the purpose of this study.

Results

Participant Characteristics

In total, 816 participants completed the web-based survey as part of the comparison group (no demographic information was collected) and 583 participants completed the web-based survey as part of the evaluation group (426 participants living with a skin condition, 97 relatives and friends of individuals living with skin conditions, and 60 dermatology professionals). The participants living with a skin condition, and the relatives and friends of individuals with a skin condition, were predominately white (394/463, 85.1%), female (407/477, 85.3%), living in the United Kingdom (465/473, 98.3%), and aged between 16 and 74 years (mean age 38.6, SD 12.6 years). The most common skin conditions reported were eczema (132/396, 33.3%), psoriasis (61/396, 15.4%), and acne (43/396, 10.9%), with some participants reporting more than one skin condition (Table 1). Health professionals included dermatologists (26/60, 43.3%), dermatology nurses (16/60, 26.7%), psychological practitioners (6/60, 10.0%), GPs and general practice nurses (3/60, 5.0%), and charity workers (2/60, 3.4%).

In addition, 37 participants took part in the focus groups (19 participants living with a skin condition, and the relatives and friends of people living with a skin condition, across the 3 focus groups, and 18 dermatology professionals across the 3 focus groups).

Psychological Well-Being

Of those participants in the evaluation group, 33.9% (132/389) reported clinically significant symptoms of depression. In addition, 37.0% (144/389) of the participants in the evaluation group reported clinically significant symptoms of anxiety. Quality of life related to the skin condition was examined in those with a skin condition in the evaluation group (those without a skin condition were not assessed on quality of life), and 88.7% (345/389) of participants indicated that their skin condition had an effect on their quality of life, ranging from a small to an extremely large effect (Table 2).

A two-tailed independent *t* test found that participants in the comparison group scored significantly higher in depression (PHQ-2: mean 2.77, SD 1.91) than participants in the evaluation group (mean 2.23, SD 1.89; t_{1203}=□4.67; $P<.001$). In addition, participants in the comparison group scored significantly higher in anxiety (GAD-2: mean 2.75, SD 1.97) than those in the evaluation group (mean 2.38, SD 1.99; t_{1203}=□3.05; $P=.002$). Finally, participants in the comparison group reported poorer quality of life related to their skin condition (DLQI: mean 13.16, SD 7.84) than participants in the evaluation group (mean 9.53, SD 7.48; t_{1207}=□7.63; $P<.001$).

Table 1. Sample characteristics from individuals with a skin condition, and the relatives and friends of individuals with a skin condition, completing the web-based survey (N=523).

Sample characteristic	Values, n (%)
Skin condition[a]	
Eczema, dermatitis, and prurigo	132 (25.2)
Acne	43 (8.2)
Psoriasis	61 (11.6)
Undiagnosed skin problems (dry, oily, itchy, or flaky skin)	31 (5.9)
Rosacea	24 (4.5)
Alopecia	13 (2.4)
Vitiligo	12 (2.3)
Scarring	12 (2.3)
Other	68 (13.0)
Total that provided skin condition information	396 (75.7)
Gender	
Male	65 (12.4)
Female	407 (77.8)
Other	5 (1.0)
Total that provided gender information	477 (91.2)
Ethnicity	
White	394 (75.3)
Asian or Asian British	39 (7.4)
Black or African or Caribbean or Black British Caribbean	9 (1.7)
Other	8 (1.5)
Preferred not to say	13 (2.4)
Total that provided ethnicity information	463 (88.5)

[a]These data are from participants with a skin condition and not relatives and friends of individuals with a skin condition.

Table 2. Dermatology quality of life scores from participants with a skin condition who completed the web-based survey (N=389).

Impact of skin condition on quality of life	Values, n (%)
No effect	44 (11.3)
Small effect	91 (23.4)
Moderate effect	110 (28.3)
Very large effect	104 (26.7)
Extremely large effect	40 (10.3)

The following information presented refers only to participants from the evaluation group, as only data on depression, anxiety, and quality of life were collected from the comparison group.

Appearance of the Website

Descriptive Statistics

Participants were asked to rate the appearance of the *SkinSupport* homepage and other pages on a scale of 0 (*not appealing*) to 100 (*very appealing*). Participants with a skin condition, and the relatives and friends of individuals with a skin condition, positively rated the appearance of the homepage (mean 74.92, SD 17.86) and the rest of the website (mean 71.49, SD 20.30). Similarly, professionals positively rated the appearance of the homepage (mean 77.32, SD 17.11) and the rest of the website (mean 76.48, SD 17.05).

The balance of pictures and text was rated on a 4-point Likert scale, ranging from poor to excellent. The majority of participants with a skin condition, and the relatives and friends of individuals with a skin condition, rated the balance of pictures and text as excellent (183/569, 32.2%) or good (309/569, 54.3%). Similarly, the majority of professionals rated the balance of text and images as excellent (18/58, 31%) or good (29/58, 50%).

Views of Individuals With Skin Conditions and the Relatives and Friends of Individuals With a Skin Condition

The appearance, layout, and images used on the website were generally viewed positively by those with a skin condition, and the relatives and friends of someone with a skin condition (Multimedia Appendix 1). The website was described as looking professional and visually appealing. The images of patients being used on the website were viewed positively, although some commented that the images were not diverse enough and omitted younger age groups and ethnic minorities. In addition, some people suggested that more pictures of the different skin conditions should be added. There were conflicting views of the balance of text and image, with some saying the balance was good and others commenting that the website was too *text heavy*. Although some participants described the colors positively (eg, as *calming*), others described the colors as bland and the words as not being distinct enough, potentially affecting readability.

Views of Dermatology Professionals

In general, professionals viewed the website positively, describing it as professional and visually appealing (Multimedia Appendix 1). As with the patient group, there were conflicting views regarding the images used on the website and the balance of images and text. Some participants commented that there was a lack of images in general, and more specifically, a lack of images representing ethnic minorities. Others commented that they liked the use of images of *real patients*. Participants suggested that adding videos to describe people's experiences could be helpful. One professional suggested that the medical information on the website was not accurate, and links to other websites needed updating. Finally, 1 dermatologist suggested that a separate area on the website for children and young people would be helpful, as the current website may not be appealing to a younger age group.

Use and Navigation

Descriptive Statistics

Participants were asked to rate the difficulty in understanding the information displayed on the website, and the language and terminology used on the website, on a scale from 0 (*very difficult to understand*) to 100 (*very easy to understand*). Those with a skin condition, and the relatives and friends of individuals with a skin condition, rated the information displayed on the website (mean 78.04, SD 20.15) and the language and terminology used (mean 77.49, SD 20.94) as easy to understand. Dermatology professionals also rated the information displayed on the website (mean 79.15, SD 20.23) and the language and terminology used (mean 77.90, SD 22.25) as easy to understand. In addition, 96.6% (504/522) of participants with a skin condition, and the relatives and friends of individuals with a skin condition, and 96.6% (56/58) of dermatology professionals, reported that the website was *easy*, or *very easy* to use.

Views of Individuals With Skin Conditions and the Relatives and Friends of Individuals With a Skin Condition

Participants reported finding the website easy to use and navigate through, even on a smartphone (Multimedia Appendix 1). However, some participants said that it was difficult to locate materials on the website and that the structure could be improved, as it was difficult to navigate to previous pages. Similarly, 1 participant commented that the navigation bar was inconsistent throughout the website and should be made consistent. Some participants also suggested that a search function should be added to each page. In addition, it was suggested that the search function should be made more intelligent so that it could predict what condition you were looking for, even if there was imprecision in the typed search term. Finally, some participants commented on the difficulty of navigating through the *A-Z* list of conditions.

Views of Dermatology Professionals

Professionals generally thought that the website was user friendly and easy to navigate (Multimedia Appendix 1). Although 1 participant felt that the use of medical jargon was avoided on the website, other participants reported that the patient information leaflets were written in unfriendly language, and some of the leaflets were too complex. It was suggested that a button that quickly navigates participants back to the home page would be useful. Finally, 1 participant was concerned about links on the website that took participants to information that did not inform or reassure sufficiently.

Information on the Website

Descriptive Statistics

Participants rated how helpful the information on the website was on a scale from 0 (*not helpful*) to 100 (*very helpful*). Participants with a skin condition had a mean score of 77.27 (SD 18.50), and the relatives and friends of someone with a skin condition had a mean score of 78.53 (SD 19.64), suggesting that they found the information helpful. In addition, 97.3% (468/481) of participants with a skin condition and the relatives and friends of someone with a skin condition and 100% (37/37) of dermatology professionals rated the self-help information on the website as clear and easy to understand, or somewhat easy to understand.

Views of Individuals With Skin Conditions and the Relatives and Friends of Individuals With a Skin Condition

Participants generally reported that the website was comprehensive and helpful (Multimedia Appendix 1). However, some commented on the fact that some information was too long and wordy. Some participants noticed missing information, for example, on different subtypes of certain skin conditions. Others commented on the fact that they learned no new information from the website. It was also suggested that the purpose of the website should be clarified. Some commented that the information should be made less medical; in particular, the use of the term *psychodermatology* should be removed. Finally, some participants said that the information was too heavily focused on adults, with too much focus on psoriasis specifically.

Views of Dermatology Professionals

The information on the website received mixed comments from dermatology professionals. Some thought the website needed more information on eczema (Multimedia Appendix 1). Others said that there was too much information on certain topics and that this may be off putting for some patients. One professional suggested that the use of videos to help with mindfulness exercises would be useful. In addition, some professionals suggested that the language of the website was overly medical in places and might benefit from revision. On certain topics, the information was said to be inaccurate. Furthermore, some professionals commented that the material was too focused on adults with a greater focus on psoriasis. Finally, 2 professionals reported being disappointed with the quality of information contained in some third-party materials on the website, including inaccurate crisis line information.

Areas for Development

Descriptive Statistics

Individuals with a skin condition, and the relatives and friends of individuals with a skin condition, were asked whether they would visit the website again; 42.3% (221/523) reported that they *definitely would* and 37.5% (196/523) reported that they *probably would*. In terms of recommending the website, 48.9% (256/523) said that they *definitely would* and 35.0% (183/523) said they *probably would* recommend the website to others living with a skin condition.

Dermatology professionals were asked whether they would recommend the website to people living with a skin condition; 75% (45/60) said that they *definitely would,* and 12% (7/60) said that they *probably would*. In terms of recommending the website to individuals supporting others with a skin condition, 65% (39/60) of dermatology professionals reported that they *definitely would,* and 18% (11/60) reported that they *probably would*.

Demographic data (ie, age, gender, and ethnicity) were compared between those individuals with a skin condition, and the relatives and friends of individuals with a skin condition, who would recommend (*definitely would* or *probably would*) the website to others and those who would not. There was no difference in age between those who would recommend the website to others (mean 38.7, SD 12.67) and those who would not recommend the website to others (mean 38.0, SD 12.45; t_{473}=4.56; *P*=.65). In addition, no differences were found in gender; 85.6% (338/395) women would recommend the website compared with 90% (69/77) women who would not recommend the website, a nonstatistically significant difference in proportions of 0.04 (*P*=.35). Similarly, no differences were found in ethnicity; 84.1% (332/395) white participants would recommend the website compared with 64.9% (61/94) white participants who would not recommend the website, a nonstatistically significant difference in proportions of 0.19 (*P*=.21).

Views of Individuals With Skin Conditions and the Relatives and Friends of Individuals With a Skin Condition

Participants were asked if there were areas of *SkinSupport* that could be developed. A total of 2 key areas were highlighted: (1) case studies and stories of people living with skin conditions, and (2) addressing the impact of stigma on people living with skin conditions (Multimedia Appendix 1). Some in 2 of the focus groups felt that the stigma surrounding skin conditions needed to be acknowledged on *SkinSupport* and could be added as another support category. Participants also thought it beneficial to have information about how skin is portrayed in the media, the view of skin conditions as contagious, and what the BAD is doing to challenge the myths around skin conditions.

Views of Dermatology Professionals

Professionals outlined several key areas that could be developed on the *SkinSupport* website. Regarding content, participants reported that information on habit reversal would be useful, and a question and answer section (Multimedia Appendix 1). One participant suggested that providing further information on common problems such as relationship issues and sleep would be beneficial, while also highlighting the connection between physical and mental health. Participants discussed having more condition-specific self-help available would be useful as a lot of the current information relates to psoriasis. Information on social stigma was also mentioned as being beneficial for patients. Finally, participants felt that the website needed further development to be applicable to young people.

Discussion

Principal Findings

This mixed methods study provides a detailed evaluation of the acceptability and usability of a psychosocial web-based support resource: *SkinSupport*. Participants included dermatology patients, and the relatives and friends of individuals with a skin condition, and professionals who work with individuals with skin conditions. Overall, *SkinSupport* was evaluated positively, and as such has the potential to be a useful resource for people living with skin conditions. For the quantitative measures of the website, the majority of participants gave positive ratings of the website's appearance, use, and navigation, and included information. In addition, participants provided positive feedback on the colors used on the website, the balance of pictures and text, and viewed the information provided as comprehensive for their condition. These quantitative results were generally supported by qualitative responses from participants in the questionnaire response boxes and in the focus groups.

Although the website was generally evaluated positively, several areas for improvement were identified. More specifically, recommendations relating to the appearance of the website include, adding more diverse images (ie, ethnic minorities, other age groups), adding more pictures of the conditions themselves, replacing text heavy sections with images, considering the use of videos, and adding further experiential accounts or stories.

Recommendations relating to the use and navigation of the website include adding a home button to each page to improve navigation, adding a search function to each page to improve navigation, improving the search function so that it is more general and intelligent (ie, specific words do not need to be typed in to find particular resources), and developing a separate area on the website for children and young people.

Recommendations relating to the information contained on the website include checking the accuracy of all the medical information on the website (including third-party links), reducing medical or unfriendly language (eg, the use of the word *psychodermatology*), making sure the information is more balanced and less focused on psoriasis, adding information that addresses the impact of stigma, relationship issues, and better signposting of the information on sleep, and adding a *question and answer* section to the website.

Some caution should be taken when generalizing the findings of the survey in this study to all users of the *SkinSupport* website. Participants who were involved in the evaluation of the website in this study demonstrated fewer symptoms of depression and anxiety and higher dermatology-related quality of life than participants in the comparison sample drawn from the existing visitors. This finding suggests that those who provided feedback on the survey may not be representative of those who typically visit the website. However, although there are some areas of the website where it could be plausible that individuals who are more distressed may evaluate the site differently (eg, self-help materials), for most areas (eg, appearance, use, and navigation), this seems unlikely. It is important to note that even those participants in the evaluation group of the website scored highly in depression (mean 2.23 SD 1.89 from a maximum of 6, the cutoff for major depression is 3; 132/389, 33.9% reached clinically significant levels of depression) and anxiety (mean 2.38 SD 1.99 from a maximum of 6, the cutoff for generalized anxiety is 3; 144/389, 37.0% reached clinically significant levels of anxiety) supporting the suggestion that such a self-help resource is needed for this population. Asking patients if they have visited this website may provide a useful rough guide for clinicians in identifying those individuals that require further psychological support.

It is important to note that 2 different constructs were being measured in this study: perceived usefulness of the website (ie, views from patients) and perceived usefulness of the website by others (ie, views from relatives, friends, and health care professionals). In general, the views of all groups aligned regarding each aspect of the website, meaning we can be confident in our conclusions on the strengths and weaknesses of the website in its current form. Indeed, many comments were repeated across groups (eg, images not diverse enough). Understandably, health care professionals were more likely to comment on the accuracy of the information and to suggest the addition of specific information (eg, on habit reversal). Overall, the website was perceived as useful (by patients) and perceived as useful by others (by relatives, friends, and health care professionals).

Limitations

A methodological limitation of this study is that participants may not have reviewed the entire website before completing the survey or being involved in the focus groups. The website contains a lot of content, and it would take a significant amount of time to review it all. As a result, participants may have been commenting only on small sections of the website that they had reviewed. We cannot comment on the areas of the website that participants visited, or the time they spent on the website, as these data were not collected. Although all visitors to the website were invited to complete questionnaires (to form the comparison group), it is not possible to comment on the overall response rate of those who visited the website as we did not collect this data. In addition, demographic data were not collected from this comparison sample to reduce the burden and increase the response rate. As a result, the comparison group may not be representative of those who visit the website. Despite these limitations, the study involved a large sample size and captured a wide range of views from patients, relatives, and friends of individuals with a skin condition, and health care professionals. The mixed methods approach meant that comprehensive responses were collected using different types of data regarding many areas of the *SkinSupport* website.

A further limitation of the study is that some of the authors of the paper (MG, AT, and NG) were also on the advisory panel for development of the website, increasing the risk of bias. However, neither the quantitative nor qualitative data were analyzed by these authors to reduce the likelihood of bias and increase the rigor of the analysis.

Future studies are needed to investigate the effectiveness of some of the untested self-help materials contained on the website, and the tested interventions [6,7] might be moved into webpage format to encourage higher usage. In addition, a brief evaluation should be carried out after the suggested changes have been implemented on the website.

Conclusions

Overall, the *SkinSupport* website is an acceptable and useful resource for people living with skin conditions, and the relatives and friends of individuals with a skin condition, and dermatology professionals. Some of the suggested changes around inaccurate information have already been implemented by BAD. Future decisions on which suggested changes to make will be made by BAD, with the help of this study, once further funding has been secured. After suggested improvements have been made, the website will serve as a valuable resource that can fit into the stepped care model of psychosocial care in dermatology, offering skin-specific self-help to people experiencing distress.

Acknowledgments

This project was created by the BAD with funding received from the UK Department of Health Voluntary Sector Investment Programme Innovation, Excellence and Strategic Development Fund (award number 251784).

References

1. The All Party Parliamentary Group on Skin. 2013. The Psychological and Social Impact of Skin Diseases on People's Lives URL: https://www.appgs.co.uk/publication/view/the-psychological-and-social-impact-of-skin-diseases-on-peoples-lives-final-report-2013/ [accessed 2019-02-12]
2. Schofield J, Fleming D, Grindlay D, Williams H. Skin conditions are the commonest new reason people present to general practitioners in England and Wales. Br J Dermatol 2011 Nov;165(5):1044-1050. [doi: 10.1111/j.1365-2133.2011.10464.x] [Medline: 21692764]
3. Grandfield T, Thompson A, Turpin G. An attitudinal study of responses to a range of dermatological conditions using the implicit association test. J Health Psychol 2005 Nov;10(6):821-829. [doi: 10.1177/1359105305057316] [Medline: 16176959]
4. Lavda A, Webb T, Thompson A. A meta-analysis of the effectiveness of psychological interventions for adults with skin conditions. Br J Dermatol 2012 Nov;167(5):970-979. [doi: 10.1111/j.1365-2133.2012.11183.x] [Medline: 22924999]
5. The All Party Parliamentary Group on Skin. 2019. Purpose and Aims URL: http://www.appgs.co.uk/wp-content/uploads/2019/02/APPGS_2019_Work_Priorities.pdf [accessed 2019-06-10]
6. Thompson A. Self-help for management of psychological distress associated with skin conditions. In: Bewley BA, Taylor RE, Reichenberg JS, Magid M, editors. Practical Psychodermatology. West Sussex: Wiley-Blackwell; 2014:60-65.
7. Beatty L, Lambert S. A systematic review of internet-based self-help therapeutic interventions to improve distress and disease-control among adults with chronic health conditions. Clin Psychol Rev 2013 Jun;33(4):609-622. [doi: 10.1016/j.cpr.2013.03.004] [Medline: 23603521]
8. Bundy C, Pinder B, Bucci S, Reeves D, Griffiths C, Tarrier N. A novel, web-based, psychological intervention for people with psoriasis: the electronic targeted intervention for psoriasis (eTIPs) study. Br J Dermatol 2013 Aug;169(2):329-336. [doi: 10.1111/bjd.12350] [Medline: 23551271]
9. British Association of Dermatologists. URL: http://www.skinsupport.org.uk/ [accessed 2020-04-26]
10. Pasterfield M, Clarke S, Thompson AR. The development of a self-help intervention to build social confidence in people living with visible skin conditions or scars: a think-aloud study. Scars Burn Heal 2019;5:1-8 [FREE Full text] [doi: 10.1177/2059513118822954] [Medline: 30675396]
11. Shah R, Hunt J, Webb TL, Thompson AR. Starting to develop self-help for social anxiety associated with vitiligo: using clinical significance to measure the potential effectiveness of enhanced psychological self-help. Br J Dermatol 2014 Aug;171(2):332-337. [doi: 10.1111/bjd.12990] [Medline: 24665869]
12. Bradbury K, Dennison L, Little P, Yardley L. Using mixed methods to develop and evaluate an online weight management intervention. Br J Health Psychol 2015 Feb;20(1):45-55. [doi: 10.1111/bjhp.12125] [Medline: 25406436]
13. Yardley L, Bishop F. Using mixed methods in health research: benefits and challenges. Br J Health Psychol 2015 Feb;20(1):1-4. [doi: 10.1111/bjhp.12126] [Medline: 25582981]
14. Yardley L, Bishop F. Mixing qualitative and quantitative methods. In: Willig C, Stainton-Rogers W, editors. The Sage Handbook Of Qualitative Research In Psychology. Thousand Oaks, CA: Sage Publications; 2007:352-369.
15. Finlay A, Khan G. Dermatology life quality index (DLQI)-a simple practical measure for routine clinical use. Clin Exp Dermatol 1994 May;19(3):210-216. [doi: 10.1111/j.1365-2230.1994.tb01167.x] [Medline: 8033378]
16. Basra M, Fenech R, Gatt R, Salek M, Finlay A. The dermatology life quality index 1994-2007: a comprehensive review of validation data and clinical results. Br J Dermatol 2008 Nov;159(5):997-1035. [doi: 10.1111/j.1365-2133.2008.08832.x] [Medline: 18795920]
17. Kroenke K, Spitzer R, Williams J. The patient health questionnaire-2: validity of a two-item depression screener. Med Care 2003 Nov;41(11):1284-1292. [doi: 10.1097/01.MLR.0000093487.78664.3C] [Medline: 14583691]
18. Kroenke K, Spitzer R, Williams J, Monahan P, Löwe B. Anxiety disorders in primary care: prevalence, impairment, comorbidity, and detection. Ann Intern Med 2007 Mar 6;146(5):317-325. [doi: 10.7326/0003-4819-146-5-200703060-00004] [Medline: 17339617]
19. Mayring P. Qualitative content analysis. In: Steinke I, Flick U, Kardoff EV, editors. A Companion to Qualitative Research. Thousand Oaks, CA: Sage Publications; 2004:266-269.
20. Braun V, Clarke V. Using thematic analysis in psychology. Qual Res Psychol 2006 Jan;3(2):77-101 [FREE Full text] [doi: 10.1191/1478088706qp063oa]
21. Glaser B, Strauss A. The Discovery of Grounded Theory. Chicago: Aldine Pub Co; 1967.

Abbreviations

BAD: British Association of Dermatologists
DLQI: dermatology quality of life index
GAD: generalized anxiety disorder
GP: general practitioner
PHQ: patient health questionnaire
QCA: qualitative content analysis

19

An mHealth App to Support Patients with Psoriasis in Relation to Follow-up Consultations

Bettina Trettin[1,2,3], MSc, RN; Dorthe Boe Danbjørg[2], RN, PhD; Flemming Andersen[2,4,5], MD, PhD; Steven Feldman[6], MD, PhD; Hanne Agerskov[2,7], RN, PhD

[1]Department of Dermatology and Allergy Centre, Odense University Hospital, Odense, Denmark

[2]Faculty of Health Science, Institute of Clinical Research, University of Southern Denmark, Odense, Denmark

[3]Centre for Innovative Medical Technology, Odense University Hospital, Odense, Denmark

[4]Department of Dermatology, Aalborg University Hospital, Aalborg, Denmark

[5]Private Hospital Molholm, Vejle, Denmark

[6]Wake Forest School of Medicine, Winston-Salem, NC, United States

[7]Department of Nephrology, Odense University Hospital, Odense, Denmark

Corresponding Author:
Bettina Trettin, MSc, RN
Department of Dermatology and Allergy Centre
Odense University Hospital
J B Winsløws Vej 4
Odense, 5000
Denmark

Email: bettina.trettin@rsyd.dk

Abstract

Background: Teledermatology has the potential to help deliver health care by transforming the relationship between patients and health care professionals (HCPs), shifting the power of consultation so that patients can become more informed, assertive, and involved in their care. Mobile health (mHealth) is a promising and reliable tool for the long-term management of patients with psoriasis on systemic treatment. In an attempt to facilitate a more patient-centered approach in clinical practice, we designed and developed an mHealth solution to support patients with self-management and empowerment.

Objective: The aim of this study is to explore the experiences and perceptions of patients and health care professionals of using an mHealth solution that was developed using a participatory design approach.

Methods: This was an exploratory qualitative study. Data were collected through semistructured interviews with patients and focus group interviews with HCPs.

Results: All participants found it easy to use the mHealth solution, and the patients found it convenient. Patients' reflexivity was improved because they could prepare ahead of consultations. Video consultations provided patients with a degree of freedom in their everyday lives, with not having to attend in-person visits. Among the HCPs, there were concerns regarding their medical responsibilities, as they could not assess the patients' skin as they used to. The mHealth solution required new workflows and procedures that were not part of the existing consultation routines.

Conclusions: The mHealth solution can strengthen the relationship between HCPs and patients and facilitate patients to become more active in their care. Alignment and structure in relation to the selection of eligible patient candidates for being offered the mHealth solution could reduce social health inequalities. In addition, video consultations changed HCPs' work practice, necessitating new types of skills to communicate with patients.

KEYWORDS

psoriasis; teledermatology; qualitative; video consultations; app; participatory design; mHealth; telehealth; patient-physician relationship; dermatology

Introduction

Background

Patient-centered health care, including patient empowerment and self-management, can enhance the care of dermatology patients. Although patients often prefer a patient-centered approach, it requires them to be more responsible for their treatment; the approach also requires a different relationship with health care professionals (HCPs) [1]. Thus, patient-centered care increases patients' responsibilities and may require changes in HCPs' interactions with their patients. For a chronic complex inflammatory disease such as psoriasis to be managed with a patient-centered approach, patients need to be informed and able to make decisions about treatment options, lifestyle behavior, and comorbidities [2]. However, patients with psoriasis may not have the necessary knowledge [3], and consultations may not fully address patients' needs [4,5].

Teledermatology (TD) has the potential to help deliver health care by transforming the relationship between patients and health care workers, shifting the power of consultation so that patients can become more informed, assertive, and involved in their care [6]. In an attempt to facilitate a more patient-centered approach in clinical practice, we designed and developed a TD solution to support patients with self-management and empowerment in relationship with HCPs [7]. TD may help optimize psoriasis treatment [8] and is well accepted by both patients and health care workers [9]. TD in the form of a mobile health (mHealth) solution could also be a promising and reliable tool for the long-term management of patients with psoriasis on systemic treatment (eg, biologics), where the course of the disease can be properly monitored and side effects of medications can be detected earlier [10].

Objectives

This study is part of a participatory design (PD) study exploring how the care and management of patients with psoriasis receiving biological treatment can be promoted by a TD solution. In the first phase of the study, patients' and HCPs' needs were identified [4,11]. In the second phase, a TD solution was designed in close collaboration with the patients, HCPs, information technology designers, and the research team [7]. The TD solution is an mHealth app designed to support needs, both during in-person consultations and by offering live interactive consultations, thereby reducing patients' in-person visits. This study reports on phase 3, in which the app was evaluated and tested in clinical practice and in patients' daily lives. Thus, the aim of this study is to explore the experiences and perceptions of patients and HCPs of using an mHealth app that was developed using a PD approach.

Methods

The Process of Developing the TD Solution

As PD was the theoretical basis of the study, the TD solution was designed with the participation of patients, HCPs, information technology designers, and researchers. The design of the solution was guided by the needs of its users and the result was the design of an app. The app included a knowledge database with information, videos, and a podcast relevant to patients. The app included 2 questionnaires for patients to complete before consultations: the Dermatology Quality of Life Index (DLQI) and a second questionnaire, which was named "preparation before consultation." It included patient-reported outcome questions and a free-text space for questions or comments to capture topics that patients wanted to discuss at consultations. Furthermore, the TD solution provided patients with the option of a video consultation. The overall aim of the TD solution was to facilitate a more patient-centered approach that would give patients the opportunity to contribute to the consultation agenda. The app was designed to support patients during their daily lives with psoriasis, when attending in person, and when offered a video consultation. Before testing the app in clinical practice, the HCPs received information about the app and its content, how to access the questionnaires and patient data, and training on how to interact during video consultations.

Design

This study was a qualitative explorative study that used a phenomenological-hermeneutic approach [12]. Semistructured telephone interviews with patients and focus group interviews with HCPs were conducted to gain insight into their experiences and perspectives of using the mHealth app in their daily lives and in clinical practice, respectively [13].

Setting

The study was conducted at an outpatient clinic at a university hospital in Denmark, where the majority of patients with psoriasis receiving biological treatment have regular follow-ups every 3 months with both a nurse and a medical doctor. However, a minority of patients were offered telephone consultations or a nursing consultation twice a year. Patients were monitored by laboratory tests; however, these were required only when patients were scheduled for an in-person visit. Laboratory tests do not require an appointment at the hospital, as the patients can choose to have them taken by their general practitioner or a local hospital close to where they live. The results of the laboratory tests were then available in the patients' personal electronic medical records at the hospital. Furthermore, patients do not have to travel to the hospital to pick up their medication; instead, they can receive it at their hospital. Patients included in the study tested the app, its content, and features for 3 months. The patients were invited by HCPs to test the solution during a scheduled in-person visit at the outpatient clinic, where the app was installed on their own devices and where they received information about the content and features by the first author and a medical secretary.

Participants

Patients

Patients were recruited in March 2020 by HCPs during in-person follow-up consultations. Inclusion criteria were as follows: Danish-speaking patients, aged >18 years, with psoriasis and patients receiving biological treatment. Of the 17 patients invited to participate, 1 patient declined because he found the TD solution to be too complicated. One patient dropped out because he found it too burdensome to answer the questionnaires. A total of 15 patients were included. The test period was 3 months and lasted until the next scheduled consultation. In total, 10 patients were scheduled for a video consultation, and 5 patients were scheduled for an in-person visit (Table 1). Moreover, 14 patients participated in the interviews, as 1 patient did not respond despite several attempts.

Table 1. Participants' characteristics (N=14).

Variables	Values
Age (years), median (range)	45 (27-67)
Sex, n (%)	
Male	12 (76)
Female	2 (14)
Employment status, n (%)	
Employed	11 (79)
Retired	2 (14)
Not working	1 (7)
Relationship, n (%)	
Single	2 (14)
In a relationship	12 (76)
Widowed	0 (0)
Treatment, n (%)	
Ustekinumab	9 (65)
Adalimumab	3 (21)
Secukinumab	2 (14)
Treatment years, median (range)	5.2 (0.5-14)
DLQI[a], median	1.8
PASI[b], median	0.7
Previously received a telephone consultation, n (%)	2 (14)
Received a video consultation, n (%)	9 (65)
Received an in-person visit, n (%)	5 (35)

[a]DLQI: Dermatology Quality of Life Index.
[b]PASI: Psoriasis Area Severity Index.

Health Care Professionals

Both nurses and medical doctors who were presumed to have used the TD solution at consultations were invited to participate in the focus group interviews. Thus, the recruitment was based on experience with the use of the mHealth solution and not on maximum variation among the participants, as this was not possible given the limited number of eligible participants. Of the 15 HCPs invited, 6 did not participate. Reasons for not participating were as follows: 2 were absent due to sickness, 1 was not able to attend due to other work, 1 had not used the app, and 2 were not present on the day the focus groups were scheduled. In total, 9 participants participated and were divided into 2 groups (Table 2). As some of the consultations in the test were performed by nurses only and some of the consultations were performed by both nurses and physicians, the focus groups were divided to match this. Therefore, 1 focus group consisted of both nurses and physicians, and 1 focus group consisted of only nurses.

Table 2. Characteristics of the health care professionals included in the focus groups (n=9).

Variables	Values
Focus group 1	
Sex, n (%)	
Male	2 (50)
Female	2 (50)
Occupation, n (%)	
Medical doctor	2 (50)
Nurse	2 (50)
Experience of treating patients with psoriasis (years), median (range)	5.6 (3-7)
Focus group 2	
Sex, n (%)	
Male	0 (0)
Female	5 (100)
Occupation, n (%)	
Medical doctor	0 (0)
Nurse	5 (100)
Experience of treating patients with psoriasis (years), medium (range)	8.2 (4-13)

Interviews

In total, 14 semistructured interviews were conducted with patients who had completed the test phase to explore their experiences and perceptions of the app and, thereby, to gain insight into their experiences of having used the solution [13]. Due to the COVID-19 pandemic and the related restrictions, the interviews were conducted by telephone. The first author recruited all the patients face-to-face before the lockdown of the society, and thus, all participants had met the researcher conducting the interviews [14]. When scheduling the interviews, patients were advised to be placed in a nondisturbed room. An interview guide was developed to explore the patients' experiences, impression, and acceptance of the app and its impact on their everyday lives. The interview guide was developed to ensure that participants could share their experiences and perspectives on the app features, function, layout, and comprehensibility, and suggestions for further development. Examples of questions asked included the following: "Please, tell me how you experienced using the app?" and "Can you describe in what way the app influenced your consultation?"

Focus Groups

The focus groups were conducted during work hours at the outpatient clinic. A semistructured interview guide was used to facilitate reflections on the use of the mHealth solution. Examples of questions asked to facilitate these reflections included the following: "How do you experience the opportunity to provide care and treatment during video consultations?" and "How do you experience the opportunity to provide care and treatment when you include the patient's app responses at in-person consultations?" Participants were asked to discuss these questions with each other, rather than addressing or answering the moderator [15]. This interaction between participants in a focus group is essential because it creates room for the interviewees to reflect, by exploring each other's perspectives [15]. The first author was the moderator, and the last author acted as an external observer; took notes on nonverbal communication; and asked questions to clarify issues raised, when necessary.

Ethical Considerations

All participants were informed about the study and received both oral and written information in accordance with the Declaration of Helsinki [16]. The patients provided written consent to participate and to be contacted after the interview. The HCPs provided written consent to participate in the focus group interviews. The study was approved by the Danish Data Protection Agency (2012-58-0018).

Data Analysis

All data were gathered into one coherent text, and the analysis was inspired by the theory of narrative and interpretation by Ricoeur [12]. The analysis followed a 3-step process: naïve reading, structural analysis and critical interpretation, and discussion. In the naïve reading step, the text was read several times to establish an initial impression of what the text was about. In the structural analysis and critical interpretation step, units of meaning (what is said) and units of significance (what the text speaks about) were identified [17]. At this stage, the transcripts were viewed objectively by abstracting the units of meaning from the text as a whole to create distanciation from the text [17,18]. In a dialectical process between explanation and understanding, 3 main themes emerged. Findings from the structural analysis step were subsequently interpreted and discussed in relation to the theory and other research results. The aim of this critical interpretation was to gain an even deeper understanding of the themes that had emerged. The findings were discussed by the entire research team. Reporting was guided by the Consolidated Criteria for Reporting Qualitative Studies [19].

Results

Overview

The naïve reading step revealed that the video consultations allowed patients a higher degree of flexibility in the everyday lives of patients, compared with in-person consultations. The patients seemed to appreciate the opportunity to prepare before attending a consultation. However, for both patients and HCPs, using an mHealth app was experienced as a new approach that required training. The structural analysis revealed 3 main themes: (1) preparation increases reflexivity, (2) video consultations increase the much-appreciated attentiveness, and (3) a new approach requires new competencies. FG1 and FG2 refer to focus group 1 and focus group 2, respectively; IIP refers to interviews with patients who had in-person visits; IV refers to interviews with patients who had video consultations; and "P" refers to participant number. The results presented focus on the specific TD solution that was tested and not on the general perception of other TD solutions.

Preparation Increases Reflexivity

Patients considered it to be able to prepare ahead of either video or in-person consultations as an advantage. The home setting gave them a chance to think about what was important for them to discuss:

> *When you arrive 10 minutes before you have to be there, you probably don't think so deeply about those things. Here you have the chance to just sit at home and think, well, maybe I could just hear a little about it or ask about.* [IIP, P1]

> *It's good to be able to set an agenda in advance, if there is something you would like to discuss. And then you are also sure to remember it.* [IV, P3]

The opportunity to contribute to the consultation agenda through the app led to reflexivity, which was not experienced when not using the app. Before patients had the app, patients had to fill out the DLQI in the waiting room, hand in a urine sample, register at the outpatient clinic, and register their transportation, all of which the patients found to be stressful. The app also assisted patients in remembering what they wanted to discuss. The patients were aware that, in advance of the consultation, the HCPs would have the patients' agenda and notes. This seemed to heighten the HCPs' focus on their duty to collaborate and engage with the patients.

The HCPs considered that the questionnaires encouraged the discussion of topics important to patients and clarified what patients wanted to address:

> *If the patient has doubts or something they would like to discuss, then these are actually good (questionnaires), so that is really good. It sets up a kind of agenda for the consultation that may also be important to them, in addition to that regarding the skin.* [Doctor, FG1]

Questionnaires used as tools for preparation created a structure for consultations that suited both parties. Despite positive acknowledgment of the questionnaires among the HCPs, it was recognized that it would take time to get used to using questionnaires in all consultations. Thus, it was beneficial to both parties that patients had the chance to reflect ahead of consultations.

Video Consultations Increase the Much-Appreciated Attentiveness

Both patients and HCPs were skeptical of video consultations and were surprised that they were easier than expected. Patients experienced attentiveness on the part of the HCPs and a sense of having a personal relationship with them:

> *That was the sense of security of it. It works. And those who sit at the other end you can feel they know what they are dealing with/what they are doing. Yes, I actually felt like I was sitting across from them.* [IV, P2]

Patients felt safe and confident during video consultations and were not distanced, as expected. However, the situation could be awkward:

> *I think you have a harder time getting started sometimes, so you sit and wait for the doctor, and then you just sit there and get filmed, like. But then we got talking about what we were supposed to talk about, and got the job done.* [IV, P6]

Some patients felt unaccustomed to video consultations. However, even those who tended to be averse preferred them over telephone consultations. They felt that visual contact avoided misunderstandings and created feelings of security. In addition, patients considered having a personal contact at in-person follow-up consultations before the video consultations as an advantage.

Attentiveness during video consultations was perceived as both unaccustomed and appreciated among HCPs. The HCPs became acutely aware during video consultations that they needed to demonstrate a different level of attentiveness, as compared with in-person meetings:

> *Well, the video consultation simply sets the stage so that now you have to look at the patient. And talk to the patient. Because they are there, right there on the table, you know? You cannot just sit there and sort through things. It requires a different preparation for us, and I think that is actually really good.* [Nurse, FG2]

HCPs were not used to having visual contact, as before video consultations became available, telephone consultations were the only option. Using a telephone gave them the opportunity to arrange other matters during these consultations, such as documenting or reviewing electronic patient records. Some HCPs appreciated being *forced* to be attentive, whereas others perceived it to be more time consuming and challenging. Thus, they felt unused to this but appreciated it.

Among the HCPs, there were some concerns regarding their medical responsibilities, given that they could not assess the patients' skin condition using the standard measuring instruments:

> *There is uncertainty, every time that there's no physical attendance. Then it is difficult to assess how the skin might look. You might only be able to relate to what it looked like in the past, or what the patients describe. Has it gotten better or worse?* [Doctor]
>
> *I sort of sit for a while and think well uncertainty in relation to how their skin is, it's also about how they feel it. Whether they are satisfied.* [Nurse, FG1]

As they did not have access to all the usual data, HCPs felt a loss of control and some felt a sense of insecurity. As a result, HCPs reflected on the importance of addressing patients' perspectives on their own skin condition, treatment, and well-being. For the HCPs, it was important that the video consultations made sense to the patients and made everyday life with psoriasis easier:

> *I don't want to be a nurse if I only get to sit and talk to patients over a video. It's a bit ambivalent, because I think it's really good for the patients. They don't have to drive for several hours to get here.* [Nurse, FG2]

The patients' needs took precedence over the HCPs' preferences to see patients at in-person visits. For some, the video consultation could fulfill this wish to some extent:

> *It just provided something completely different, being able to see him. Because you don't know, when you call them. You have no idea, if it is someone you don't know, how they are feeling. And it just provided something, that one could talk and laugh a little and so I am also positive about it.* [Nurse, FG2]

Furthermore, HCPs emphasized that video consultations should be based on patients' needs and that patients should be made to feel safe and confident.

Although the HCPs had some concerns regarding their medical responsibilities, patients felt a sense of confidence related to there being no need to attend quarterly follow-ups:

> *I'm following a course of treatment and I can of course see on my own body. I don't need to see what the numbers and all that say.* [IV, P6]

As patients had lived with a chronic disease for many years and were now on treatment with a significantly higher effect (biological treatment), they felt confident and were capable of self-assessing their needs at either a follow-up in person or by video. In this way, patients expressed independence and were willing to take on responsibility.

Giving patients the chance to have video consultations provided them with a degree of freedom related to everyday life and work:

> *I experienced it like going to a meeting where you have to show up, but within parameters where you can do what suits you. I was at home so it was super easy...so I could just be by myself. I have to use a whole day more or less [for in-person visits]. So I can save 2 days and spend them on something else. That's what's positive about having these video consultations.* [IV, P3]

When patients attended video consultations, there was peace and quiet during and around the consultations. Not having to take a day off work and spend a day on traveling was regarded as an advantage, both personally and financially. Thus, using the app allowed for flexibility, which was highly appreciated by the patients. That said, patients used it when they needed to and when it was beneficial to their everyday lives. Along with the unaccustomed and appreciated attentiveness through video consultations, the mHealth solution was experienced as an improvement in the management of psoriasis.

A New Approach Requires New Competencies

Using a new technology during follow-up consultations required that the HCPs acquire new competencies and working procedures. Regardless of whether the consultations were conducted by video or in person, they had to manage the digital responses to the questionnaires:

> *I have to say as well that it is still so new for me, I looked at the questionnaires and then I forgot everything about what they wrote.* [Nurse, FG1]

The new workflows and procedures were not a part of the existing consultation routines, and this meant that some completed questionnaires were not addressed or were not followed up. For the patients, this was somewhat annoying, although they recognized that it was a new workflow, and thus, they seemed to be prepared for difficulties during the test:

> *I had also written all my numerical values/data and things like that, but I don't know if it wasn't up and running or something, but in any case they had not checked them, but I'm sure it will come.* [IIP, P2]

Another difficulty during the test was that not all the HCPs seemed familiar with all of the app's content and features. If patients were not told about the app capabilities, they did not know to register their personal data, such as blood pressure, pulse, and weight. The focus was on the questionnaires, and during a busy workday, HCPs forgot to inform patients about all of the app's features. However, they also expressed the need to become much more familiar with the technology and its possibilities.

For the HCPs, it seemed important that the video consultations required more structure and that there should be some considerations about how many patients should be booked and at what time during the day:

> *Yes, if one had all telemedicine patients gathered on one day. Or one morning, or late in the day. Then you can take them one after the other. However, if they are booked in between the other patients, there is always a great risk of getting delayed. Because you don't know, just before, what kind of patient you are getting. Then you get more pressured.* [Doctor, FG1]

The pressure on workflow was caused by the fact that video consultations were not part of the routine, and therefore, the HCPs did not know what to expect. In addition, because consultation by video had not yet become routine, they were not sure how best to round off consultations, which also added some pressure:

> *When it is a video, it takes longer, because the patients have such a desire to talk. So, maybe it has opened up more. And for some [HCPs] it has also been a bit hard to round off.* [Nurse, FG2]

There was overall agreement between HCPs that the app should be offered to all patients with psoriasis; however, there were reflections on which patients should be offered video consultations. HCPs were reluctant to offer video consultations to the patients categorized as complicated:

> *But if it is a complicated patient, then I don't want to mention it.* [Doctor, FG1]

The HCPs' individual and subjective assessments of the patient would define whether the patient was complicated. This could be related to patients with social challenges or lifestyle-related diseases. Nevertheless, if a complicated patient requested a video consultation, the HCPs said they would offer it. When they first started recruiting patients for video consultations, there was a tendency to include patients who lived far away from the hospital. With time, however, there was a growing recognition that this was not an optimal strategy:

> *Yes, yes, but that about not even offering it because one thinks they are over 75 and can't work it out. I've had someone who himself requested it. He was 86.* [Nurse, FG1]

The quoted text shows that it was impossible to predict who wanted, who could benefit from, and who could manage a video consolation. This created an awareness that all patients should be considered eligible candidates, and the opportunities should be discussed with patients to identify their thoughts and perspectives on future video consultations.

Discussion

Principal Findings

In this qualitative study, patients experienced that their reflection on what was important for them to discuss at consultations was improved, through preparation using questionnaires that were filled out electronically at home. The questionnaires gave them the opportunity to ask questions ahead of a consultation. In a Cochrane review, interventions that helped patients ask questions and gather information before consultations resulted in small increases in questions asked and patient satisfaction [20]. Being able to ask questions and take responsibility for your health is an important part of self-management. The consultation, and thus the relationship between patients and their HCPs, is essential and should facilitate patient participation in decision making. Including patients' agendas in consultations is important, but the limited communication between patients and HCPs seems to challenge this [21] and needs to be strengthened [22]. Using an app that included preparation and contributed to the agenda, had a positive effect on patients' perceptions of the collaboration between HCPs and patients. This is consistent with another study that found that patients' reflection and collaboration with HCPs was improved by the use of an app that used questions as a preparation for consultations, as it gave patients a voice in consultations [23]. The use of questions to prepare ahead of consultations allowed patients to contribute to their individual experiences and gave them the opportunity to address aspects other than medical ones [23]. This could indicate that patients' involvement before and during video consultations could be a way to strengthen the relationship.

This study found that video consultations provided patients with a degree of freedom to better balance everyday life with psoriasis. In relation to other chronic conditions, telehealth is perceived by patients to be convenient and leads to them feeling more involved in decisions about their care and greater confidence in managing their own health [24]. Our patient participants experienced independence and were willing to take on responsibility for not having to physically attend follow-ups every 3 months. By allowing them to decide whether they wanted to participate in video consultations, patients were encouraged to become active in their care. Supporting patients in this active role or active engagement can be seen as a step toward a more patient-centered approach [25].

Some patients and HCPs were unaccustomed to video consultations and required more adaptation, which is consistent with other findings [26]. According to postphenomenology, as described by Ihde [27], dealing with technology in the field of health care is a process. There must be room for resistance and adaptation of the technology in the interaction with humans in practice. Ihde [27] uses the term embodiment to describe the integration of a technology. It refers to the process that occurs when a given technology becomes integrated as a useful tool for those who use it. Thus, postphenomenology deals with how a technology shapes the relationship between humans, where technology is not regarded as a neutral force [28]. Technological mediation, constitution, and multistability are the concepts used to describe this relationship [28]. The mHealth solution in this study enabled both preparation ahead of consultations and video consultations that mediated a new way of interaction between patients and HCPs. Although most patients felt confident in video consultations, some HCPs were concerned about the limited access to patient data and that they could not measure and assess patients in the usual way. In this way, the technology mediated a reflection on the importance of addressing the patients' perspectives on how they experience their skin, treatment, and well-being. Sometimes, the completed questionnaires were not addressed by HCPs during the consultation, leading to the risk of a lack of patient-centeredness. This supports the postphenomenological concept of multistability, in that the mHealth solution can have different meanings and purposes for different users in different contexts.

Patients undergoing biological treatment are closely monitored with blood tests, skin examination, and quality of life measurements. Although the DLQI questionnaire was embedded in the TD solution and access to patients' blood samples was available, we found that the missing skin examination was a concern for HCPs. Patients' safety is an important aspect in the field of TD, especially when a TD solution, such as the one in this study, may replace some routine consultations. However, decreasing in-person visits for patients receiving biologics has shown no harm in patient safety or monitoring, but instead, it provides patients with more flexibility [29]. In this study, we did not focus on replacing routine in-person consultations, but on facilitating a more patient-centered approach in clinical practice through the use of technology. In our study, the use of video consultations was requested by patients during phase 2 of a PD process [7].

Another finding was that HCPs offered the mHealth solution to patients they perceived as not complicated or to patients living far away from the hospital. It is often argued that telehealth reduces inequality in health by increasing access to health services [30]. Furthermore, the use of a PD, as in this study, is recommended to further reduce these inequalities [31]. However, if HCPs subjectively choose eligible candidates, this could increase social health inequalities, as it automatically excludes a certain group of patients. During the test period, some HCPs became aware that their approach to patient selection might have been wrong, as they found that certain patients, who they would not have considered including, asked for a video consultation. In this way, the HCPs were confronted with some of their existing prejudices and reflected on how to solve this problem. Nevertheless, this is a barrier for the full embodiment of the mHealth solution, and a clear structure and alignment regarding who to include is required.

Limitations

A limitation of this study is that it was a single-center study that included 14 patients and 9 HCPs, which is a rather small sample size. However, this was an evaluation of an mHealth solution whose aim was to explore the experiences and perceptions of patients and HCPs who used it. This lends itself to a qualitative approach, and thus, the sample size seems adequate, as qualitative research is concerned with the deepening and understanding of a phenomenon, rather than with numerical representability [32]. In addition, we aimed for maximum variation during participant recruitment and included patients aged 27-67 years, which is considered a strength [33]. Telephone interviews used in qualitative research are not the most common method for data generation because of the loss of contextual data, such as nonverbal communication. However, there seems to be limited evidence that telephone interviews, with certainty, lead to data loss [14]. Furthermore, this study did not collect sensitive data, and the participants were familiar with the author conducting the interviews.

Implications for Practice

An mHealth app for patients with psoriasis receiving biological treatment can be used at follow-up consultations. However, it should be used as a solution to support both HCPs and patients to facilitate a patient-centered approach and increase patients' self-management. Thus, an mHealth solution has the potential to improve health management of this patient group.

Conclusions

The mHealth solution, in the form of an app, has the potential to strengthen the relationship between HCPs and patients and for patients to become more involved in their care. The mHealth solution was considered easy to use and facilitated support and reflection among patients, as it gave patients the opportunity to prepare ahead of consultations. Video consultations provided patients with a degree of freedom to better balance their everyday life with psoriasis. However, alignment and a clear structure with regard to patient selection as eligible candidates for video consultations are required to reduce social health inequalities. In addition, video consultations changed the HCPs' work practice, necessitating new types of skills to communicate with patients.

Future Study

The mHealth solution has an impact on clinical practice, and to ensure its sustainability and increase its use, initiatives need to be designed to start the implementation process.

Acknowledgments

The authors thank all participants in the study: the patients for testing the app and sharing their experiences and the HCPs for their engagement and commitment to the study.

References

1. Scambler S, Newton P, Asimakopoulou K. The context of empowerment and self-care within the field of diabetes. Health (London) 2014 Nov 01;18(6):545-560. [doi: 10.1177/1363459314524801] [Medline: 24695383]
2. Nelson PA, Barker Z, Griffiths CE, Cordingley L, Chew-Graham CA, IMPACT Team. 'On the surface': a qualitative study of GPs' and patients' perspectives on psoriasis. BMC Fam Pract 2013 Oct 20;14(1):158 [FREE Full text] [doi: 10.1186/1471-2296-14-158] [Medline: 24138455]
3. Cordingley L, Nelson P, Griffiths C, Chew-Graham C. Beyond skin: the need for a new approach to the management of psoriasis in primary care. Br J Gen Pract 2012 Nov;62(604):568-569 [FREE Full text] [doi: 10.3399/bjgp12X658133] [Medline: 23211152]
4. Trettin B, Feldman S, Andersen F, Danbjørg DB, Agerskov H. Improving management of psoriasis patients receiving biological treatment: a qualitative approach. Nurs Open 2021 Jan 01;8(3):1283-1291 [FREE Full text] [doi: 10.1002/nop2.745] [Medline: 33385301]
5. Khoury L, Skov L, Møller T. Facing the dilemma of patient-centred psoriasis care: a qualitative study identifying patient needs in dermatological outpatient clinics. Br J Dermatol 2017 Aug 04;177(2):436-444. [doi: 10.1111/bjd.15292] [Medline: 28032892]

6. Finch T, Mort M, Mair F, May C. Future patients? Telehealthcare, roles and responsibilities. Health Soc Care Community 2008 Jan;16(1):86-95. [doi: 10.1111/j.1365-2524.2007.00726.x] [Medline: 18181818]
7. Trettin B, Danbjørg DB, Andersen F, Feldman S, Agerskov H. Development of an mHealth app for patients with psoriasis undergoing biological treatment: participatory design study. JMIR Dermatol 2021 May 10;4(1):e26673. [doi: 10.2196/26673]
8. Hayn D, Koller S, Hofmann-Wellenhof R, Salmhofer W, Kastner P, Schreier G. Mobile phone-based teledermatologic compliance management - preliminary results of the TELECOMP study. Stud Health Technol Inform 2009;150:468-472. [Medline: 19745356]
9. Frühauf J, Schwantzer G, Ambros-Rudolph C, Weger W, Ahlgrimm-Siess V, Salmhofer W, et al. Pilot study on the acceptance of mobile teledermatology for the home monitoring of high-need patients with psoriasis. Australas J Dermatol 2012 Feb;53(1):41-46. [doi: 10.1111/j.1440-0960.2011.00852.x] [Medline: 22309330]
10. Koller S, Hofmann-Wellenhof R, Hayn D, Weger W, Kastner P, Schreier G, et al. Teledermatological monitoring of psoriasis patients on biologic therapy. Acta Derm Venereol 2011 Oct;91(6):680-685 [FREE Full text] [doi: 10.2340/00015555-1148] [Medline: 21879250]
11. Trettin B, Feldman S, Andersen F, Danbjørg DB, Agerskov H. A changed life: the life experiences of patients with psoriasis receiving biological treatment. Br J Dermatol 2020 Sep 12;183(3):516-523. [doi: 10.1111/bjd.18876] [Medline: 31953845]
12. Ricoeur P. Interpretation Theory: Discourse and the Surplus of Meaning. Fort Worth, Texas: Texas Christian University Press; 1976:1-118.
13. Kvale S, Brinkmann S. InterViews: Learning the Craft of Qualitative Research Interviewing. Thousand Oaks, California, United States: Sage Publications Inc; 2008:1-376.
14. Novick G. Is there a bias against telephone interviews in qualitative research? Res Nurs Health 2008 Aug;31(4):391-398 [FREE Full text] [doi: 10.1002/nur.20259] [Medline: 18203128]
15. Kitzinger J. The methodology of Focus Groups: the importance of interaction between research participants. Sociol Health Illn 1994 Jan;16(1):103-121. [doi: 10.1111/1467-9566.ep11347023]
16. World Medical Association. World Medical Association Declaration of Helsinki: ethical principles for medical research involving human subjects. J Am Med Assoc 2013 Nov 27;310(20):2191-2194. [doi: 10.1001/jama.2013.281053] [Medline: 24141714]
17. Pedersen B. Nursing practice language and cognition. PhD Thesis, The Faculty of Health Science, University of Aarhus, Denmark. 1999. URL: https://www.worldcat.org/title/sygeplejepraksis-sprog-erkendelse-ph-d-afhandling/oclc/468093806 [accessed 2021-05-31]
18. Dreyer P, Pedersen B. Distanciation in Ricoeur's theory of interpretation: narrations in a study of life experiences of living with chronic illness and home mechanical ventilation. Nurs Inq 2009 Mar;16(1):64-73. [doi: 10.1111/j.1440-1800.2009.00433.x] [Medline: 19228305]
19. Tong A, Sainsbury P, Craig J. Consolidated criteria for reporting qualitative research (COREQ): a 32-item checklist for interviews and focus groups. Int J Qual Health Care 2007 Dec 16;19(6):349-357. [doi: 10.1093/intqhc/mzm042] [Medline: 17872937]
20. Kinnersley P, Edwards A, Hood K, Ryan R, Prout H, Cadbury N, et al. Interventions before consultations to help patients address their information needs by encouraging question asking: systematic review. Br Med J 2008 Jul 16;337(jul16 1):a485 [FREE Full text] [doi: 10.1136/bmj.a485] [Medline: 18632672]
21. Marvel MK, Epstein RM, Flowers K, Beckman HB. Soliciting the patient's agenda: have we improved? J Am Med Assoc 1999 Jan 20;281(3):283-287. [doi: 10.1001/jama.281.3.283] [Medline: 9918487]
22. Larsen MH, Hagen KB, Krogstad AL, Wahl AK. Shared decision making in psoriasis: a systematic review of quantitative and qualitative studies. Am J Clin Dermatol 2019 Feb 15;20(1):13-29. [doi: 10.1007/s40257-018-0390-5] [Medline: 30324563]
23. Nielsen C, Agerskov H, Bistrup C, Clemensen J. Evaluation of a telehealth solution developed to improve follow-up after kidney transplantation. J Clin Nurs 2020 Apr 17;29(7-8):1053-1063. [doi: 10.1111/jocn.15178] [Medline: 31889357]
24. Odeh B, Kayyali R, Nabhani-Gebara S, Philip N, Robinson P, Wallace CR. Evaluation of a telehealth service for COPD and HF patients: clinical outcome and patients' perceptions. J Telemed Telecare 2015 Mar 11;21(5):292-297. [doi: 10.1177/1357633x15574807]
25. Michie S, Miles J, Weinman J. Patient-centredness in chronic illness: what is it and does it matter? Patient Educ Couns 2003 Nov;51(3):197-206. [doi: 10.1016/s0738-3991(02)00194-5]
26. Ariens LF, Schussler-Raymakers FM, Frima C, Flinterman A, Hamminga E, Arents BW, et al. Barriers and facilitators to eHealth use in daily practice: perspectives of patients and professionals in dermatology. J Med Internet Res 2017 Sep 05;19(9):e300 [FREE Full text] [doi: 10.2196/jmir.7512] [Medline: 28874336]
27. Ihde D. Postphenomenologyays in the Postmodern Context. Evanston, Illinois: Northwestern University Press; 1995:1-162.
28. Rosenberger R, Verbeek P. Postphenomenological Investigationsays on Human-technology Relations. Lanham, MD: Lexington Books; 2017:1-281.
29. Khoury L, Møller T, Zachariae C, Skov L. A prospective 52-week randomized controlled trial of patient-initiated care consultations for patients with psoriasis. Br J Dermatol 2018 Aug 23;179(2):301-308. [doi: 10.1111/bjd.16369] [Medline: 29363093]

30. Dodson S, Good S, Osborne R. Health literacy toolkit for low and middle-income countries: a series of information sheets to empower communities and strengthen health systems. In: World Health Organization, Regional Office for South-East Asia. Regional Office for South-East Asia: World Health Organization; 2015.
31. Latulippe K, Hamel C, Giroux D. Social health inequalities and eHealth: a literature review with qualitative synthesis of theoretical and empirical studies. J Med Internet Res 2017 Apr 27;19(4):e136 [FREE Full text] [doi: 10.2196/jmir.6731] [Medline: 28450271]
32. Queirós A, Faria D, Almeida F. Strengths and limitations of qualitative and quantitative research methods. Eu. J Educ Stud 2017;3(9):887089. [doi: 10.5281/zenodo.887089]
33. Polit D, Beck C. Essentials of Nursing Research: Appraising Evidence for Nursing Practice. Philadelphia, Pennsylvania, United States: Lippincott Williams and Wilkins; 2017:1-512.

Abbreviations

DLQI: Dermatology Quality of Life Index
HCP: health care professional
mHealth: mobile health
PD: participatory design
TD: teledermatology

20

College Students' Attitudes and Behaviors Related to Sun Safety and Appearance in Relation to Health Information-Seeking Behavior and Social Media Use

Corey H Basch[1], EdD, MPH; Grace C Hillyer[2], EdD, MPH; Rachelle-Ann Romero[1]; Sarah A MacLean[3], BA; Danna Ethan[4], MSW, EdD

[1]William Paterson University, Department of Public Health, Wayne, NJ, United States

[2]Mailman School of Public Health, Department of Epidemiology, Columbia University, New York, NY, United States

[3]The Icahn School of Medicine at Mount Sinai, New York, NY, United States

[4]Lehman College, CUNY, New York, NY, United States

Corresponding Author:
Corey H Basch, EdD, MPH
William Paterson University
Department of Public Health
366 University Hall
Wayne, NJ, 07470
United States

Email: baschc@wpunj.edu

Abstract

Background: Skin cancer is the most common type of cancer in the United States. Rates of melanoma, a malignant form of skin cancer, are on the rise and are high among people under 30 years of age.

Objective: This study aims to explore factors related to sun protection and tanning behavior and examine the influence of social media use and health information-seeking behaviors (HISB) on sun protection actions among a group of college students.

Methods: In this cross-sectional study, students (N=258) at a large public university completed a survey that included questions on sun safety and tanning attitudes and behaviors, as well as HISB. A sun protection behavior score was created on the basis of behaviors related to seeking shade, using sunscreen, tanning booth and bed use, and the number of lifetime blistering sunburns. Multivariate logistic regression analyses were performed to assess associations between high and low sun protection behavior and sun safety and tanning attitudes and HISB.

Results: The majority of participants were females (164/258, 63.8%), 31.0% (80/258) were white, and the mean age was 20.3 (SD 4.1) years. Females (odds ratio [OR] 0.42, 95% CI 0.22-0.81) and believers that suntan improves appearance (OR 0.25, 95% CI 0.10-0.66) were less likely to have "high" sun protection behaviors.

Conclusions: The cultural belief that having a suntan improves appearance, especially among female college students, results in low sun protection behaviors. Interventions can be developed to improve skin cancer-related HISB among college students with the aim of developing better cognizance of skin cancer and sun protection behaviors.

KEYWORDS

United States; universities; students; skin neoplasms; ultraviolet rays

Introduction

Skin cancer is the most common type of cancer in the United States [1]. Rates of melanoma, a malignant form of skin cancer, have risen over the years [1,2]. The American Cancer Society estimates there will be 99,550 new cases of skin cancer in 2018, excluding basal and squamous types (as there is no requirement to report these to cancer registries), of which, 91,270 (92%) are melanoma [3]. In addition, a recent study suggested that the number of individuals diagnosed with melanoma will nearly double in 2026-2031 [4]. Melanoma is among the most common cancers in people under 30 years of age [4]. Ultraviolet exposure is a well-known risk factor for the development of melanoma [5]. College students tend to have high levels of sun exposure, low levels of concern for sun protection, and a strong desire to suntan [6-10].

Behaviors can be influenced by a number of factors, one of which is social media. The use of digital platforms, particularly social media, is at an all-time high [11]. The emergence of social media has allowed individuals opportunities in networking, navigation, and real-time connection [11,12]. College-aged individuals, who are part of a technologically adapted generation, frequently use social media, with 88% of those aged 18-29 years reporting that they are using social media [13]. College-aged individuals (age: 18-24 years) are markedly more likely to use Twitter, Snapchat, and Instagram, highly popular social media platforms [13]; of individuals in this age bracket, 51% reported that social media would be difficult for them to give up [13]. These young consumers are regularly productive through social media (eg, messaging, searching, sharing, and discussing various topics) [12]. As individuals continue to embrace social media, public health professionals should be aware of the potential health implications in nature of the information and messages that are accessed or shared.

One study specifically examined social media use and indoor tanning behavior and determined that social media is a medium that could increase peer pressure to partake in indoor tanning [14]. College-aged individuals, particularly women, are among individuals that frequently tan [15,16] and use social media [13]. As social media is so widespread, there are potential risks in spreading messages that could endanger health. As active information and image sharing on these platforms may be encouraging indoor tanning [14], a concern should be raised as indoor tanning is a major risk factor for skin cancer [17].

With the use of social media on the rise, there is a heightened sensitivity to self-image and physical appearance among younger age groups [18-20]. Many of these individuals associate tanned skin to attractiveness. Recent studies indicated that appearance dissatisfaction and tanning intentions strongly associated with social media use [18,21]. Current literature regarding social media [18,22] is consistent with research on traditional media in that images are often pro-tan and lack focus on skin cancer prevention [23-27].

As social media is reportedly used to promote tanning activity [28], it can also be used to promote health and can be highly effective as a medium for disseminating information in this population and promoting prevention efforts [29,30]. There remains a gap in the literature in terms of health information-seeking behaviors (HISB) of college students when it comes to skin cancer. Therefore, this study aims to explore factors related to sun protection and tanning behavior and examine the influence of health information seeking on sun protection behaviors among a group of college students.

Methods

This cross-sectional study, conducted in March-May of 2018, was ancillary to a larger study that focused on HISB of college students in general [31]. Instructors of 9 sections of a personal health course at a large public university in New Jersey distributed surveys to all students who were present (n=329) in class and voluntarily participated (n=258). The response rate was 78.4%. Of note, the course is part of the University Core Curriculum in which all students must take a personal health course, and this course is one of the offerings. Survey questions were adapted from the Health Information National Trends Survey questionnaire, and from our prior study on sun safety [6]. The survey questions pertinent to this study are described below.

Sun safety and tanning behaviors were captured in 5 questions. Sun safety behaviors were measured in 2 questions aimed at the likelihood that respondents would (1) seek shade; and (2) use sunblock on a sunny day. In addition, tanning behaviors were captured in 2 questions that encompassed the likelihood that respondents would go indoor tanning and specifically how many times they have used a tanning booth and bed in the past 12 months. The overall exposure was measured by asking how many blistering sunburns respondents experienced in their lives.

When looking at reasons for tanning and sun protection, we queried students regarding their perceived satisfaction in appearance and whether they believed that having a tan improves appearance. Moreover, we included questions concerning self-esteem and stress to further investigate the influence of social factors and individual thoughts and beliefs about the tanned skin. Appearance-based questions included the following: *Have you ever been dissatisfied with your appearance? Are you currently satisfied with your physical appearance?Do you think having a suntan improves your appearance?Do you think having a suntan improves your self-esteem?Do you think sun-tanning or sunbathing is a way to relieve stress?*

Respondents were asked questions related to HISB, specifically how many hours per day they were engaged on social media. Furthermore, questions were posed to assess respondents' attitudes toward the accuracy of information on social media, in general, and beliefs related to the helpfulness of social media as resources for health issues.

Descriptive analyses included frequency distributions, mean, median, and range. To construct the outcome variable, "sun protection behaviors," the following variables were recoded and summed: seek shade on sunny days ("likely" or "very likely"), use sunscreen on sunny days ("likely" or "very likely"), use a tanning booth and bed ("very unlikely" or "unlikely"), zero times using a tanning booth and bed in the past 12 months, and zero blistering sunburns in one's lifetime. The potential range of the 5 variables was 0-5; mean and median scores were 3.1 (SD 1.0) and 3.0, respectively. The sun protection behavior score was dichotomized with values of 0-3 coded as "low" sun protection behaviors and values of 4-5 as "high" sun protection behaviors. The race was recoded as black or African American individuals versus all other races and college year as "freshmen" versus "upper classmen." Variables coded on a 5-point Likert scale "very inaccurate" through "very accurate" were collapsed and recorded as "inaccurate" versus "accurate" and "strongly disagree" through "strongly agree" as "disagree" versus "agree." Univariate analyses were performed to test the association between sun protection behaviors (low vs high) using the chi-square test for categorical variables and the analysis of variance for continuous variables.

The unadjusted logistic regression was conducted for all variables with *P*<.05 in the univariate analysis followed by the backward, stepwise multivariable regression. Because the number of variables in each family examined (eg, demographics, attitudes toward tanning and sun protection, use of internet, social media, and attitudes toward internet, social media) were relatively few and a single comparison (low vs high sun protection behaviors) was conducted, Bonferroni correction for multiple analyses was not judged to be necessary. All analyses were conducted using IBM SPSS version 25. In addition, *P*<.05 was considered statistically significant. This study was approved by the Institutional Review Board at William Paterson University.

Results

Table 1 outlines the demographic characteristics, sun protection attitudes and behaviors, and health information-seeking beliefs and attitudes. Of 258 respondents, 63.8% (164/258) were females. The race was fairly equally distributed with 25.2% (65/258) black or African American, 28.3% (73/258) Hispanic, and 31.0% (80/258) white individuals. The mean age of a respondent was 20.3 (SD 4.1) years, and most were freshmen (156/258, 60.5%). Slightly more than half of the respondents declared a health-related major (135/258, 52.3%). No respondents reporting personally having had skin cancer, and few had a friend or family member with skin cancer (36/258, 14.0%). Approximately one-third of respondents reported they were "likely" to seek shade (93/258, 36.1%) and use sunscreen on a sunny day (71/258, 27.5%). The majority (225/258, 87.2%) were "very unlikely" or "unlikely" to use a tanning booth and bed, with 92.2% (238/258) stating they have not used a tanning booth and bed in the past 12 months. Nearly two-thirds were dissatisfied with their appearance at some time in the past, but 57.4% (148/258) were currently satisfied with their appearance. One-third believed that tanning improved their appearance (87/258, 33.7%), whereas roughly one-quarter believed it improved their self-esteem (66/258, 25.6%) or felt that sun tanning was a way to relieve stress (60/258, 23.3%). The use of social media was limited to about 4.5 hours per day with many (125/258, 48.4%) believing that social media is accurate to some degree and a helpful resource for health information (108/258, 41.9%).

Table 1. Demographic characteristics, sun protection attitudes and behaviors, and health information-seeking beliefs and attitudes among college students.

Characteristics	Value (n=258)
Demographics	
Gender, n (%)	
Female	164 (63.8)
Male	92 (35.7)
Other	1 (0.4)
Race, n (%)	
American Indian or Alaskan Native individuals	1 (0.4)
Asian individuals	28 (10.9)
Black or African American individuals	65 (25.2)
Hispanic individuals	73 (28.3)
Nat Haw or Other Pacific Islander individuals	1 (0.4)
White individuals	80 (31.0)
Mixed-race individuals	3 (1.2)
Other individuals	7 (2.7)
Age	
Mean (SD)	20.3 (4.1)
Median	19.0
Range	18-59
Health-related major, n (%)	
Yes	135 (52.3)
No	122 (47.3)
Missing	1 (0.4)
College year, n (%)	
Freshmen	156 (60.5)
Sophomore	38 (14.7)
Junior	41 (15.9)
Senior	20 (7.8)
Graduate student	0 (0.0)
Other	3 (1.2)
Relative with skin cancer, n (%)	
Yes	36 (14.0)
No	215 (83.3)
Missing	7 (2.7)
Self-skin cancer, n (%)	
Yes	252 (97.7)
No	0 (0.0)
Missing	6 (2.3)
Sun safety and tanning behaviors	
Seek shade on sunny days, n (%)	
Very unlikely	12 (4.7)
Unlikely	50 (19.4)

Characteristics	Value (n=258)
Neutral	100 (38.8)
Likely	67 (26.0)
Very likely	26 (10.1)
Missing	3 (1.2)
Use sunscreen on a sunny day, n (%)	
Very unlikely	58 (22.5)
Unlikely	60 (23.3)
Neutral	65 (25.2)
Likely	45 (17.4)
Very likely	26 (10.1)
Missing	4 (1.6)
Use of a tanning bed, n (%)	
Very unlikely	203 (78.7)
Unlikely	22 (8.5)
Neutral	20 (7.8)
Likely	7 (2.7)
Very likely	2 (0.8)
Missing	4 (1.6)
Number of times tanning booth and bed used in the past 12 mo, n (%)	
0	238 (92.2)
1-2	8 (3.1)
3-5	3 (1.2)
≥6	8 (3.1)
Missing	1 (0.4)
Number of lifetime blistering sunburns	
Mean (SD)	1.0 (2.3)
Median	0.0
Range	0-15
Reasons for tanning and sun protection, n (%)	
Dissatisfied with appearance	
Yes	163 (63.2)
No	93 (36.0)
Missing	2 (0.8)
Currently satisfied with the appearance	
Yes	148 (57.4)
No	110 (42.6)
Tanning improves appearance	
Yes	87 (33.7)
No	171 (66.3)
Tanning improves self-esteem	
Yes	66 (25.6)
No	191 (74.0)
Sun tanning relieves stress	

Characteristics	Value (n=258)
Yes	60 (23.3)
No	193 (74.8)
Missing	5 (1.9)
Use of social media	
Social media use (hours per day)	
Mean (SD)	4.5 (3.6)
Median	4.0
Range	0-24
Social media attitudes, n (%)	
How accurate is social media	
Very inaccurate	38 (14.7)
Inaccurate	93 (36.0)
Somewhat accurate	105 (40.7)
Accurate	15 (5.8)
Very accurate	5 (1.9)
Missing	2 (0.8)
Social media provides helpful health resource	
Strongly disagree	34 (13.2)
Disagree	74 (28.7)
Somewhat agree	108 (41.9)
Agree	34 (13.2)
Strongly agree	4(1.6)
Missing	4 (1.6)

Table 2 presents a comparison of demographic characteristics, sun protection attitudes, and health information-seeking attitudes and behaviors by the level of sun protection behavior. Those who reported "low" sun protection behaviors (153/241, 63%) more often stated that tanning improves one's appearance (43.1% vs 17.8%, *P*<.001), that tanning improves their self-esteem (31.4% vs 15.7%, *P*=.01), and that sun tanning relieves stress (29.1% vs 12.6%, *P*=.004) compared with those with "high" sun protection behaviors. In addition, individuals with "low" sun protection behaviors more often believed that social media was an accurate source of health information (10.5% vs 3.3%, *P*=.046) and a helpful resource for health information (62.5% vs 46.7%, *P*=.02) compared with those with a "high" sun protection behavior score. More often females (76.7% vs 57.2%, *P*=.01) and those who were in a health-related major (60.7% vs 47.7%, *P*=.05) had a "high" sun protection behavior score.

Table 2. The comparison of demographic characteristics, sun protection attitudes, and health information-seeking attitudes and behaviors by the level of sun protection behavior.

Characteristics	Total (n=258)	Sun protection behaviors (n=241)		*P* value[a]
		Low (n=153)	High (n=90)	
Demographics				
Gender, n (%)				*.01*
Female	156 (64.5)	87 (57.2)	*69 (76.7)*	
Male	85 (35.1)	64 (42.1)	21 (23.3)	
Other	1 (0.4)	1 (0.7)	0 (0.0)	
Race, n (%)				.18
Black or African American individuals	61 (25.1)	34 (22.2)	27 (30.0)	
All other races	182 (74.9)	119 (77.8)	63 (70.0)	
Age in years, mean (SD)	20.3 (4.1)	20.5 (4.7)	19.7 (2.7)	.17
Health-related major concern, n (%)				*.05*
Yes	127 (52.5)	73 (47.7)	*54 (60.7)*	
No	115 (47.5)	80 (52.3)	35 (39.3)	
College year, n (%)				.12
Freshman	152 (62.6)	90 (58.8)	62 (68.9)	
Upper classmen	91 (37.4)	63 (41.2)	28 (31.1)	
Relative with skin cancer, n (%)				.54
Yes	35 (14.8)	24 (15.9)	11 (12.9)	
No	201 (85.2)	127 (84.1)	74 (87.1)	
Reasons for tanning and sun protection				
Dissatisfied with appearance, n (%)				.68
Yes	153 (63.5)	95 (62.5)	58 (65.2)	
No	88 (36.5)	57 (37.5)	31 (34.8)	
Currently satisfied with the appearance, n (%)				.25
Yes	137 (56.4)	82 (53.6)	55 (61.1)	
No	106 (43.6)	71 (46.4)	35 (38.9)	
Tanning improves appearance, n (%)				*<.001*
Yes	82 (33.7)	*66 (43.1)*	16 (17.8)	
No	161 (66.3)	87 (56.9)	74 (82.2)	
Tanning improves self-esteem, n (%)				*.01*
Yes	62 (25.6)	*48 (31.4)*	14 (15.7)	
No	180 (74.4)	105 (68.6)	75 (84.3)	
Sun tanning relieves stress, n (%)				*.004*
Yes	55 (23.1)	*44 (29.1)*	11 (12.6)	
No	183 (76.9)	107 (70.9)	76 (87.4)	
Use of social media (hours/day), mean (SD)	4.5 (3.6)	4.4 (3.2)	5.0 (4.4)	.22
Social media attitudes, n (%)				
How accurate is social media				*.046*
Inaccurate	224 (92.2)	137 (89.5)	87 (96.7)	
Accurate	19 (7.8)	*16 (10.5)*	3 (3.3)	
Social media provides helpful health resource				*.02*

Characteristics	Total (n=258)	Sun protection behaviors (n=241)		*P* value[a]
		Low (n=153)	High (n=90)	
Disagree	105 (43.4)	57 (37.5)	48 (53.3)	
Agree	137 (56.6)	*95 (62.5)*	42 (46.7)	

[a]Italicized *P* values indicate significance (*P*<.05).

Table 3. Factors associated with high sun protection behaviors.

Characteristics	Unadjusted OR[a]		Adjusted OR	
	OR (95% CI)	*P* value	OR (95% CI)	*P* value[b]
Gender				
Male	1.00	Referent	1.00	Referent
Female	*0.41 (0.23-.74)*	*.003*	*0.42 (0.22-0.81)*	*.01*
Race				
Black or African American individuals	1.00	Referent	1.00	Referent
All other races	0.67 (0.37-1.20)	.18	0.92 (0.47-1.82)	.82
Health-related major concern				
No	1.00	Referent	1.00	Referent
Yes	0.59 (0.35-1.00)	.052	0.63 (0.35-1.15)	.14
Suntan improves appearance				
No	1.00	Referent	1.00	Referent
Yes	*0.28 (0.15-0.53)*	*<.001*	*0.25 (0.10-0.66)*	*.01*
Suntan improves self-esteem				
No	1.00	Referent	1.00	Referent
Yes	*0.41 (0.21-0.79)*	*.01*	1.31 (0.41-3.13)	.81
Sun tanning relieves stress				
No	1.00	Referent	1.00	
Yes	*0.35 (0.17-0.73)*	*.01*	0.61 (0.27-1.38)	.24
Social media is accurate				
Disagree	1.00	Referent	1.00	Referent
Agree	0.30 (0.08-1.04)	.06	0.61 (0.15-2.49)	.49
Social media is helpful				
Disagree	1.00	Referent	1.00	Referent
Agree	*0.53 (0.31-0.89)*	*.02*	0.60 (0.33-1.09)	.09

[a]OR: odds ratio.

[b]Italicized *P* values indicate significance (*P*<.05).

In the unadjusted logistic regression (Table 3), females (odds ratio, OR, 0.41, 95% CI 0.23-0.74) and individuals who believed a suntan improves appearance (OR 0.28, 95% CI 0.015-0.53), suntan improves self-esteem (OR 0.41, 95% CI 0.21-0.79), sun tanning relieves stress (OR 0.35, 95% CI 0.17-0.73), and that social media is a helpful resource for health information were all less likely to have "high" sun protection behaviors. After including all variables in the multivariate model, females (OR 0.42, 95% CI 0.22-0.81) and believers that suntan improves appearance (OR 0.25, 95% CI 0.10-0.66) remained less likely to have "high" sun protection behaviors.

Discussion

This study revealed that white female respondents were less likely to have a high sun protection behavior; this is consistent with the literature [16] and remains troubling, as this is a high-risk group for the development of melanoma [3]. In addition, this study corroborates previous research reporting that college students tan for psychosocial reasons, namely appearance [9,32]. In addition, this study revealed that those who were dissatisfied with their appearance were markedly more likely to believe that suntan improves self-esteem. Interestingly, those who spent more time on the internet were more likely to be dissatisfied with their appearance.

Research indicates that knowledge does not necessarily result in the adoption of healthy behaviors [9]. Reportedly, college students who understand the dangers of tanning and sun exposure, but also feel having a tan is important, often still desire to tan and forego means of sun protection [9,32]. Students in this study reported that they, by and large, felt that information related to health on the internet was accurate. Our ancillary study on HISB delves deeper into how these respondents use the internet to seek health information [31]. A tenet of HISB is that as an individual utilizes technology and understands more about how to use it, the person is more likely to use that specific technology as a source to search and gather health-related information [33,34]. Future studies can focus on interventions to ascertain the rate at which college students follow best practices in skin cancer-related HISBs.

Although social media is linked to risky behaviors, this source can incite opportunities for interventions promoting behavioral changes. Key issues can be communicated through popular social media platforms, such as Instagram, Twitter, and Facebook. To effectively address issues related to using Web-based methods, the target population must also understand the purpose of interventions. On the topic of skin cancer, interventions should inform college students regarding the influence of social media on knowledge and attitudes, and how this may lead to the adoption of risky health behaviors. Much like electronic health literacy, media literacy should be carefully utilized to increase the understanding of skin cancer; however, it must be strategic, as audience members may respond differently to an array of communication platforms. For instance, research confirms that young women, in particular, are visually oriented social media users, thus using images with prevention messages may be more effective [18,30]. By improving the methods of Web-based skin cancer prevention, college students may be motivated to appropriately and efficiently engage in HISB and, in turn, adopt healthier behaviors in the long term.

This study has several limitations that warrant mention. First, the cross-sectional design creates the inability to generalize these results. Second, the data were based on self-report and, thus, subject to recall bias. Third, the timing of the survey could influence thoughts and ideas related to sun safety. Despite these limitations, this study contributes to the literature on an important topic.

In sum, sharing content on social media is common. Personal stories of this nature can spark public engagement and result in Web-based search related to skin cancer and prevention [29]. By incorporating personal stories and graphic images with skin cancer prevention messages, this may improve message recall. The degree to which this incites a behavioral change warrants further study. Given that knowledge alone may not necessarily influence behaviors, effective interventions focused on skin cancer prevention and sun protection behaviors must be multifaceted. Furthermore, future research may be able to present critical data on seeking information about health topics (skin cancer, particularly) in social media, an underrecognized area of study.

References

1. National Cancer Institute 2018. Skin cancer (including melanoma) URL: https://www.cancer.gov/types/skin [accessed 2018-05-07] [WebCite Cache ID 6zE0jaiDD]
2. Chang C, Murzaku EC, Penn L, Abbasi NR, Davis PD, Berwick M, et al. More skin, more sun, more tan, more melanoma. Am J Public Health 2014 Nov;104(11):e92-e99. [doi: 10.2105/AJPH.2014.302185] [Medline: 25211764]
3. American Cancer Society 2018. Cancer facts and figures 2018 URL: https://www.cancer.org/content/dam/cancer-org/research/cancer-facts-and-statistics/annual-cancer-facts-and-figures/2018/cancer-facts-and-figures-2018.pdf [accessed 2018-05-07] [WebCite Cache ID 6zE0CDZM8]
4. Whiteman DC, Green AC, Olsen CM. The Growing Burden of Invasive Melanoma: Projections of Incidence Rates and Numbers of New Cases in Six Susceptible Populations through 2031. J Invest Dermatol 2016 Dec;136(6):1161-1171 [FREE Full text] [doi: 10.1016/j.jid.2016.01.035] [Medline: 26902923]
5. Fabbrocini G, Triassi M, Mauriello MC, Torre G, Annunziata MC, De VV, et al. Epidemiology of skin cancer: role of some environmental factors. Cancers (Basel) 2010 Nov 24;2(4):1980-1989 [FREE Full text] [doi: 10.3390/cancers2041980] [Medline: 24281212]
6. Basch CH, Cadorett V, MacLean SA, Hillyer GC, Kernan WD. Attitudes and Behaviors Related to Sun-Safety in College Students. J Community Health 2017 Aug;42(4):757-762. [doi: 10.1007/s10900-017-0314-y] [Medline: 28243774]
7. Glanz K, Jordan A, Lazovich D, Bleakley A. Frequent Indoor Tanners' Beliefs About Indoor Tanning and Cessation. Am J Health Promot 2018 Jan 01:890117118784235. [doi: 10.1177/0890117118784235] [Medline: 29973065]
8. Fabbrocini G, Triassi M, Mauriello MC, Torre G, Annunziata MC, De VV, et al. Epidemiology of skin cancer: role of some environmental factors. Cancers (Basel) 2010 Nov 24;2(4):1980-1989 [FREE Full text] [doi: 10.3390/cancers2041980] [Medline: 24281212]
9. Dennis LK, Lowe JB, Snetselaar LG. Tanning behavior among young frequent tanners is related to attitudes and not lack of knowledge about the dangers. Health Educ J 2009 Sep;68(3):232-243 [FREE Full text] [doi: 10.1177/0017896909345195] [Medline: 22707763]

10. Zhang M, Qureshi AA, Geller AC, Frazier L, Hunter DJ, Han J. Use of tanning beds and incidence of skin cancer. J Clin Oncol 2012 May 10;30(14):1588-1593 [FREE Full text] [doi: 10.1200/JCO.2011.39.3652] [Medline: 22370316]
11. Duggan M. 2015. Pew Research Center, Int Tech URL: http://www.pewinternet.org/2015/08/19/mobile-messaging-and-social-media-2015/ [accessed 2018-05-07] [WebCite Cache ID 6zE1DMH1f]
12. Smith A. U.S. Smartphone Use in 2015. 2015. Pew Research Center: Internet & Technology URL: http://www.pewinternet.org/2015/04/01/us-smartphone-use-in-2015/ [accessed 2018-10-29] [WebCite Cache ID 6zE1TTVb9]
13. Smith A, Anderson M. Social media use in 2018. 2018. Pew Research Center: Internet & Technology URL: http://www.pewinternet.org/2018/03/01/social-media-use-in-2018/ [accessed 2018-05-07] [WebCite Cache ID 6zE29BciM]
14. Stapleton JL, Hillhouse J, Coups EJ, Pagoto S. Social media use and indoor tanning among a national sample of young adult nonHispanic white women: A cross-sectional study. J Am Acad Dermatol 2016 Jul;75(1):218-220 [FREE Full text] [doi: 10.1016/j.jaad.2016.01.043] [Medline: 27317521]
15. Guy GP, Berkowitz Z, Watson M, Holman DM, Richardson LC. Indoor tanning among young non-Hispanic white females. JAMA Intern Med 2013 Nov 11;173(20):1920-1922 [FREE Full text] [doi: 10.1001/jamainternmed.2013.10013] [Medline: 23959651]
16. Basch CH, Basch CE, Rajan S, Ruggles KV. Use of sunscreen and indoor tanning devices among a nationally representative sample of high school students, 2001-2011. Prev Chronic Dis 2014 Aug 21;11:E144 [FREE Full text] [doi: 10.5888/pcd11.140191] [Medline: 25144679]
17. Boniol M, Autier P, Boyle P, Gandini S. Cutaneous melanoma attributable to sunbed use: systematic review and meta-analysis. BMJ 2012 Jul 24;345:e4757 [FREE Full text] [Medline: 22833605]
18. Mingoia J, Hutchinson AD, Gleaves DH, Corsini N, Wilson C. Use of social networking sites and associations with skin tone dissatisfaction, sun exposure, and sun protection in a sample of Australian adolescents. Psychol Health 2017 Dec;32(12):1502-1517. [doi: 10.1080/08870446.2017.1347788] [Medline: 28691513]
19. McLean SA, Paxton SJ, Wertheim EH, Masters J. Photoshopping the selfie: Self photo editing and photo investment are associated with body dissatisfaction in adolescent girls. Int J Eat Disord 2015 Dec;48(8):1132-1140. [doi: 10.1002/eat.22449] [Medline: 26311205]
20. Meier EP, Gray J. Facebook photo activity associated with body image disturbance in adolescent girls. Cyberpsychol Behav Soc Netw 2014 Apr;17(4):199-206. [doi: 10.1089/cyber.2013.0305] [Medline: 24237288]
21. Myrick JG, Noar SM, Kelley D, Zeitany AE. The Relationships Between Female Adolescents' Media Use, Indoor Tanning Outcome Expectations, and Behavioral Intentions. Health Educ Behav 2017 Dec;44(3):403-410. [doi: 10.1177/1090198116667251] [Medline: 27590838]
22. Banerjee SC, Rodríguez VM, Greene K, Hay JL. Trending on Pinterest: an examination of pins about skin tanning. Transl Behav Med 2018 Apr 10. [doi: 10.1093/tbm/iby036] [Medline: 29648613]
23. Basch CH, Hillyer GC, Basch CE. Descriptive analysis of articles and advertisements pertaining to skin cancer prevention in 2 popular US parenting magazines, 2000-2010. Prev Chronic Dis 2013 Apr 04;10:E48 [FREE Full text] [doi: 10.5888/pcd10.120200] [Medline: 23557639]
24. Basch CH, Mongiovi J, Hillyer GC, Fullwood MD, Ethan D, Hammond R. An Advertisement and Article Analysis of Skin Products and Topics in Popular Women's Magazines: Implications for Skin Cancer Prevention. Health Promot Perspect 2015 Jan;5(4):261-268 [FREE Full text] [doi: 10.15171/hpp.2015.031] [Medline: 26933645]
25. Basch CH, Ethan D, Hillyer GC, Berdnik A. Skin cancer prevention coverage in popular US women's health and fitness magazines: an analysis of advertisements and articles. Glob J Health Sci 2014 Apr 02;6(4):42-48 [FREE Full text] [doi: 10.5539/gjhs.v6n4p42] [Medline: 24999136]
26. Basch CH, Hillyer GC, Ethan D, Berdnik A, Basch CE. Tanning Shade Gradations of Models in Mainstream Fitness and Muscle Enthusiast Magazines: Implications for Skin Cancer Prevention in Men. Am J Mens Health 2015 Jul;9(4):301-306. [doi: 10.1177/1557988314543511] [Medline: 25038234]
27. Cho H, Lee S, Wilson K. Magazine exposure, tanned women stereotypes, and tanning attitudes. Body Image 2010 Sep;7(4):364-367 [FREE Full text] [doi: 10.1016/j.bodyim.2010.04.002] [Medline: 20573553]
28. Ricklefs CA, Asdigian NL, Kalra HL, Mayer JA, Dellavalle RP, Holman DM, et al. Indoor tanning promotions on social media in six US cities #UVTanning #tanning. Transl Behav Med 2016 Dec;6(2):260-270 [FREE Full text] [doi: 10.1007/s13142-015-0378-0] [Medline: 27356996]
29. Noar SM, Leas E, Althouse BM, Dredze M, Kelley D, Ayers JW. Can a selfie promote public engagement with skin cancer? Prev Med 2018 Jun;111:280-283. [doi: 10.1016/j.ypmed.2017.10.038] [Medline: 29109014]
30. Falzone AE, Brindis CD, Chren M, Junn A, Pagoto S, Wehner M, et al. Teens, Tweets, and Tanning Beds: Rethinking the Use of Social Media for Skin Cancer Prevention. Am J Prev Med 2017 Sep;53(3S1):S86-S94 [FREE Full text] [doi: 10.1016/j.amepre.2017.04.027] [Medline: 28818251]
31. MacLean SA, Basch CH, Clark A, Basch CE. Readability of information on colonoscopy preparation on the internet. Health Promot Perspect 2018 Apr;8(2):167-170 [FREE Full text] [doi: 10.15171/hpp.2018.22] [Medline: 29744314]
32. Harrington CR, Beswick TC, Leitenberger J, Minhajuddin A, Jacobe HT, Adinoff B. Addictive-like behaviours to ultraviolet light among frequent indoor tanners. Clin Exp Dermatol 2011 Jan;36(1):33-38. [doi: 10.1111/j.1365-2230.2010.03882.x] [Medline: 20545951]

33. Britt RK, Collins WB, Wilson K, Linnemeier G, Englebert AM. eHealth Literacy and Health Behaviors Affecting Modern College Students: A Pilot Study of Issues Identified by the American College Health Association. J Med Internet Res 2017 Dec 19;19(12):e392 [FREE Full text] [doi: 10.2196/jmir.3100] [Medline: 29258979]
34. Norman CD, Skinner HA. eHEALS: The eHealth Literacy Scale. J Med Internet Res 2006 Nov;8(4):e27 [FREE Full text] [doi: 10.2196/jmir.8.4.e27] [Medline: 17213046]

Abbreviations

HISB: health information-seeking behaviors
OR: odds ratio

21

Development of an mHealth App for Patients with Psoriasis Undergoing Biological Treatment: Participatory Design Study

Bettina Trettin[1,2,3], RN, MSc; Dorthe Boe Danbjørg[3], RN, MSc, PhD; Flemming Andersen[3,4,5], PhD, MD; Steven Feldman[6], PhD, Prof Dr, MD; Hanne Agerskov[3,7], RN, MSc, PhD

[1]Centre for Innovative Medical Technology, Odense University Hospital, Odense, Denmark

[2]Department of Dermatology and Allergy Centre, Odense University Hospital, Odense, Denmark

[3]Department of Clinical Research, University of Southern Denmark, Odense, Denmark

[4]Private Hospital Molholm, Vejle, Denmark

[5]Department of Dermatology, Aalborg University Hospital, Aalborg, Denmark

[6]Center for Dermatology Research, Wake Forest School of Medicine, Winston-Salem, NC, United States

[7]Department of Nephrology, Odense University Hospital, Odense, Denmark

Corresponding Author:
Bettina Trettin, RN, MSc
Centre for Innovative Medical Technology
Odense University Hospital
Kløverværnget 8C, entrance 101, 3rd fl
Odense, 5000
Denmark

Email: bettina.trettin@rsyd.dk

Abstract

Background: In Denmark, patients with psoriasis undergoing biological treatment have regular follow-ups, typically every 3 months. This may pose a challenge for patients who live far away from the hospital. Mobile health (mHealth) is a promising and reliable tool for the long-term management of patients with psoriasis undergoing biological treatment because the disease course can be properly monitored. Despite recent developments in mHealth, the full potential of teledermatology remains to be tapped by newer, more attractive forms of services focused on patients' needs.

Objective: This study aims to design and develop an mHealth app to support the self-management of patients with psoriasis using a participatory design.

Methods: Using participatory design, we conducted 1 future workshop, 4 mock-up workshops, and 1 prototype test with patients and health care professionals to co-design a prototype. The process was iterative to ensure that all stakeholders would provide input into the design and outcome; this approach enabled continuous revision of the prototype until an acceptable solution was agreed upon. Data were analyzed according to the steps—plan, act, observe, and reflect—in the methodology of participatory design.

Results: Health care professionals and patients emphasized the importance of a more patient-centered approach, focusing on the communication and maintenance of relationships. Patients perceived consultations to be impersonal and repetitive and wanted the opportunity to contribute to the agenda while attending a consultation. Patients also stated they would prefer not to attend visits in person every 3 months. On the basis of these findings, we designed an mHealth app that could replace in-person visits and support patients at in-person visits. Video consultations, self-monitoring, and registration of patient-reported outcome data were embedded in the app.

Conclusions: Using participatory design facilitated mutual learning and democratic processes that gave end users a significant influence over the solution. Despite the advantages of using participatory design in developing mHealth solutions, organizational conditions may still represent a barrier to the optimization of solutions.

KEYWORDS

mHealth; psoriasis; biologics; participatory design; teledermatology; mobile phone

Introduction

Background

Psoriasis is a chronic, complex inflammatory disease that requires long-term management. In Denmark, patients with psoriasis receiving biological treatment have in-person follow-ups every 3 months. Patients are frustrated by these quarterly mandatory checkups and do not always benefit from consultations, which they experience as time consuming and rigidly structured, in a way that is not targeted to patients' individual needs [1,2]. Hence, this may present an opportunity to improve the current clinical practice.

The application of telemedicine in dermatology is referred to as teledermatology (TD). TD has the potential to transform health care delivery to better meet patients' needs [3]. TD improves access to specialist care, diagnostic accuracy, and treatment adherence while also reducing costs [4]. Attempts have been made within TD to develop *mobile* solutions, also referred to as mobile health (mHealth), using new-generation smartphones. Mobile TD has been used to treat patients with acute and chronic skin diseases [5-7]. Mobile TD may help in optimizing psoriasis treatment [8] and has been accepted by both patients and health care professionals (HCPs). It reduces in-person visits and augments person-centered care [9]. Mobile TD could be a promising tool for the long-term management of patients with psoriasis on systemic treatment (eg, biologics), where the disease course can be properly monitored and medication side effects can be detected earlier [10].

A TD solution is as effective as the in-person management of patients with psoriasis, as assessed by objective clinical outcomes [11]. TD can increase access to specialized care and reduce commuting and in-office waiting times [12]. Patients and HCPs acknowledge the benefits of telemedicine solutions; however, there are still several barriers to TD (eg, economic factors, reliability, availability, and reluctance to use it) that need to be addressed [13]. Another challenge in implementing telemedicine [14] is the limited understanding of the requirements for optimal clinical effectiveness [15]. The full potential of TD remains to be tapped by newer, more attractive forms of services that closely focus on patients' needs [16]. One method to develop a TD solution adapted to patients' and HCPs' requirements is to use participatory design (PD). In PD, the focus is on designing and developing a technology that forecasts the possibilities of future technology before the solution is developed [17]. Mutual learning is the core element of PD. Through participation, the intention is to equalize the power between end users and designers by sharing knowledge. Researchers and designers need in-depth knowledge about end users' needs and daily lives, whereas end users need knowledge about technical aspects and possibilities, together with clinical opportunities and limitations. This approach reflects the democratic aspects of PD, as it offers end users a voice in the design and development of a technology that will affect patients' daily life and HCPs' current clinical practice.

Objective

The aim of this study is to design and develop a patient-centered TD solution based on patients' and HCPs' needs. This paper describes the design and development of an mHealth app and the involvement of patients, HCPs, researchers, and information technology (IT) designers in a PD study.

Methods

Overview

The PD study was conducted in 3 phases [18]. In phase 1, we identified end users' needs by exploring their experiences. We used ethnographic methods to explore patients' everyday life experiences with the disease and the HCPs' experiences of clinical practice. Previous studies have reported the results from phase 1 [1,2]. In phase 2, we designed and developed a telemedicine solution to meet the needs identified in phase 1. In phase 3, we tested the prototypes in clinical practice. All phases were conducted as iterative processes throughout the study (Figure 1). Literature studies were conducted continuously in all phases to broaden our understanding of the emerging findings [19]. This paper reports reflections on phase 2 and describes and critically discusses the iterative process of the design and development of an mHealth app. In this paper, the terms high- and low-fidelity prototypes are used to visualize the design process. Design fidelity refers to the level of detail and functionality of a prototype. Low-fidelity prototypes are often created using no technology but instead a drawing, which enables the collection and analysis of feedback in the early stages of the design phase. High-fidelity prototypes are highly functional, interactive, and close to the final product [20].

Figure 1. The three phases in the teledermatology solution design and development.

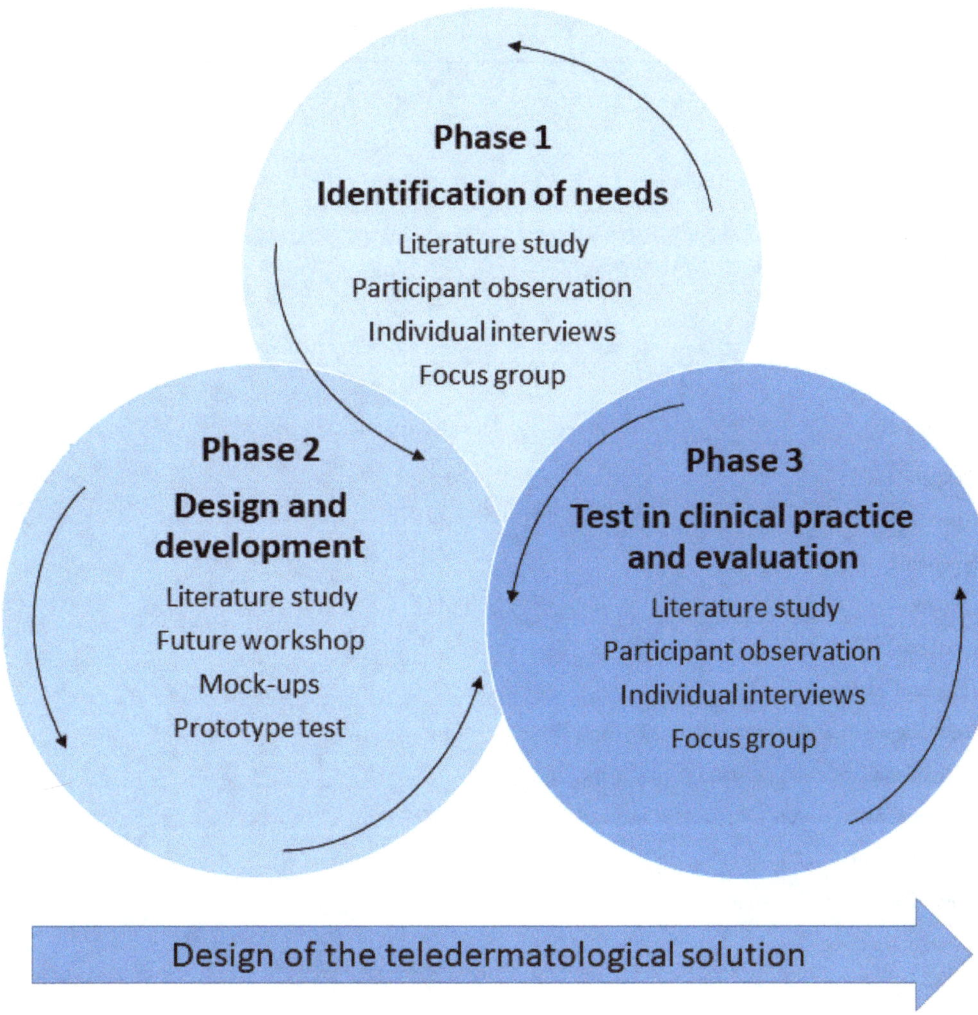

Setting

The study was conducted at an outpatient clinic of a university hospital in Denmark. Workshops and prototype testing were conducted between April and December 2019. We conducted several workshops: (1) 1 future workshop in which ideas were generated based on the needs assessment of phase 1; (2) 2 mock-up workshops with patients to discuss the initial prototype; (3) 2 mock-up workshops with HCPs to discuss the initial prototype and patients' suggestions and corrections; and (4) 1 prototype test, where the initial prototype was tested in a real-life setting. At the time of data collection, patients were obliged to attend quarterly follow-ups to receive their biological medication, in accordance with national health policies.

Participants

Participants in the workshops included nurses (n=9) and physicians (n=4) with several years of experience in dermatology as well as the care and management of patients with psoriasis undergoing biological treatment. Participants' characteristics and overview of attendance are shown in Table 1. The same patients (n=3) participated in all the workshops. The patient participants were familiar with the first author, as they had contributed to their experiences of living with psoriasis in phase 1 of this study, and gave their consent to be contacted for further participation in the study. Patients were contacted by phone. In addition, a medical secretary, an IT designer, and a research team also participated. The research team consisted of a senior researcher within dermatology; a senior researcher within PD; a senior researcher within qualitative research; and the first author, who was the project leader.

Table 1. Participants' characteristics and attendance at the workshops and prototype test (N=23).

Participants and characteristics	Overview of attendance		
	Future workshop	Mock-up workshop	Prototype test
Nurse, f[a], >3 years' experience	✓	✓	
Nurse, f, >6 years' experience	✓	✓	✓
Nurse, f, >2 years' experience	✓	✓	✓
Nurse, f, >4 years' experience	✓		
Nurse, f, >13 years' experience	✓	✓	✓
Nurse, f, >3 years' experience	✓		
Nurse, f, >7 years' experience		✓	✓
Nurse, f, >3 years' experience			✓
Nurse, f, >8 years' experience			✓
Doctor, m[b], >20 years' experience	✓		
Doctor, m, >5 years' experience			✓
Doctor, f, >10 years' experience		✓	
Doctor, f, >8 years' experience			✓
Doctor, f, >5 years' experience			✓
Medical secretary, f, >15 years' experience			✓
Patient, f, aged 54 years; moderate to severe psoriasis for 31 years	✓	✓	
Patient, f, aged 28 years; moderate to severe psoriasis for 13 years	✓	✓	
Patient, m, aged 36 years; moderate to severe psoriasis for 18 years	✓	✓	✓
Information technology designer, m	✓	✓	✓
Researcher, f, experienced in participatory design	✓		✓
Researcher, m, experienced in psoriasis	✓		✓
Researcher, f, experienced in qualitative research	✓		✓
Researcher, f, PhD student	✓	✓	✓

[a]f: female.

[b]m: male.

Data Collection and Analysis

Before the workshops and prototype testing, a detailed script describing the various steps and responsibilities was prepared and delivered to the research team and IT designers. The script included the aim of the workshops and the introduction to group exercises and plenary discussions. The study data comprised recorded transcripts from the future workshop and photographs, along with a number of written notes from all participants. Field notes taken at each mock-up workshop and the content of the discussions and suggestions for designing a prototype at the workshops were summarized in a document. Suggestions from the patients and HCPs were added to the low-fidelity prototype and served as data. During the prototype testing, all participants were given observational guides to observe and note during the test. The observational guide asked the participants to observe and note both the patients' preparation before a consultation and the interaction during the consultation. These field notes served as data along with photographs and written field notes from one of the researchers (HA).

The analysis of the data material from the workshops and prototype test was inspired by the PD approach. The steps plan, act, observe, and reflect were followed in the data analysis in an iterative process [18]. It was not possible to plan or predict the number of iterations required to develop the final prototype. Each workshop was planned by the research group based on how the previous workshop had transpired. After each workshop, the research team shared their reflections as a part of the data analysis. On the basis of this process, the next step in the design and development phase was planned, thus facilitating mutual learning through shared experiences and perspectives. As member checking is a natural part of the PD process, participants were presented with findings from the previous activity, thus allowing them to comment on and contribute to the findings and further development of the prototype. Reporting was guided by the Consolidated Criteria for Reporting Qualitative Studies [21].

Future Workshop

A 2-hour future workshop was conducted to identify new approaches in clinical practice through a joint critique of the existing approach [22]. The future workshop comprised 3 phases: phase 1, a critique phase; phase 2, a vision phase; and phase 3, a reality phase. In the critique phase, participants were informed about the aim of the workshop and then presented with findings from ethnographic field studies [1]. Selected findings were available in writing, together with photographs of the consultations taken during the participant observation from phase 1. The participants were then divided into 2 groups and encouraged to select the critique findings that they considered most suitable. They were also encouraged to write down additional critiques. Notes were written on post-it labels and placed on posters. Each phase of the future workshop had its own poster. In groups, they were asked to prioritize and select which points of critique they would proceed with. In the second phase of the future workshop, the vision phase, the participants were asked to convert the critique into positive ideas by asking "What if...?" They were asked to be creative and use their thoughts, visions, and dreams and to discuss categories and select the most important and significant topics. In the third phase, the reality phase, participants were asked to come up with ideas by asking "We do that by..." to create more specific and clear strategies to realize the visions. The words "What if...?" and "We do that by..." were printed on cards for the participants to fill out. The workshop was audio-recorded and further documented using notes and photos.

Mock-up Workshops

The research group created a low-fidelity prototype, and several mock-up workshops were conducted to explore its content and detail it further. At the mock-up workshops, the aim was to further design the solution based on the results of the future workshop. The solution was an app to empower the patients. It aimed to give them the opportunity to prepare ahead of follow-up consultations and allow for video consultations. Due to organizational circumstances, it was not possible for patients and HCPs to meet at the workshops. Therefore, they were conducted iteratively with HCPs and patients separately to achieve a continuous feedback and ensure the true emancipation of PD. The various features of the app were presented to the participants, and suggestions and critiques were written down on a poster.

Prototype Test

A high-fidelity prototype was developed based on the results from the previous workshops. As this prototype also allowed for video consultations and for patients to fill out 2 questionnaires before consultations, a prototype test was required. The 2-hour prototype test was conducted at the outpatient clinic, in the usual consultation rooms, to ensure that the setting was a realistic environment. The aim was to ensure a continued co-design with users and to test the technology. First, the participants were introduced to the prototype. They were then asked to play out a follow-up consultation based on the completed questionnaires. The set-up was planned so that it was as close to reality as possible. For this reason, doctors, nurses, and patients represented themselves. The remaining participants were equipped with observational guides and asked to make notes and write down questions, suggestions, and reflections during the consultation. Two consultations were performed simultaneously. Subsequently, the video consultations were conducted. Again, each participant represented themselves in their usual role in clinical practice, apart from one HCP, who acted as a patient, as only one patient showed up. This HCP is referred to as a patient in the following *Results* section. One video consultation was conducted during a plenary session. Those who did not participate in the consultations were asked to fill out the observational guides. The process was documented by field notes from all participants as well as photos taken by the research group. The prototype test was finalized with an evaluation of all the participants.

Ethics

All participants received oral and written information about the study, in accordance with the applicable ethical rules [23], and gave their written consent. The Danish Data Protection Agency (2012-58-0018) approved the study.

Results

Future Workshop

The most common suggestion for change in clinical practice was the inclusion of a more patient-centered approach. In this approach, patients would be given the opportunity to contribute to the agenda of the consultations, which were perceived as being impersonal and repetitive. Patients expressed that they wanted to have a say in what would be discussed, rather than "just answering the same questions over and over again.":

> *I know you have to inform about smoking, but don't say it to me every time. There must be some information missing in your IT system, or something.* [Patient]

Patients also requested flexibility and that they would not have to attend in person every 3 months. General information regarding psoriasis and comorbidities was considered important. However, even though participants were asked about their weights or smoking habits, no strategies for how to improve, for example, lifestyle behavior, were proffered. Both patients and HCPs emphasized that the future care and management of patients with psoriasis should focus on communication and mutual relations:

> *Up here, I haven't had a regular nurse, so I actually have no relationship with anyone.* [Patient]

Another significant issue for patients was the lack of continuity in meeting HCPs. One patient pointed out that she had been a patient at the outpatient clinic for 8 years but always met new medical doctors at consultations. The workshop further revealed that not all patients were offered the same services, for example, an appointment with a dietitian. These services or opportunities should be made visible and offered equally to all patients. This would give them the opportunity to discuss, for example, their nutrition habits with the HCP. In the reality phase of the future workshop, participants proposed that some of the abovementioned items could be offered in video consultations and prepared at home ahead of consultations:

> *What if maybe we only need to see them physically twice a year?* [Nurse]

What if the patient was given the opportunity in advance to fill in a form from home electronically [about] some areas they would like to talk about. Then you could run the consultation based on that. [Nurse]

Patients also questioned having to attend in-person to collect their medication. The findings from the future workshop were depicted in a drawing, whose purpose was to serve as a design artifact for further elaboration at the mock-up workshops (for the English version, see Multimedia Appendix 1).

Mock-up Workshops

On the basis of the results from the future workshop, it was decided to design an app for patients with psoriasis undergoing biological treatment, with the intention of meeting their needs and requests related to daily life with psoriasis and follow-up visits. HCPs acknowledged this move as a possible and appropriate solution. A low-fidelity prototype (for the English version, see Multimedia Appendix 2) was designed, and features and possible content were discussed with patients, HCPs, and an IT designer. Patients pointed out the importance of using the *good stories* to communicate knowledge and information about disease and treatment and that written knowledge and information should highlight that "you can have a good life with psoriasis.":

I think it is insanely important that patients are also told that you can actually have or get a good life with psoriasis, it gives, like, hope. [Patient]

The low-fidelity prototype included the registration of patient data, such as the self-monitoring of blood pressure, pulse, and weight. The Dermatology Quality of Life Questionnaire (DLQI) was embedded in the app. Normally, these measurements are taken at all in-person consultations. The low-fidelity prototype would make it possible for patients to complete the DLQI at home and register their patient data, meaning that this information would be automatically digitally received at the hospital. The HCPs discussed the importance of integrating the opportunity for patients to prepare ahead of consultations and that the main focus of consultations would be what is important to the patients. An existing questionnaire developed by the nurses was presented, evaluated, and adjusted by 5 new patients who did not participate in the workshops. This was done to ensure that it was also comprehensible for patients not involved in the design process. The questionnaire called preparation before consultation gave the patients several topics that could be discussed at their next consultation, including a free-text space for questions or comments. A feature in the app called preparation before consultation was designed, and the questionnaires and patient data were gathered to help patients prepare before a consultation. Furthermore, HCPs requested the development of a medication function that would allow them to order, distribute, and track patients' medication, using a track and trace feature. Likewise, patients requested a track and trace function of their medication.

Prototype Testing

On the basis of the suggestions, corrections, and further development, a high-fidelity prototype app called *Psoriasis* was designed (for the English version, see the Multimedia Appendix 3). It was based on an existing platform at the university hospital called *My Hospital*. *My hospital* is a digital platform developed to facilitate communication between the hospital and patients and is integrated in the patients' personal electronic medical records. For prototype testing in December 2019, *Psoriasis* was activated in a real-life setting. In testing the preparation feature, patients were asked to fill out the self-monitoring data, the DLQI questionnaire, and the preparation before consultation questionnaire before attending a face-to-face consultation. The HCPs were instructed on how to conduct a consultation based on the feature data and responses. There was an overall agreement that whenever the questionnaire preparation before consultation was used during the consultations, it changed the content of and approach to the consultations in a positive way, by focusing on the patients' needs and requests:

The doctor refers to a form on which the patient has noted sadness—and they talk about it. The doctor asks what the patient has been done about it and the patient says he has started seeing a psychologist. The nurse enters the dialogue and confirms the patient's problems (has known the patient for several years). Eye contact is maintained throughout. [Field note]

However, for HCPs, it was challenging to change their practice and not return to their previous routines and questions:

The doctor asks direct questions about psoriasis and treatment. They talk back and forth about the treatment and the doctor asks, "Do you have any side effects?" To which the patient replies, "No, I have a bit on my scalp." They talk about possible treatment. The patient refers to the form and the doctor asks: "Where?" The doctor finds it and addresses what has been ticked. [Field note]

One patient mentioned including a question about travel plans, as this is important due to traveling with biological medication.

In testing the video function, patients and HCPs were instructed as described above. For the video test, we used an iPad (Apple Inc) and a regular workstation in the outpatient clinic. Patients used their own devices. The functionality was good for both sound and picture. Patients were positive and expressed the personal advantages of video consultations. However, they suggested providing a guide in the app regarding how to initiate video consultations. Some HCPs were more reluctant and emphasized the need to meet and get to know patients before offering a video consultation because observing reactions, signs, and nonverbal communication was found to be challenging. Despite this, they acknowledged the patients' perspectives.

Final Design

HCPs and patients (including those who did not attend the prototype test) were asked to comment on the interface, usability, and content of the high-fidelity prototype. Small adjustments were made based on these comments, for example, the inclusion of more pictures to visualize the different types of psoriasis and a podcast on living with psoriasis (Table 2).

Table 2. Overview of the features in the app based on the identified needs.

Identified needs	Features in the app	Potential impact
Information about psoriasis and treatment	Knowledge database contains information about • Psoriasis • What psoriasis looks like • Comorbidities • Medications • Video recording of how to inject oneself • Video recording of emollient treatment	To support patients with psoriasis by providing them with knowledge
Information about biological treatment	Knowledge database contains information about • Biological treatment • Biosimilar treatment • Decision on treatment start • Addressing patients' fear of discontinuance	To support patients and include them in the process of receiving biologics and encourage them in addressing their concerns
Information about living with psoriasis	Knowledge database contains information about • Diet, exercise, smoking, alcohol, and stress • Being together with others • A podcast about living with psoriasis	To provide patients with information about lifestyle-related issues and addressing psychological aspects
Preparation before attending a consultation	Information to prepare the patients before attending a consultation, including patient data • DLQI[a] questionnaire and the questionnaire "prepare before consultation" • Self-monitoring of blood pressure, pulse, weight, and urine • Free-text space	To support patients in self-management, preparation before a consultation, and contributing to the agenda
Reducing in-person consultations	• Video consultations for Android and IOS • Guidance on how to attend a video consultation • Messages to the Department of Dermatology to address nonurgent questions • Information about where to pick up the biological treatment (link to map)	To support communication between the patients and HCPs[b] and provide care and management based on the patients' everyday life perspectives

[a]DLQI: Dermatology Quality of Life Questionnaire.

[b]HCP: health care professional.

Discussion

Principal Findings

In this study, an mHealth app for patients with psoriasis undergoing biological treatment was designed, adjusted, and tested through a PD process in close collaboration with patients, HCPs, IT designers, and fellow researchers. The future workshop revealed that users' needs could be met by an app. Its use could replace in-person follow-up visits; it can be used at in-person visits and can facilitate person-centered care. The iterative process enabled us to continuously revise, redesign, and test the app until a solution that reflected the needs of the end users emerged. This highlights the importance of using PD, in which users, designers, and researchers collaborate in the design and development of new health care services. The use of PD and thus the importance of user participation and democratic processes in the medical field have been acknowledged for many years [24].

mHealth interventions have been widely used in the management of chronic conditions [25-27] and have the potential to successfully support the process. However, the use of interdisciplinary team–based approaches in the process of designing and developing mHealth solutions is essential, given that it facilitates an understanding of the context in which the solution will be used by patients and HCPs and ensures that the solution is compatible with patients' needs and clinical demands [28].

For this study, we established a team that represented patients and stakeholders from all levels within the field, that is, the management of patients with psoriasis undergoing biological treatment. Thus, they were all familiar with the health care context and daily life with psoriasis. However, the prototype test revealed that HCPs were somewhat reluctant to use video consultations, as they were concerned about not being able to observe the patients' nonverbal communication. Conversely, the patients experienced video consultations as suitable and convenient. This highlights not only the important democratic aspects of PD but also the shift of power dynamics in the PD process [29]. Giving patients a voice as to how they prefer the management of their condition in daily life provides HCPs with new insights and understanding, and this mutual understanding may have had a significant impact on the acceptability and implementation of the app in this study.

Likewise, the future workshop contributed to mutual learning, as it revealed that usual consultations were perceived as impersonal and repetitive. In addition, it emerged that patients would actually like to *have a say* in what to discuss and have the chance to contribute to the agenda for follow-up visits. Future workshops emphasize critique, learning, teamwork, democracy, and empowerment, which make them suitable for use in PD [22]. Future workshops were developed by Jungk [22], who believed that utopian and fantasy-based ideas and strategies for the future could be created through critique. Being creative is naturally accompanied by open mindedness; however, in practice, mental blocks often occur, thus hindering creative thinking [30]. The use of "What if..." and "We do that by..." cards in our future workshop supported the participants in being creative and share their ideas and visions for their future consultations. The use of this tool and technique engaged the participants in telling, making, and enacting [31]. Despite striving for the true emancipation and engagement of all end users, not all of the needs and requests of the end users could be met. The design and development of a technological medication delivery system have failed. Biological medication and its management are highly regulated, as this is an expensive medication that is prescribed free of charge for patients. For this reason, it was not possible to prescribe the existing web-based system in the region of Southern Denmark. However, an agreement was made among local hospitals in the region. In the future, the biological medicine will be sent to the hospital closest to the patient for distribution. The prescription and ordering of medication would continue to be made as usual on paper, which made it impossible to deliver push messages to patients when their medication had arrived. This was presented to the participants at the mock-up workshops, followed by an explanation of the existing technology and policy practices regarding biological medicine. Kyhn [32] argues that by providing end users with details about the structure and content of the emerging system, we support them in developing an understanding of the opportunities and limitations that go beyond the present interface. Therefore, mutual learning can be fostered, as we develop a shared understanding of the practice and potentials.

While engaging in a PD project, user activities are often creative and experimental, involving all stakeholders [17]. As, in our study, it was not possible for both patients and HCPs to attend a mock-up workshop at the same time, we decided to conduct several small mock-up workshops in iterative processes. The reason for this was to ensure that all stakeholders would *have a say* in the design and could influence the outcome, thereby staying true to one of the core elements of PD. Expanding the creativity in the PD process itself, for example, conducting *one-to-one* workshops, may be acceptable and may still facilitate empowerment among patients and HCPs [33].

This study was a small, single-center study connected to a clinical setting, which may put transferability in question. However, this is not an uncommon setting for qualitative research. In addition, the design process was based on findings from previous qualitative field and interview studies, thus including experiences and perspectives from other groups of patients with psoriasis and experienced HCPs. A limitation of this study was that only one patient was included in the prototype test. All 3 patients were invited, but 2 of them canceled a few hours before the test. Limited user participation is a known practical limitation in PD [34]; however, because the patients were a part of the other workshops and had planned for the mHealth solution to be tested in clinical practice, we decided to conduct the prototype test. Again, creativity and readjustment were necessary, and a HCP acted as a patient during the prototype test. To overcome this barrier, the mHealth solution was tested further in clinical practice, but it will be reported in a separate paper.

Conclusions

Results from the future workshop, mock-up workshops, and the prototype test, based on findings from ethnographic field studies, led to the design of an app for patients with psoriasis receiving biological treatment. By using PD that facilitated mutual learning and democratic processes, end users exerted a significant impact on the solution, given that it was customized to both clinical practice and end users' needs. The app provided both HCPs and patients the opportunity to facilitate a new approach in clinical practice. Despite the advantages of using PD in the development of mHealth solutions, organizational factors may still represent a barrier to the most desirable solution.

Acknowledgments

Funding for this project was provided by The University of Southern Denmark, Odense University Hospital, Kirsten Wehnerts og Robert Wehnerts Fond, and Novartis (grant DK1809880731). The authors would like to thank all the participants for their time, creativity, and effort throughout this project.

References

1. Trettin B, Feldman SR, Andersen F, Danbjørg DB, Agerskov H. A changed life: the life experiences of patients with psoriasis receiving biological treatment. Br J Dermatol 2020 Sep;183(3):516-523. [doi: 10.1111/bjd.18876] [Medline: 31953845]
2. Trettin B, Feldman S, Andersen F, Danbjørg DB, Agerskov H. Improving management of psoriasis patients receiving biological treatment: a qualitative approach. Nurs Open 2021 Jan 01:745 [FREE Full text] [doi: 10.1002/nop2.745] [Medline: 33385301]

3. Finch TL, Mort M, Mair FS, May CR. Future patients? Telehealthcare, roles and responsibilities. Health Soc Care Community 2008 Jan;16(1):86-95. [doi: 10.1111/j.1365-2524.2007.00726.x] [Medline: 18181818]
4. Bashshur RL, Shannon GW, Tejasvi T, Kvedar JC, Gates M. The empirical foundations of teledermatology: a review of the research evidence. Telemed J E Health 2015 Dec;21(12):953-979 [FREE Full text] [doi: 10.1089/tmj.2015.0146] [Medline: 26394022]
5. Massone C, Lozzi GP, Wurm E, Hofmann-Wellenhof R, Schoellnast R, Zalaudek I, et al. Cellular phones in clinical teledermatology. Arch Dermatol 2005 Oct;141(10):1319-1320. [doi: 10.1001/archderm.141.10.1319] [Medline: 16230577]
6. Ebner C, Wurm EM, Binder B, Kittler H, Lozzi GP, Massone C, et al. Mobile teledermatology: a feasibility study of 58 subjects using mobile phones. J Telemed Telecare 2008;14(1):2-7. [doi: 10.1258/jtt.2007.070302] [Medline: 18318921]
7. Schreier G, Hayn D, Kastner P, Koller S, Salmhofer W, Hofmann-Wellenhof R. A mobile-phone based teledermatology system to support self-management of patients suffering from psoriasis. Annu Int Conf IEEE Eng Med Biol Soc 2008;2008:5338-5341. [doi: 10.1109/IEMBS.2008.4650420] [Medline: 19163923]
8. Hayn D, Koller S, Hofmann-Wellenhof R, Salmhofer W, Kastner P, Schreier G. Mobile phone-based teledermatologic compliance management - preliminary results of the TELECOMP study. Stud Health Technol Inform 2009;150:468-472. [Medline: 19745356]
9. Frühauf J, Schwantzer G, Ambros-Rudolph CM, Weger W, Ahlgrimm-Siess V, Salmhofer W, et al. Pilot study on the acceptance of mobile teledermatology for the home monitoring of high-need patients with psoriasis. Australas J Dermatol 2012 Feb;53(1):41-46. [doi: 10.1111/j.1440-0960.2011.00852.x] [Medline: 22309330]
10. Koller S, Hofmann-Wellenhof R, Hayn D, Weger W, Kastner P, Schreier G, et al. Teledermatological monitoring of psoriasis patients on biologic therapy. Acta Derm Venereol 2011 Oct;91(6):680-685 [FREE Full text] [doi: 10.2340/00015555-1148] [Medline: 21879250]
11. Armstrong AW, Chambers CJ, Maverakis E, Cheng MY, Dunnick CA, Chren M, et al. Effectiveness of online vs in-person care for adults with psoriasis: a randomized clinical trial. JAMA Netw Open 2018 Oct 05;1(6):e183062 [FREE Full text] [doi: 10.1001/jamanetworkopen.2018.3062] [Medline: 30646223]
12. Ford AR, Gibbons CM, Torres J, Kornmehl HA, Singh S, Young PM, et al. Access to dermatological care with an innovative online model for psoriasis management: results from a randomized controlled trial. Telemed J E Health 2019 Jul;25(7):619-627 [FREE Full text] [doi: 10.1089/tmj.2018.0160] [Medline: 30222518]
13. Ariens LF, Schussler-Raymakers FM, Frima C, Flinterman A, Hamminga E, Arents BW, et al. Barriers and facilitators to ehealth use in daily practice: perspectives of patients and professionals in dermatology. J Med Internet Res 2017 Sep 05;19(9):e300 [FREE Full text] [doi: 10.2196/jmir.7512] [Medline: 28874336]
14. Jennett P, Yeo M, Pauls M, Graham J. Organizational readiness for telemedicine: implications for success and failure. J Telemed Telecare 2003 Dec 02;9 Suppl 2(2_suppl):27-30. [doi: 10.1258/135763303322596183] [Medline: 14728753]
15. Armfield NR, Edirippulige SK, Bradford N, Smith AC. Telemedicine-is the cart being put before the horse? Med J Aust 2014 May 19;200(9):530-533. [doi: 10.5694/mja13.11101] [Medline: 24835716]
16. Greis C, Meier Zürcher C, Djamei V, Moser A, Lautenschlager S, Navarini AA. Unmet digital health service needs in dermatology patients. J Dermatolog Treat 2018 Nov;29(7):643-647. [doi: 10.1080/09546634.2018.1441488] [Medline: 29455570]
17. Clemensen J, Larsen SB, Kyng M, Kirkevold M. Participatory design in health sciences: using cooperative experimental methods in developing health services and computer technology. Qual Health Res 2007 Jan;17(1):122-130. [doi: 10.1177/1049732306293664] [Medline: 17170250]
18. Clemensen J, Rothmann MJ, Smith AC, Caffery LJ, Danbjorg DB. Participatory design methods in telemedicine research. J Telemed Telecare 2016 Jan 01. [doi: 10.1177/1357633X16686747] [Medline: 28027678]
19. Clemensen J. Pervasive healthcare: home treatment of patients with diabetic foot ulcers. 2006. URL: https://tinyurl.com/5bm2cheu [accessed 2021-04-24]
20. Rudd J, Stern K, Isensee S. Low vs. high-fidelity prototyping debate. interactions 1996 Jan 02;3(1):76-85. [doi: 10.1145/223500.223514]
21. Tong A, Sainsbury P, Craig J. Consolidated criteria for reporting qualitative research (COREQ): a 32-item checklist for interviews and focus groups. Int J Qual Health Care 2007 Dec 16;19(6):349-357. [doi: 10.1093/intqhc/mzm042] [Medline: 17872937]
22. Jungk R, Müllert N, Institute for Social Inventions. Future Workshops : How to Create Desirable Futures. London: Institute for Social Inventions; 1987:1-126.
23. World Medical Association. World Medical Association Declaration of Helsinki: ethical principles for medical research involving human subjects. J Am Med Assoc 2013 Nov 27;310(20):2191-2194. [doi: 10.1001/jama.2013.281053] [Medline: 24141714]
24. Palmer VJ, Weavell W, Callander R, Piper D, Richard L, Maher L, et al. The Participatory Zeitgeist: an explanatory theoretical model of change in an era of coproduction and codesign in healthcare improvement. Med Humanit 2019 Sep;45(3):247-257 [FREE Full text] [doi: 10.1136/medhum-2017-011398] [Medline: 29954854]
25. Lim S, Kang SM, Shin H, Lee HJ, Won Yoon J, Yu SH, et al. Improved glycemic control without hypoglycemia in elderly diabetic patients using the ubiquitous healthcare service, a new medical information system. Diabetes Care 2011 Feb 26;34(2):308-313 [FREE Full text] [doi: 10.2337/dc10-1447] [Medline: 21270188]

26. Nguyen HQ, Wolpin S, Chiang KC, Cuenco D, Carrieri-Kohlman V. Exercise and symptom monitoring with a mobile device. AMIA Annu Symp Proc 2006:1047 [FREE Full text] [Medline: 17238666]
27. Bellamy N, Wilson C, Hendrikz J, Whitehouse SL, Patel B, Dennison S, EDC Study Group. Osteoarthritis Index delivered by mobile phone (m-WOMAC) is valid, reliable, and responsive. J Clin Epidemiol 2011 Feb;64(2):182-190. [doi: 10.1016/j.jclinepi.2010.03.013] [Medline: 20609562]
28. Matthew-Maich N, Harris L, Ploeg J, Markle-Reid M, Valaitis R, Ibrahim S, et al. Designing, implementing, and evaluating mobile health technologies for managing chronic conditions in older adults: a scoping review. JMIR Mhealth Uhealth 2016 Jun 09;4(2):e29 [FREE Full text] [doi: 10.2196/mhealth.5127] [Medline: 27282195]
29. Bratteteig T, Bødker K, Dittrich Y, Mogensen PH, Simonsen J. Methods: organising principles and general guidelines for Participatory Design projects. In: Routledge International Handbook of Participatory Design. Milton, UK: Routledge; 2013:137-164.
30. Troxler P, Kuhnt B. Future workshops - the unthinkable and how to make it happen. Hands-On Knowledge Co-Creation and Sharing: Practical Methods and Techniques. 2007. URL: https://surfsharekit.nl/objectstore/515a2c91-e9e6-4bd8-acfe-d7431a8f13e0 [accessed 2021-04-24]
31. Brandt E, Binder T, Sanders E. Tools and techniques: ways to engage telling, making and enacting. In: Routledge International Handbook of Participatory Design. Milton, UK: Routledge; 2013:145-181.
32. Kyng M. Making representations work. Commun ACM 1995 Sep;38(9):46-55. [doi: 10.1145/223248.223261]
33. Jensen CM, Overgaard S, Wiil UK, Smith AC, Clemensen J. Bridging the gap: a user-driven study on new ways to support self-care and empowerment for patients with hip fracture. SAGE Open Med 2018 Sep 07;6 [FREE Full text] [doi: 10.1177/2050312118799121] [Medline: 30210796]
34. Spinuzzi C. The methodology of participatory design. Technical Communication. 2005. URL: https://repositories.lib.utexas.edu/bitstream/handle/2152/28277/SpinuzziTheMethodologyOfParticipatoryDesign.pdf [accessed 2021-04-24]

Abbreviations

DLQI: Dermatology Quality of Life Questionnaire
HCP: health care professional
IT: information technology
mHealth: mobile health
PD: participatory design
TD: teledermatology

22

Analysis of Keywords Used in Internet Searches for Melanoma Information

Japbani K Nanda[1], BS; Jennifer L Hay[2], PhD; Michael A Marchetti[1], MD

[1]Dermatology Service, Department of Medicine, Memorial Sloan Kettering Cancer Center, New York, NY, United States

[2]Department of Psychiatry and Behavioral Sciences, Memorial Sloan Kettering Cancer Center, New York, NY, United States

Corresponding Author:
Michael A Marchetti, MD
Dermatology Service
Department of Medicine
Memorial Sloan Kettering Cancer Center
530 E 74th St
New York, NY, 10021
United States

Email: marchetm@mskcc.org

Abstract

Background: The internet is an accessible resource for health care information and is often used by patients to learn about melanoma. The keywords that are used in internet searches can reflect internet users' interest in specific topics and the public's awareness of health-related issues.

Objective: This study aims to describe the most frequently used keywords, questions, and corresponding websites in internet searches for melanoma.

Methods: This is an observational study using data retrieved from Google Trends, Alexa Internet, SEMrush, Ahrefs, and SE Ranking for the keywords "melanoma" and "skin cancer."

Results: Average search interest as per Google Trends was greater for the keyword "skin cancer" than for the keyword "melanoma." Searches for the top 25 keywords in 3 databases resulted in 34 unique melanoma keywords and 33 unique skin cancer keywords. Melanoma keywords were most frequently related to clinicopathologic classification (n=11, 32%), and skin cancer keywords were most frequently about diagnosis (n=14, 42%). Questions about the prognosis of melanoma appeared most frequently among the most popular melanoma questions, but general questions or questions about the diagnosis of melanoma contributed the greatest proportion of searches by search volume. Skin cancer question searches were most commonly about diagnosis. The highest proportion of searches for popular melanoma and skin cancer keywords most frequently sent traffic to websites from nonprofit organizations and media companies, respectively.

Conclusions: We identified common keywords, questions, and websites used to access information about melanoma on the internet. These data may help health care providers and public health professionals when educating and counseling patients and the public about skin cancer.

KEYWORDS

internet; melanoma; skin cancer; health information; search; keyword; question; website; cost-per-click

Introduction

In 2017, there were an estimated 1.2 million people living with invasive melanoma in the United States [1]. People may choose from a number of information sources to learn about melanoma, including the internet. In 2019, 90% of US adults used the internet, and 72% reported that they looked for medical or health information for themselves using a smartphone, computer, or other electronic means [2,3]. Although 95% of patients with melanoma at the University of Michigan reported that their physician provided sufficient information, 83% still looked to the internet for more information about melanoma [4]. Younger respondents, females, those with a higher level of education, and those diagnosed with melanoma were found to be more likely to search the internet for information about their diagnosis [4]. Although the majority of patients described their use of the internet as a positive experience, one-third of patients with melanoma have reported higher anxiety after internet use [4].

Researchers have previously studied trends in internet searches related to skin cancer. Using Google Trends, Bloom et al [5] found that internet searches for the terms "melanoma" and "skin cancer" in the United States increased each summer from 2010 to 2014. The peak for skin cancer searches occurred in May, which is skin cancer awareness month, suggesting a possible association with outreach programs [6]. German studies of Google search volume spanning 2013-2018 found that the most frequently used keywords for internet searches related to skin cancer were "skin cancer," "white skin cancer," "basalioma," and "melanoma" [7,8]. Internet users searched for information about skin cancer types, identification, and skin changes [8]. The variety of search terms and questions used by internet users and the resulting websites accessed for information related to melanoma are not well characterized, particularly in the United States. Given the widespread use of the internet for health information broadly and skin cancer information specifically, our objective is to describe the keywords and questions used in melanoma internet searches. We also seek to identify the most frequently accessed websites for corresponding keyword searches.

Methods

Databases

This study was exempt from Institutional Review Board review because the data were publicly available. Data were obtained from multiple online databases: Google Trends [9], Alexa Internet [10], SEMrush [11], Ahrefs (URL Rating and Ahrefs Top) [12], and SE Ranking [13]. Google Trends provides keyword search interest data. Alexa, SEMrush, Ahrefs, and SE Ranking provide keyword or website analysis tools. Data from Alexa originates from the use of one of more than 25,000 browser extensions by millions of global internet users and from sites that install an Alexa script and permit Alexa to measure site traffic [14,15]. SEMrush uses third-party data providers to collect Google's search results for the 500 million most popular keywords and collects information about websites in the top 100 positions [16]. Ahrefs uses independently obtained data across 10 different search engines (ie, does not use output from Alexa, Google, etc), processes clickstream data, and has the world's largest third-party search query database [17,18]. SE Ranking is a cloud-based search engine optimization and marketing tool that tracks real-time website rankings for major search engines [19]. Data were extracted from databases on June 21, 2020, and analyzed using descriptive statistics.

Keyword Search Interest and Search Volume

We defined a keyword as a term that is entered into a search engine (like Google), which subsequently lists websites on a results page. As internet users may initially search for information about melanoma with a more general term such as skin cancer, we performed searches and analyses for both melanoma and skin cancer. To determine search term interest (ranging from 0 to 100), we extracted US and worldwide web search data using Google Trends' term comparison functionality to compare the terms "melanoma" and "skin cancer." Search interest at a given time is presented relative to the peak popularity for a search term, which is indicated by a score of 100. We also recorded average monthly keyword search volumes over a 12-month period using SEMrush and Ahrefs.

Keyword Popularity and Search Volume Analysis

We extracted the 25 most popular keywords related to melanoma and skin cancer searches using Alexa, SEMrush, and Ahrefs. For keywords that appeared in the first 25 consecutively listed keywords for one database but not another, the corresponding ranking in each database was recorded, if available. In Alexa, we determined the website with the highest share of voice for the keyword "melanoma." Share of voice refers to the proportion of searches made for a keyword that result in traffic receipt by a specific website. Within the "Keyword Clusters" tool for organic keywords, we selected the melanoma cluster and ranked keywords by popularity (ranging from 0 to 100), which is updated monthly and indicates the relative frequency of searches for that keyword. In SEMrush, we searched for "melanoma" in the "Keyword Magic Tool" (US database) using the exact match filter, sorted by average monthly volume of searches during a 1-year period. In Ahrefs, we searched for "melanoma" in the "Keywords explorer" (Google, US database) using the phrase match filter, sorted by average monthly volume of searches. This process was similarly performed for the keyword "skin cancer" using Alexa, SEMrush, and Ahrefs. Keywords were classified into one of eight categories: general, diagnosis, clinicopathologic classification, etiology, prognosis, treatment, prevention, or screening.

Keyword Advertising and Associated Websites

Keyword cost-per-click (CPC; USD) was recorded, if available, using SEMrush (based on Google Ads) and Ahrefs (based on multiple search engines). CPC is the average price paid by advertisers when their advertisement is clicked on in the results for that keyword. We recorded Alexa's indicator of paid competition (ranging from 0 to 100), which is updated monthly and reflects the amount of advertisements that appear on major search engines for a searched keyword. We recorded the websites with the highest keyword share of voice per Alexa for each popular keyword. The organizations associated with popular websites were classified as nonprofit, media company, government, charity, or medical practice [20-35].

Melanoma and Skin Cancer–Related Questions

The first 25 consecutively listed search questions related to melanoma and skin cancer were recorded using SEMrush's "Keyword Magic Tool" (US database) and Ahrefs's "Keywords explorer" (Google, US database). In SEMrush, questions were identified using the exact match filter and ranked based on average monthly volume of searches during a 1-year period. In Ahrefs, questions were ranked based on the average monthly volume of searches. Questions were classified into the same categories as keywords (previously mentioned).

Popular Websites for Highest Ranked Melanoma and Skin Cancer Keywords

For the single most popular melanoma and skin cancer keywords, we used Alexa, Ahrefs, and SE Ranking to determine the 10 websites that received the highest share of voice of organic traffic or were the highest ranked. Alexa provided the websites with the highest share of voice during the prior 6 months. In Ahrefs, the websites were ranked by monthly estimated search traffic (Google, US). SE Ranking provided websites ranked on data from April 2020 (Google, US). For websites that appeared in the top 10 for one database and not another, the corresponding ranking for that website in each database was noted if available.

Results

Search Interest and Search Volume

"Skin cancer" was more frequently used than "melanoma" as a search term per Google Trends. From January 2004 to June 2020, average search term interest in the United States was 62 (min-max: 39-100) for "skin cancer" and 49 (min-max: 32-76) for "melanoma." In June 2020 specifically, search term interest was 71 for "skin cancer" and 48 for "melanoma." Worldwide, "skin cancer" was also more frequently used than "melanoma" (data not shown). The average US monthly search volume for the keyword "melanoma" was 246,000 (SEMrush) and 243,000 (Ahrefs); global estimates were 585,500 (SEMrush) and 644,000 (Ahrefs). The average US monthly search volume for the keyword "skin cancer" was 301,000 (SEMrush) and 190,000 (Ahrefs); global estimates were 547,300 (SEMrush) and 356,000 (Ahrefs).

Popular Keywords

There were 34 unique keywords among the top 25 melanoma-related keywords in Alexa, SEMrush, and Ahrefs (Multimedia Appendix 1, Table S1). Keywords that appeared in the top 10 of all 3 databases were "melanoma," "malignant melanoma," "ocular melanoma," "metastatic melanoma," "melanoma symptoms," "melanoma cancer," "nodular melanoma," and "melanoma pictures." Keywords were most frequently related to melanoma clinicopathologic classification (n=11, 32%). There were 33 unique keywords among the top 25 skin cancer–related keywords in Alexa, SEMrush, and Ahrefs (Multimedia Appendix 1, Table S2). Keywords that appeared in the top 10 of all 3 databases were "skin cancer," "skin cancer types," "skin cancer pictures," "what does skin cancer look like," "skin cancer symptoms," "skin cancer images," and "signs of skin cancer." Keywords were most frequently related to skin cancer diagnosis (n=14, 42%).

Keyword Advertising and Commonly Accessed Websites

Using advertising competition data (paid competition and CPC) from multiple databases for the most popular keywords and questions in internet searches for melanoma and skin cancer, the keyword or question associated with the highest or one of the highest indicators of advertising competition (in the case of a tie) was related to treatment in 7 out of 10 cases. The keyword or question associated with the lowest indicator of advertising competition was related to diagnosis in 8 out of 10 cases.

A total of 11 unique websites had the highest share of voice per Alexa for the 34 melanoma keywords, and cancer.org (nonprofit; n=10, 29%) was the most frequent (Multimedia Appendix 1, Table S1). A total of 5 unique websites had the highest share of voice for the 33 skin cancer keywords, and webmd.com (media company; n=18, 55%) was the most frequent (Multimedia Appendix 1, Table S2).

Popular Question Searches

The top 25 question searches about melanoma are shown in Multimedia Appendix 1, Table S3. Questions related to melanoma that appeared in the top 5 of SEMrush or Ahrefs were "what is melanoma," "what does melanoma look like," "does melanoma itch," "what causes melanoma," "what is melanoma cancer," "what is the first sign of melanoma," "what does early signs of melanoma look like," and "where does melanoma spread to first." Among the top 25 melanoma questions, the most frequent category was prognosis (16/50, 32%). Per SEMrush, general melanoma questions contributed the greatest proportion of searches by search volume (14,440/33,400, 43.2%). Per Ahrefs, questions about the diagnosis of melanoma contributed the greatest proportion of searches by search volume (16,200/41,100, 39.4%).

The top 25 question searches about skin cancer are shown in Multimedia Appendix 1, Table S4. Questions in the top 5 were "what does skin cancer look like," "does skin cancer itch," "is skin cancer itchy," "can you die from skin cancer," "is skin cancer deadly," "how serious is basal cell skin cancer," "what is skin cancer," "what do the early stages of skin cancer look like," and "what causes skin cancer." Among the top 25 skin cancer questions, the most frequent category was diagnosis (27/50, 54%). Per SEMrush and Ahrefs, questions about diagnosis contributed the greatest proportion of searches by search volume (63,700/82,040, 77.6% and 30,400/43,400, 70.0%, respectively).

Popular Websites for Highest Ranked Keywords

The 5 most popular or highest ranked websites for the keyword "melanoma" in Alexa, Ahrefs, and SE Ranking were skincancer.org (nonprofit), cancer.org (nonprofit), wikipedia.org (nonprofit), medicalnewstoday.com (media company), and mayoclinic.org (nonprofit). The 5 most popular or highest ranked websites for the keyword "skin cancer" were webmd.com (media company), skincancer.org (nonprofit), cancer.org (nonprofit), mayoclinic.org (nonprofit), and medicinenet.com (media company; Multimedia Appendix 1, Table S5).

Discussion

Principal Findings

Herein, we described the volume of searches, popular keyword search strategies, and popular websites accessed for information about melanoma and skin cancer on the internet. The most popular melanoma and skin cancer keywords were related to clinicopathologic classification and diagnosis, respectively. Queries about diagnosis often pertained to images, signs, or symptoms of skin cancer, suggesting a greater need for publicly available high-quality images of skin cancer. Our findings suggest that internet users are interested in online resources to learn about skin cancer diagnosis. This may also reflect awareness of the importance of skin cancer detection. Similarly, an analysis of internet search terms related to skin cancer in Germany found that keyword searches were often related to skin cancer identification via images or symptoms [7]. We also found that keyword searches related to prevention were uncommon. This may represent a need for increased awareness about the importance of primary prevention. Alternatively, this may suggest that the public already has adequate knowledge about preventative measures or that different, less technical terms are used, which were not captured in our study design.

With regard to searched questions, interest was directed toward melanoma prognosis, general information about melanoma, diagnosis of melanoma, and diagnosis of skin cancer. This may reflect internet users' concerns regarding prognosis and the importance of prognostic and staging information in the determination of treatment options for melanoma. These findings further support the need for online resources with information about the detection of melanoma and skin cancer. Keyword searches related to treatment were less common for both melanoma and skin cancer. Our findings parallel the results of a German study that investigated topics of interest in internet searches related to melanoma and nonmelanoma skin cancer [8]. The study found that searches related to the treatment of skin cancer were made less frequently, while searches related to the forms of skin cancer were more common [8].

Our findings based on CPC data suggest that there is greater advertising competition for keywords related to the treatment of skin cancer than for the diagnosis of skin cancer. Nonprofit or charity-associated websites comprised 71% (24/34) and 36% (12/33) of the websites with the highest share of voice for popular melanoma and skin cancer keywords, respectively. Although cancer.org, a website of the nonprofit American Cancer Society [33], most frequently received traffic from the highest proportion of searches made for popular melanoma keywords, the highest proportion of searches for the great majority of popular skin cancer keywords sent traffic to webmd.com (WebMD LLC), which is a consumer health information brand under media company Internet Brands [31,32]. The type of website that receives a high share of traffic from internet searches may be affected by the specificity of a given keyword search as determined by the topic of interest, topic complexity, or the chosen keyword vocabulary. This is important to note because the quality and readability of health information can vary between websites associated with media companies, governmental organizations, and nonprofit groups [36-39].

An internet search for health information can affect treatment plans and serve as a topic of discussion between patients and health care providers. The majority (71%) of Canadian patients with melanoma found that information from the internet affected their decisions regarding treatment [40]. Most found the internet to be useful, albeit difficult to understand to various degrees [40]. Websites resulting from "melanoma" searches in 2017 demonstrated variability in quality and available content, as well as a higher than recommended reading level [41]. Therefore, physicians continue to play an important role by encouraging patients to discuss the findings of their internet searches for health information and addressing potential misinformation from online sources. Health care providers should be prepared to address questions or concerns that arise from patients' health-related internet searches and guide patients toward reliable online sources of information. In this way, patients can better serve as active participants and advocates for their own health.

Limitations

Our study is limited by its observational design using retrospective data and an inability to comment on the proportion of internet searches made by patients with or survivors of skin cancer or internet users at high risk for skin cancer. Nonetheless, our use of multiple keyword and website analysis services allowed us to evaluate the most popular keywords and websites accessed by the public. It is possible that internet users who searched for melanoma keywords may have been diagnosed with melanoma and sought to learn more about their diagnosis, while those who performed searches for skin cancer information may have been looking for general skin cancer information. A survey of 31 patients with melanoma found that 96% used the internet to acquire information about melanoma treatment [40]. Bloom et al [5] found a positive correlation between skin cancer search volume index and increased mortality due to melanoma, postulating that this may have been due to a higher volume of searches performed by individuals with advanced melanoma or others who were indirectly affected. Future research would be invaluable to study associations between the characteristics of internet users and specific keyword internet searches. Our study is also limited to analysis of the data as reported by keyword databases. Internet users can choose to learn about specific topics of interest or enhance their understanding of a given topic by directly clicking on links within an accessed webpage instead of performing a keyword search. Although keywords related to prevention were uncommon in our study, internet users may perform searches related to prevention using other keywords. For example, searches for sunburn prevention or sunscreen are relevant for skin cancer prevention but do not contain the keywords "melanoma" or "skin cancer."

Conclusions

Skin cancer is a public health issue that was highlighted in the US Surgeon General's call for preventative action [42]. As a highly accessible resource, the internet is a valuable educational tool for skin cancer. Our study sheds light on internet users' interests and awareness of topics related to melanoma and skin cancer. Our findings suggest that efforts should be made to ensure that the public has access to high quality information to address general concerns about melanoma and other interests related to the clinicopathologic classification, prognosis, and diagnosis of melanoma, as well as the diagnosis of skin cancer in general. This may also be an opportunity for public health professionals and clinicians to emphasize the importance of sun protective measures and skin cancer prevention. Public health professionals can create educational materials and initiate campaigns that effectively address topics of interest as expressed in internet searches while using keyword analysis to improve access to high quality resources. By understanding topics of interest, popular search queries, and frequently accessed websites for health information, clinicians can better prepare themselves to offer options for preferred information sources or critically evaluate the quality of online content accessed by patients. Familiarity with the types of skin cancer–related information that are of interest to the public and the most frequently accessed internet sources for this information may assist health care providers and public health professionals as they counsel and educate patients and the public on skin cancer.

Acknowledgments

This research is funded in part by a grant from the National Cancer Institute/National Institutes of Health (P30-CA008748).

References

1. Howlader N, Noone AM, Krapcho M, Miller D, Brest A, Yu M, et al. SEER Cancer Statistics Review 1975-2017. Surveillance, Epidemiology, and End Results Program. Bethesda, MD: National Cancer Institute; 2020 Apr. URL: https://seer.cancer.gov/csr/1975_2017/ [accessed 2020-07-08]
2. Internet/broadband fact sheet. Pew Research Center. URL: https://www.pewresearch.org/internet/fact-sheet/internet-broadband/ [accessed 2020-06-08]
3. In the past 12 months, have you used a computer, smartphone, or other electronic means to look for health or medical information for yourself? Health Information National Trends Survey. URL: https://hints.cancer.gov/view-questions-topics/question-details.aspx?PK_Cycle=12&qid=1606 [accessed 2020-07-11]
4. Ludgate MW, Sabel MS, Fullen DR, Frohm ML, Lee JS, Couper MP, et al. Internet use and anxiety in people with melanoma and nonmelanoma skin cancer. Dermatol Surg 2011 Sep;37(9):1252-1259. [doi: 10.1111/j.1524-4725.2011.02124.x] [Medline: 22988988]
5. Bloom R, Amber KT, Hu S, Kirsner R. Google search trends and skin cancer: evaluating the US population's interest in skin cancer and its association with melanoma outcomes. JAMA Dermatol 2015 Aug;151(8):903-905. [doi: 10.1001/jamadermatol.2015.1216] [Medline: 26061357]
6. Kantor J. Association of Google search volume index peaks for skin cancer with skin cancer awareness month. JAMA Dermatol 2016 Jan;152(1):113. [doi: 10.1001/jamadermatol.2015.3814] [Medline: 26762257]
7. Tizek L, Schielein MC, Rüth M, Szeimies RM, Philipp-Dormston WG, Braun SA, et al. Interest in skin cancer in urban populations: a retrospective analysis of Google search terms in nine large German cities. Acta Derm Venereol 2019 Jul 01;99(9):797-804 [FREE Full text] [doi: 10.2340/00015555-3214] [Medline: 31073622]
8. Seidl S, Schuster B, Rüth M, Biedermann T, Zink A. What do Germans want to know about skin cancer? A nationwide Google search analysis from 2013 to 2017. J Med Internet Res 2018 May 02;20(5):e10327 [FREE Full text] [doi: 10.2196/10327] [Medline: 29698213]
9. Google Trends. URL: https://trends.google.com/trends/?geo=US [accessed 2020-06-21]
10. Alexa. URL: https://www.alexa.com/ [accessed 2020-06-21]
11. Semrush. URL: https://www.semrush.com/ [accessed 2020-06-21]
12. Ahrefs. URL: https://ahrefs.com/ [accessed 2020-06-21]
13. SE Ranking. URL: https://seranking.com/ [accessed 2020-06-21]
14. Yesbeck J. Your top questions about Alexa data and ranks, answered. Alexa Blog. URL: https://blog.alexa.com/top-questions-about-alexa-answered/ [accessed 2020-07-11]
15. How do I get my site's metrics Certified? Alexa. URL: https://support.alexa.com/hc/en-us/articles/200450354-How-do-I-get-my-site-s-metrics-Certified- [accessed 2020-07-11]
16. Where does Semrush data come from? Semrush. URL: https://www.semrush.com/kb/998-where-does-semrush-data-come-from [accessed 2020-07-11]
17. Ahrefs by the numbers. Ahrefs. URL: https://ahrefs.com/big-data [accessed 2020-07-11]
18. Helen. Where do you get the data from? Ahrefs. URL: https://help.ahrefs.com/en/articles/78119-where-do-you-get-the-data-from [accessed 2020-07-11]
19. Getting started. SE Ranking. URL: https://help.seranking.com/getting-started/ [accessed 2020-07-11]
20. The Skin Cancer Foundation. URL: https://www.skincancer.org/ [accessed 2020-07-02]
21. Frequently asked questions. Mayo Clinic. URL: https://www.mayoclinic.org/giving-to-mayo-clinic/contact-us/frequently-asked-questions [accessed 2020-07-02]
22. You're on a journey to health and wellness. And we're right there with you. Healthline. URL: https://www.healthline.com/about#mission [accessed 2020-07-02]
23. Wikipedia. URL: https://www.wikipedia.org/ [accessed 2020-07-02]

24. About this website. National Cancer Institute. URL: https://www.cancer.gov/about-website [accessed 2020-07-02]
25. Frequently asked questions. DermNet NZ. URL: https://dermnetnz.org/faq/ [accessed 2020-07-02]
26. Why have a skin cancer check? Bondi Junction Skin Cancer Clinic. URL: https://www.skincancer.net.au/why-have-a-skin-check [accessed 2020-07-02]
27. Vision, mission and core values. Texas Oncology. URL: https://www.texasoncology.com/who-we-are/who-is-texas-oncology/vision-mission-core-values [accessed 2020-07-02]
28. About Dotdash. Verywell Health. URL: https://www.verywellhealth.com/about-us#AboutDotdash [accessed 2020-07-02]
29. Our story. Cancer Treatment Centers of America. URL: https://www.cancercenter.com/community/about-us/our-story [accessed 2020-07-02]
30. Academy values. American Academy of Dermatology Association. URL: https://www.aad.org/employment [accessed 2020-07-02]
31. Our business. WebMD. URL: https://www.webmd.com/corporate/our-business [accessed 2020-07-01]
32. Internet Brands. URL: https://www.internetbrands.com/ [accessed 2020-07-02]
33. Facts about the American Cancer Society. American Cancer Society. URL: https://www.cancer.org/about-us/who-we-are/fact-sheet.html [accessed 2020-07-01]
34. About us. MedicineNet. URL: https://www.medicinenet.com/script/main/art.asp?articlekey=12510 [accessed 2020-07-11]
35. About Medical News Today. Medical News Today. URL: https://www.medicalnewstoday.com/about [accessed 2020-07-11]
36. Promislow S, Walker JR, Taheri M, Bernstein CN. How well does the internet answer patients' questions about inflammatory bowel disease? Can J Gastroenterol 2010 Nov;24(11):671-677 [FREE Full text] [doi: 10.1155/2010/957264] [Medline: 21157582]
37. Pusz MD, Brietzke SE. How good is Google? The quality of otolaryngology information on the internet. Otolaryngol Head Neck Surg 2012 Sep;147(3):462-465. [doi: 10.1177/0194599812447733] [Medline: 22597577]
38. Laplante-Lévesque A, Brännström KJ, Andersson G, Lunner T. Quality and readability of English-language internet information for adults with hearing impairment and their significant others. Int J Audiol 2012 Aug;51(8):618-626. [doi: 10.3109/14992027.2012.684406] [Medline: 22731921]
39. Storino A, Castillo-Angeles M, Watkins AA, Vargas C, Mancias JD, Bullock A, et al. Assessing the accuracy and readability of online health information for patients with pancreatic cancer. JAMA Surg 2016 Sep 01;151(9):831-837. [doi: 10.1001/jamasurg.2016.0730] [Medline: 27144966]
40. Hamilton SN, Scali EP, Yu I, Gusnowski E, Ingledew PA. Sifting through it all: characterizing melanoma patients' utilization of the internet as an information source. J Cancer Educ 2015 Sep;30(3):580-584. [doi: 10.1007/s13187-014-0711-1] [Medline: 25077770]
41. Alshaikh EA, Almedimigh AF, Alruwaili AM, Almajnoni AH, Alhajiahmed A, Almalki TS, et al. Patient-focused online resources for melanoma: highly variable content and quality. J Cancer Educ 2019 Aug;34(4):775-781. [doi: 10.1007/s13187-018-1372-2] [Medline: 29732480]
42. US Department of Health and Human Services. The Surgeon General's call to action to prevent skin cancer. HHS.gov. Washington, DC: US Dept of Health and Human Services, Office of the Surgeon General; 2014. URL: https://www.hhs.gov/sites/default/files/call-to-action-prevent-skin-cancer.pdf [accessed 2020-04-13]

Abbreviations

CPC: cost-per-click

23

LesionMap: A Method and Tool for the Semantic Annotation of Dermatological Lesions for Documentation and Machine Learning

Bell Raj Eapen[1], MD, MSc; Norm Archer[1], PhD; Kamran Sartipi[2], PhD

[1]Information Systems, McMaster University, Hamilton, ON, Canada

[2]Department of Computer Science, East Carolina University, Greenville, NC, United States

Corresponding Author:
Bell Raj Eapen, MD, MSc
Information Systems
McMaster University
DSB - 211
1280 Main Street West
Hamilton, ON, L8S 4L8
Canada

Email: eapenbp@mcmaster.ca

Abstract

Diagnosis and follow-up of patients in dermatology rely on visual cues. Documentation of skin lesions in dermatology is time-consuming and inaccurate. Digital photography is resource-intensive, difficult to standardize, and has privacy concerns. We propose a simple method—LesionMap—and an electronic health software tool—LesionMapper—for semantically annotating dermatological lesions on a body wireframe. We discuss how the type, distribution, and progression of lesions can be represented in a standardized way. The tool is an open-source JavaScript package that can be integrated into web-based electronic medical records. We believe that LesionMapper will facilitate documentation in dermatology that can be used for machine learning in a privacy-preserving manner.

KEYWORDS

LesionMap; LesionMapper; digital imaging; machine learning; dermatology

Introduction

Documenting the origin, distribution, and nature of dermatological lesions in a textual form is inefficient and imprecise. Dermatologists often document the images of the patient or draw the lesions on a body wireframe for later reference. Digital photography for clinical documentation is time-consuming and resource intensive to capture, organize, and maintain [1]. Additionally, there is a growing privacy-related concern over the use of these images [2].

Capturing a detailed account of dermatological lesions in a privacy-preserving way is becoming increasingly important in the era of machine learning and artificial intelligence (AI). Documentation in electronic medical records (EMRs) requires a simple and efficient tool that fits into the clinical workflow. There is a growing need for a standardized methodology and an annotation schema to facilitate the capture of rich data related to dermatological conditions for machine learning. For this, we propose a simple method—LesionMap (LM)—and an electronic health (eHealth) software tool—LesionMapper (LMR)—that fits into the clinical workflow.

The sharing of clinical images between dermatologists for learning purposes is common, and most images are published with the consent of the patient [2]. However, increasingly, social media platforms are used for the easy sharing of such resources, with the associated implications on privacy [3]. Machine learning and AI applications need access to a large volume of data to build machine learning models for clinical decision support. Emerging techniques in machine learning and AI such as convolutional neural networks (CNN) and transfer learning [4] have several applications in dermatology [5]. Interestingly, some computer-vision methods can be applied to machine-generated images in addition to digital images [6].

In this paper, we describe common skin lesions, the semantic annotation methodology (LM), and a software tool (LMR) that can be used for semantic annotations. The tool is designed as an extensible software library (JavaScript) that can be incorporated into web-based EMRs. We briefly describe two such integrations with open-source EMRs—OpenMRS and OSCAR EMR.

Classification of Skin Lesions

Dermatologists use numerous descriptive terms to identify and describe skin lesions [7]. Flat skin lesions that are small are called macules, and when they exceed 1 cm in size, they are called patches. An elevated dome-shaped lesion is called a nodule, whereas a flat elevated lesion is called a plaque. Small fluid-filled lesions are called vesicles, and if they exceed 1 cm, they are called bullae. If vesicles are filled with pus instead of clear fluid, they are called pustules.

Scales refer to a thickened outer layer of skin while the crust is a liquid debris. An ulcer is an irregularly shaped, deep loss of skin, and if it is superficial it is called an erosion. Atrophy is a thinning of skin, and a fissure is a linear cleft. Necrosis is dead skin tissue, and the scar is the replacement of lost skin by connective tissue. Localized hemorrhage into the skin is called purpura, and petechiae, when the hemorrhagic lesions are small.

The color of the lesion can provide diagnostic cues, along with the shape, arrangement, and distribution. Discoid and annular are terms used to describe the shape. The distribution can be grouped, discrete, linear, serpiginous, reticular, generalized, symmetrical, or photodistributed. The size, location, and severity are also important. Although this is not an exhaustive list of dermatological descriptions, the most common descriptions are included here. Discrepancies in the terminology of dermatological lesions exist in the literature [8]. LM does not attempt to formalize the ontology, but proposes a pragmatic standard using the iconographic method.

Iconographic Representations of Skin Lesions

Most descriptive terms used in dermatology can be represented by iconographic images representative of the lesion or feature. The use of iconography in clinical documentation has been demonstrated in the context of pain [9]. The type of lesion can be easily represented by icons due to their visual similarity. The list of icons can be supplemented with custom icons for representing descriptive characteristics, such as the site of onset. LMR provides a set of icons for representing visual and nonvisual characteristics of common skin lesions and additional icons for descriptive characteristics (see Figure 1A and B).

Figure 1. The LesionMapper interface: (A,B) icons for descriptive characteristics; (C) large nodule; (D) ulcer on lateral side; (E) multiple discrete plaques; (F) Christmas tree pattern in pityriasis rosea; (G) vitiligo patch showing variation in opacity.

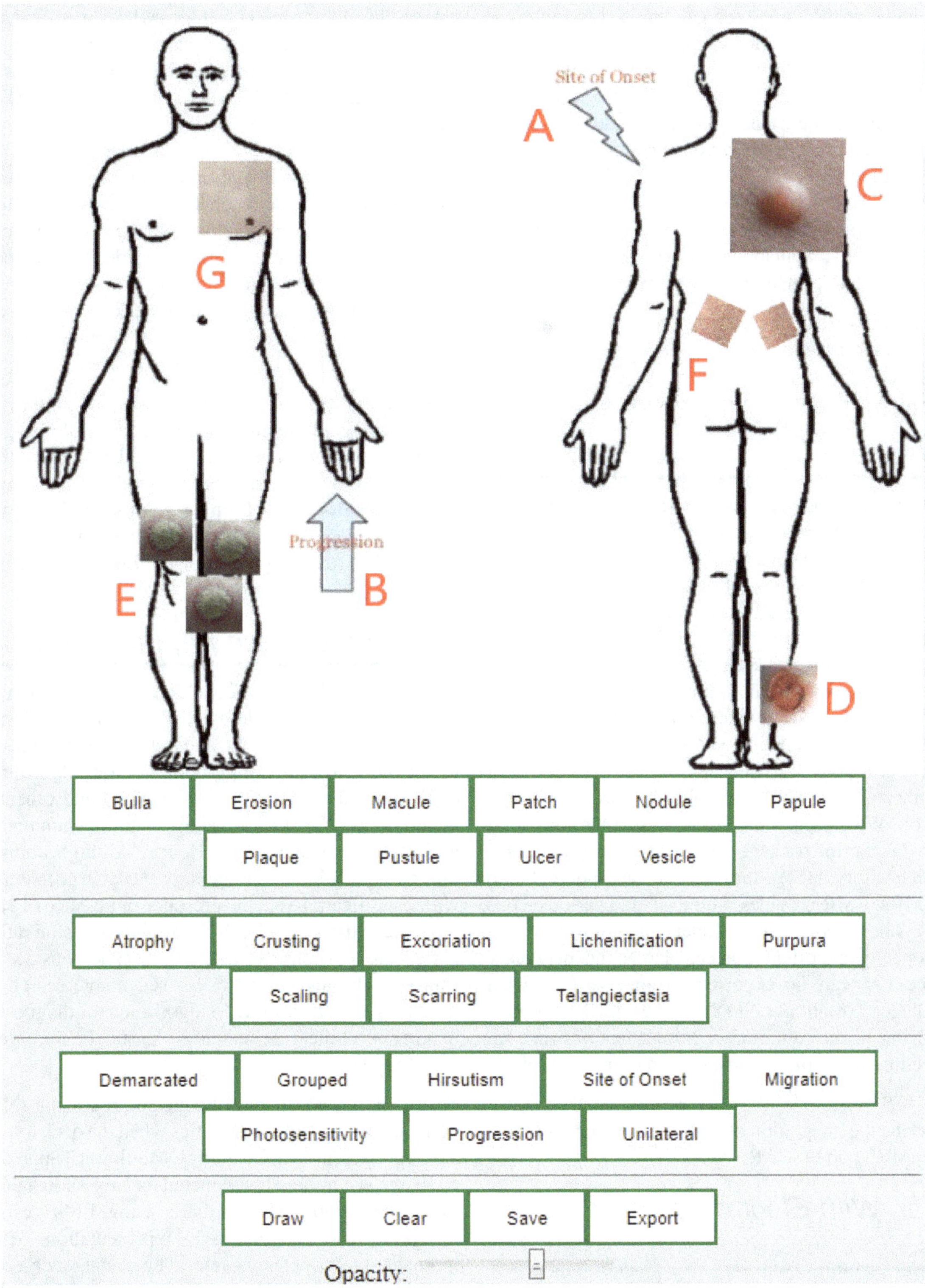

In addition to the type of lesions, there are five other characteristics of each icon that can be changed: size, position, number, orientation, and opacity. Additional information pertaining to the lesion can be encoded using the following characteristics:

- The size of the icon can be used to indicate the average size of the lesion in conditions where lesion size points toward a diagnosis or a particular subtype of the primary diagnosis. For example, the size of the plaques can be a differentiating feature for small-plaque and large-plaque parapsoriasis. The original size of the icon, when placed on the LM, can be used for comparison (see the large nodule in Figure 1C).
- The position of icon placement indicates the distribution of the lesions. The front and back of the body are depicted in the LM. The lateral view is not included to simplify the interface. To represent lateral distribution, the icons can be

placed in the corresponding edge of the wireframe with an overlap of 50% (see the ulcer on the legs in Figure 1D).

- Multiple icons of the same type can be used to represent discrete lesions, and a single large icon can be used to represent confluent distribution (see discrete plaques in Figure 1E).
- The orientation can be used to indicate a pathognomonic distribution, such as the Christmas tree pattern in pityriasis rosea (see Figure 1F).
- The opacity of the lesion can be used to indicate the severity of the presentation. For example, it can be used to represent the degree of depigmentation in a vitiligo patch or the severity of contact dermatitis (see Figure 1G).

Mapping lesions consistently and accurately requires a tool that supports the various functions described above. In addition, from a design perspective, the tool should have the capability to integrate with other health information systems and EMRs.

LesionMapper

LMR is a prototype implementation of the LM method described above. We adopted the design science principles of Hevner et al [10] for information systems to design LMR. We searched the literature for similar approaches and available tools to address the problem of lesional documentation. Based on the success of similar approaches (Pain-QuILT for annotating pain [9]), we chose iconography as the method and standardized it based on our domain expertise in dermatology. Thereafter, we distinguished some of the easily identifiable characteristics of icons that can be programmatically controlled, such as size, orientation, and transparency. Subsequently, we converged on a popular framework (VueJS JavaScript framework [11]) for implementation. We designed the artifact adopting a modular pattern—as a JavaScript package shared as open source (see the GitHub repository [12])—that can be incorporated into web-based EMRs. LMR provides buttons to add various icons to the canvas. These icons can be independently moved and resized. The opacity and orientation can also be independently modified. The LM can be exported as an image or as a JavaScript Object Notation (JSON) string. LMR supports freehand drawing in the canvas to represent features that are not represented by icons though machine interpretation of the freehand drawing is challenging.

Next, we describe the integration of LMR into two open-source EMRs—OpenMRS and OSCAR.

Integration With Electronic Medical Records

The modular design helps in the integration of LMR into web-based EMRs. The prototype is created using the VueJS JavaScript framework following the Universal Module Definition (UMD) pattern [13] that can be imported by different module loaders into other browser-based applications. The icons are converted into Base64 strings and included in the JavaScript files.

Open Medical Records System (OpenMRS) is an open-source, Java-based EMR for developing countries with a modular and extensible architecture [14]. OpenMRS supports the Open Web Apps (OWA) specifications that make it possible to design external applications that extend the core functions. The OWA communicates with OpenMRS using REST APIs (representational state transfer application programming interfaces), a software architectural style used for creating Web services, and is embedded in the same server instance. OpenMRS has a custom concept dictionary that helps map data points to a uniform terminology. Nontextual data such as images are stored as "complex concepts" outside the relational database. LMR can easily fit into an OWA design pattern, and the exported LM images can be stored as complex observations in the patient record. We have a prototype integration that can be used as an example [15].

OSCAR EMR is a web-based EMR system initially developed for primary care practitioners in Canada. OSCAR EMR has a complex data model, and additional data points are supported by an electronic form (eForm) module that stores data as key-value pairs [16]. eForms do not support images or other nontextual data. The ability of LMR to save LMs as a JSON string makes the integration of the LMR module into eForms possible.

Machine Learning Applications

Dermatological diseases have diverse presentations, with skin type and skin color adding to this variation. Some of these diseases involve hair, nails, and mucous membranes in addition to the skin. Traditional computer-vision algorithms such as convolutional neural networks (CNNs) and other variants of neural networks have limited application when there are many decision alternatives [17]. Hence, AI algorithms have had limited application in dermatology except in problems associated with classification (eg, the presence or absence of cancer) [18]. Such algorithms can classify only a given lesion rather than the patient as a whole (ie, a lesion is cancerous vs patient has cancer). Although few CNN-based image search algorithms have proven to be useful, AI algorithms for diagnostic decision making in clinical dermatology lag far behind areas such as radiology [17].

Text analytics and natural language processing (NLP) can be more useful than image analytics when the decision alternatives are numerous, as in dermatology. Multimodal approaches where an image is combined with metadata have shown promise [19]. Machine learning models built using LMs—especially the models created using the JSON representation—resemble text more than an image. Some relevant metadata such as the position and distribution of the lesions, which are difficult to be captured in text and hard to precisely decipher with NLP, are implicitly captured in LMs. The icons represent ontological concepts from dermatology and can map to any standard terminology system [7]. We posit that LMs are semantically rich enough to be used for machine learning applications. Machine learning models from LMs are likely to be more "explainable" than traditional black box algorithms [20]. The implicit metadata captured by

LMs can supplement regular digital images, leading to better machine learning models.

Advantages and Limitations

LMs may save time for busy practitioners while capturing the type, distribution, and characteristics of the lesion; these data can be used to assess clinical progress. The LM exported as JSON resembles a markup language amenable to data mining and machine learning methods [21]. LMs are portable and can be easily and safely exchanged without privacy concerns.

LMR can export LMs as images. These images can be used as a proxy for patient images in some computer vision–based applications. Computer vision has been successfully applied to identify metabolic defects from gene expression maps [22]. MNIST (Modified National Institute of Standards and Technology database), a dataset widely used in machine learning, consists of images of handwritten digits [23].

It is widely accepted that machine learning can reinforce some health care disparities in dermatology [24]. Skin color is a significant background noise that needs to be accounted for in any machine learning model. It is possible that some of the existing models are biased toward particular skin types that predominate in the training data set. Such models tend to be less sensitive in making predictions on different skin types [25]. The LMs are not affected by such bias.

LMs, however, do not capture all the features, both explainable and unexplainable, captured by a digital image. Hence, LMs are not useful in scenarios where accurate and sensitive extraction of features from an image is important for prediction. For example, LMs are not appropriate for skin cancer classification [5] and mole mapping [26]. LMs do not support annotating dermatopathology images [27]; they are also not applicable for dermatoscopic images that rely on pixel-level analysis [28]. Examination findings such as fluctuation, consistency, and tenderness are not represented by icons at present to keep the interface simple. More icons can be added if the user community requires them.

LMR and the LM method have not been clinically tested. The integration of LMR into existing EMRs may be difficult. Despite its anticipated ease of use, the actual impact of LMR on physician workflow, if any, needs to be investigated further.

Discussion

The skin is the largest organ in the human body, and as such, skin conditions are commonly encountered in any health care practice. Although dermatology is a specialization within clinical medicine, 50% of skin conditions are assessed and documented by nondermatologists [29].

There is no universal standard for pictographic documentation of the type, distribution, progression, and severity of lesions in dermatology, as in dentistry [30] and ophthalmology [31]. The LM standardizes visual representation using icons that can be extended to accommodate different use cases in clinical and cosmetic dermatology. The simplicity of the mapping rules facilitates use by nondermatologists in the skincare industry; LMs are also semantically rich enough to capture most relevant information about a skin condition with minimal effort.

Image analytics in dermatology is not as popular, as it is in visually oriented medical specialties such as radiology and pathology; the exception is the field of skin cancer diagnostics. This is because of the privacy concerns associated with dermatological images and the difficulties in standardizing image capture. The LM is not a replacement for a digital image of the lesion. However, some of the diagnostic aspects that are difficult to be captured in images, such as distribution and progression, can be useful for machine learning applications, especially when combined with the textual representation of a patient's history. Such multimodal approaches mimic the clinical workflow more so than CNN-based algorithms [32]. New computer-vision algorithms are proving to be capable of learning from computer-generated images [22]. We believe that LMs can be similarly used with computer-vision methods. Finally, we urge the open-source community to help us improve LMR and potential users to report issues on the repository [12] so that we can fix them. We will work on a 3D wireframe for better accuracy, and we welcome other feature requests from the user community.

References

1. Aspres N, Egerton IB, Lim AC, Shumack SP. Imaging the skin. Australas J Dermatol 2003 Feb;44(1):19-27. [doi: 10.1046/j.1440-0960.2003.00632.x]
2. Kunde L, McMeniman E, Parker M. Clinical photography in dermatology: Ethical and medico-legal considerations in the age of digital and smartphone technology. Australasian Journal of Dermatology 2013 May 29;54(3):192-197. [doi: 10.1111/ajd.12063]
3. Ventola CL. Social media and health care professionals: benefits, risks, and best practices. P & T 2014 Jul;39(7):491-520 [FREE Full text] [Medline: 25083128]
4. Shin H, Roth HR, Gao M, Lu L, Xu Z, Nogues I, et al. Deep Convolutional Neural Networks for Computer-Aided Detection: CNN Architectures, Dataset Characteristics and Transfer Learning. IEEE Trans. Med. Imaging 2016 May;35(5):1285-1298. [doi: 10.1109/tmi.2016.2528162]

5. Esteva A, Kuprel B, Novoa RA, Ko J, Swetter SM, Blau HM, et al. Dermatologist-level classification of skin cancer with deep neural networks. Nature 2017 Jan 25;542(7639):115-118. [doi: 10.1038/nature21056]
6. Levine MD, Nazif AM. Dynamic Measurement of Computer Generated Image Segmentations. IEEE Trans Pattern Anal Mach Intell 1985 Mar;PAMI-7(2):155-164. [doi: 10.1109/tpami.1985.4767640]
7. Eapen BR. ONTODerm--a domain ontology for dermatology. Dermatol Online J 2008 Jun 15;14(6):16. [Medline: 18713597]
8. Cardili RN, Roselino AM. Elementary lesions in dermatological semiology: literature review. An Bras Dermatol 2016 Oct;91(5):629-633. [doi: 10.1590/abd1806-4841.20164931]
9. Lalloo C, Kumbhare D, Stinson JN, Henry JL. Pain-QuILT: clinical feasibility of a web-based visual pain assessment tool in adults with chronic pain. J Med Internet Res 2014 May 12;16(5):e127 [FREE Full text] [doi: 10.2196/jmir.3292] [Medline: 24819478]
10. Hevner AR, March ST, Park J, Ram S. Design Science in Information Systems Research. MIS Quarterly 2004;28(1):75. [doi: 10.2307/25148625]
11. Street M, Passaglia A, Halliday P. Complete Vue. In: Complete Vue.js 2 Web Development: Practical Guide To Building End-to-end Web Development Solutions With Vue.js 2. Birmingham: Packt Publishing; 2018.
12. Eapen BR. GitHub. 2020. LesionMapper - Vue component for standardized mapping of lesions in dermatology URL: https://github.com/dermatologist/lesion-mapper [accessed 2020-01-16]
13. Rich H. Dismantling the barriers to entry. Queue 2015;13(5):37 [FREE Full text] [doi: 10.1145/2742580.2742813]
14. Mamlin BW, Biondich PG, Wolfe BA, Fraser H, Jazayeri D, Allen C, et al. Cooking up an open source emr for developing countries: OpenMRS, a recipe for successful collaboration. In: American Medical Informatics Association. 2006 Presented at: AMIA Annual Symposium Proceedings; 2006; Washington p. 529.
15. Eapen BR. OpenMRS. 2017. Dermatology LesionMapper URL: https://addons.openmrs.org/show/org.openmrs.module.dermatology-lesionmapper [accessed 2020-01-18]
16. Safadi H, Chan D, Dawes M, Roper M, Faraj S. Open-source health information technology: A case study of electronic medical records. Health Policy and Technology 2015 Mar;4(1):14-28. [doi: 10.1016/j.hlpt.2014.10.011]
17. Li C, Shen C, Xue K, Shen X, Jing Y, Wang Z, et al. Artificial intelligence in dermatology. Chinese Medical Journal 2019;132(17):2017-2020. [doi: 10.1097/cm9.0000000000000372]
18. Sidey-Gibbons JAM, Sidey-Gibbons CJ. Machine learning in medicine: a practical introduction. BMC Med Res Methodol 2019 Mar 19;19(1). [doi: 10.1186/s12874-019-0681-4]
19. Wang H, Wang Y, Liang C, Li Y. Assessment of Deep Learning Using Nonimaging Information and Sequential Medical Records to Develop a Prediction Model for Nonmelanoma Skin Cancer. JAMA Dermatol 2019 Nov 01;155(11):1277. [doi: 10.1001/jamadermatol.2019.2335]
20. Andreas H, Chris B, Constantinos SP, Douglas BK. What do we need to build explainable AI systems for the medical domain? arXiv.org 2017 [FREE Full text]
21. Guazzelli A, Lin W, Jena T. PMML in action: unleashing the power of open standards for data mining and predictive analytics. California: Createspace Independent Publishing Platform; 2020.
22. Zhang J, Naik HS, Assefa T, Sarkar S, Reddy RVC, Singh A, et al. Computer vision and machine learning for robust phenotyping in genome-wide studies. Sci Rep 2017 Mar 8;7(1). [doi: 10.1038/srep44048]
23. Li Deng. The MNIST Database of Handwritten Digit Images for Machine Learning Research [Best of the Web]. IEEE Signal Process. Mag 2012 Nov;29(6):141-142. [doi: 10.1109/msp.2012.2211477]
24. Adamson AS, Smith A. Machine Learning and Health Care Disparities in Dermatology. JAMA Dermatol 2018 Nov 01;154(11):1247. [doi: 10.1001/jamadermatol.2018.2348]
25. Kamulegeya LH, Okello M, Bwanika JM, Musinguzi D, Lubega W, Rusoke D, et al. Using artificial intelligence on dermatology conditions in uganda: A case for diversity in training data sets for machine learning. bioRxiv.org 2019 [FREE Full text] [doi: 10.1101/826057]
26. Berk-Krauss J, Polsky D, Stein JA. Mole Mapping for Management of Pigmented Skin Lesions. Dermatologic Clinics 2017 Oct;35(4):439-445. [doi: 10.1016/j.det.2017.06.004]
27. Toro P, Corredor G, Romero E, Arias V. A visualization, navigation, and annotation system for dermatopathology training. In: International Society for Optics and Photonics. 2018 Presented at: 14th International Symposium on Medical Information Processing and Analysis, volume 10975; 2018; Mazatlán, Mexico. [doi: 10.1117/12.2511638]
28. Ferreira B, Barata C, Marques JS. What is the role of annotations in the detection of dermoscopic structures? In: Iberian Conference on Pattern Recognition and Image Analysis. 2019 Presented at: 9th Iberian Conference, IbPRIA 2019; 2019; Madrid, Spain p. 3-11. [doi: 10.1007/978-3-030-31321-0_1]
29. Ahiarah A, Fox C, Servoss T. Brief intervention to improve diagnosis and treatment knowledge of skin disorders by family medicine residents. Fam Med 2007;39(10):720-723 [FREE Full text] [Medline: 17987414]
30. Wu M, Koenig L, Lynch J, Wirtz T. Spatially-oriented EMR for Dental Surgery. In: American Medical Informatics Association. 2006 Presented at: AMIA Annual Symposium Proceedings; 2006; Washington p. 1147.
31. Chiang MF, Boland MV, Brewer A, Epley KD, Horton MB, Lim MC, American Academy of Ophthalmology Medical Information Technology Committee. Special Requirements for Electronic Health Record Systems in Ophthalmology. Ophthalmology 2011 Aug 1;118(8):1681-1687. [doi: 10.1016/j.ophtha.2011.04.015] [Medline: 21680023]

32. Baltrusaitis T, Ahuja C, Morency L. Multimodal Machine Learning: A Survey and Taxonomy. IEEE Trans Pattern Anal Mach Intell 2019 Feb 1;41(2):423-443. [doi: 10.1109/tpami.2018.2798607]

Abbreviations

AI: artificial intelligence
API: application programming interface
CNN: convolutional neural network
eForm: electronic form
eHealth: electronic health
EMR: electronic medical record
JSON: JavaScript Object Notation
LM: LesionMap
LMR: LesionMapper
MNIST: Modified National Institute of Standards and Technology database
NLP: natural language processing
OWA: Open Web Apps
REST: representational state transfer
UMD: Universal Module Definition

24

The Feasibility and Acceptability of Using a Wearable UV Radiation Exposure Monitoring Device in Adults and Children

Elizabeth Sela Nagelhout[1*], MPH, PhD; Riley Lensink[2*], BS; Angela Zhu[2*], BS; Bridget G Parsons[2*], MSPH; Jakob D Jensen[3*], PhD; Yelena P Wu[2,4*], PhD

[1]Department of Family and Preventive Medicine, University of Utah, Salt Lake City, UT, United States

[2]Huntsman Cancer Institute, Salt Lake City, UT, United States

[3]Department of Communications, University of Utah, Salt Lake City, UT, United States

[4]Department of Dermatology, University of Utah, Salt Lake City, UT, United States

[*]all authors contributed equally

Corresponding Author:
Yelena P Wu, PhD
Huntsman Cancer Institute
2000 Circle of Hope
Salt Lake City, UT, 84112
United States

Email: yelena.wu@utah.edu

Abstract

Background: In the United States, melanoma is the fifth most common type of cancer. Reducing UV radiation (UVR) exposure is essential for the prevention of melanoma. The assessment of individual-level UVR exposure using wearable technology is a promising method to monitor and reduce UVR exposure. However, the feasibility and acceptability of using wearable UVR monitoring devices have not been assessed.

Objective: This study aimed to assess the feasibility and acceptability of using a commercially available UVR monitoring wearable device in adults and children.

Methods: We recruited families (1 parent and 1 child) to test a new, commercially available UVR monitoring device (namely, Shade). Participants wore Shade for 2 weeks and completed questionnaires assessing the feasibility and acceptability of wearing the device. Qualitative analyses were conducted to summarize participants' open-ended responses regarding device feasibility.

Results: A total of 194 individuals (97 adults and 97 children) participated in this study. The participating children were aged, on average, 12.7 years. Overall, adults and children reported moderate satisfaction with wearing Shade. The feasibility of the use of Shade was adequate, with 73% (65/89) of adults and 61% (54/89) of children reporting that they wore the device "all of the time they were outside." Through open-ended responses, participants reported that the device was easy to use, was compact, and increased their awareness about their exposure to UVR.

Conclusions: Adults and children can feasibly use a wearable UVR monitoring device, and the use of the device was acceptable to participants. The device could be integrated into melanoma preventive interventions to increase individuals' and families' awareness of UVR exposure and to facilitate the use of recommended melanoma preventive strategies.

KEYWORDS

ultraviolet radiation exposure; wearable device; melanoma; melanoma prevention

Introduction

Background

In the United States, melanoma is the fifth most common type of cancer [1]. Over the past three decades, overall melanoma incidence has increased by 1.5% each year; the incidence in pediatric populations is increasing, and these trends are expected to continue [1]. Individual UV radiation (UVR) exposure is the primary modifiable risk factor related to melanoma development [2]. The reduction of UVR exposure through the use of sun protection strategies (eg, wearing a sunscreen, wearing long sleeves, and avoiding peak UVR hours from 10 AM to 4 PM) is essential for the prevention of melanoma. Decreasing UVR exposure during childhood is especially critical because 25% of one's lifetime UVR exposure occurs during childhood, a key period of skin cell development and susceptibility [3,4]. Children and adolescents often rely on their parents to engage in sun-safe habits (eg, helping apply a sunscreen, providing long-sleeved shirts for children to wear, and buying a sunscreen for the household), thereby decreasing their UVR exposure, and are more likely to be successful in engaging in these behaviors if their parents model sun-safe habits [5-7]. However, many parents do not provide sufficient sun protection for their children [7]. Furthermore, children often do not use the recommended sun protection strategies to decrease UVR exposure, and they receive multiple sunburns, which can double their lifetime risk of melanoma [8,9].

Typically, the assessment of an individual's UVR exposure has relied on self-reported questionnaires and diaries of sun protection, time spent outdoors, and the number of sunburns [10-13]. However, self-reported measurements of UVR exposure can be upwardly biased because of inaccurate recall and social desirability effects [14-17]. There are few objective assessments of UVR exposure available. The most common method for assessing objectively measured UVR exposure has been through the use of personal electronic dosimeters, which are worn as wristwatches or fixed to clothing and collect individual UVR exposure at instantaneous readings (eg, every second) [18-24]. Previous studies using electronic dosimeters have been limited by the use of dosimeters that detect UV-B only, are not commercially available and thus have a lower likelihood for broader dissemination, have low sensitivity and specificity, and are unable to filter out visible light that could overestimate actual UVR measurements [25-27].

The Shade UVR sensor is a newly developed wearable radiometer, which records both instantaneous readings and accumulated UVR doses over time [26]. The device is capable of measuring both UV-B and UV-A, filtering out visible light, and is weighted according to the erythemal action spectra, which is standardized by the International Commission on Illumination and adopted by the World Health Organization [26,28,29]. Using a standardized unit of UVR exposure allows for the comparability of exposure measurements among study populations. In addition, Shade has documented excellent sensitivity and accuracy, including when compared with other UVR monitoring devices [26]. For example, the accuracy of Shade is roughly 80%, whereas the accuracy of the Band wearable device is roughly 20% [26].

Objectives

Commercially available UVR monitoring devices have the potential to be integrated into melanoma preventive interventions aimed at reducing UVR exposure. For example, such devices could facilitate the self-monitoring of UVR exposure and increase an individual's awareness of their overall UVR exposure levels. In other areas of research and practice, including those focused on increasing physical activity to prevent or treat obesity, self-monitoring of health behaviors (eg, time spent engaging in physical activity) has been shown to be beneficial for positive health behavior changes [30,31]. However, previous studies have not yet assessed the feasibility and acceptability of using a commercially available UVR monitoring device, from participants' perspectives [19,21,32]. Establishing the adequate feasibility and acceptability of such devices is essential before being used in skin cancer preventive interventions aimed at decreasing UVR exposure. The purpose of this study was to examine the feasibility and acceptability of using a newly developed, commercially available UVR monitoring wearable device (ie, Shade) in children and adults.

Methods

Study Sample

All study participants were recruited within the state of Utah, which has the highest incidence of melanoma in the United States [33]. Adults were eligible to participate in the study if (1) they were at least aged 18 years, (2) were residents of Utah, (3) had at least one child aged 8 to 17 years who was willing to participate in the study, (4) did not have a pacemaker (because of the strong magnet in the UVR monitoring device), (5) had and were willing to use a Bluetooth or Wi-Fi–enabled mobile phone for research purposes (to communicate with the research staff and synchronized the device), (6) were willing to download and use a free mobile phone app that shared their UVR exposure data with the research team, and (7) were able to read and speak English. Children were eligible to participate if (1) they were aged 8 to 17 years, (2) lived with a primary caretaker in Utah, and (3) did not have a pacemaker. Children who did not have a Bluetooth or Wi-Fi–enabled device that allowed them to share their UVR exposure data with the research team were loaned one for the duration of the study.

A total of 194 participants (97 parent-child dyads) were enrolled in the study. Of the adults who completed eligibility screening, 34 were ineligible. The reasons for ineligibility included the parent not having children aged between 8 and 17 years (n=28), not having a mobile phone with Bluetooth and Wi-Fi (n=5), and being unable to read English (n=1). Of the 116 eligible adults, 7 decided not to participate and 12 were unable to participate because of a limited number of devices available for use within the context of this study. There were no parent-child dyads excluded because of child ineligibility after it was determined that the parent was eligible to participate. Data were collected between June 2018 and October 2018 to capture the experiences of adults and children wearing the device during the summer months and once school had started. An institutional review board approved all the study procedures.

Study Procedures

Before their study enrollment, parental consent, parental permission, and child assent forms were emailed to participants, and Shade was mailed to participants. Once participants received the devices, they provided informed consent by phone. During the consent call, research assistants reviewed instructions on the use and care for the device. Parents and children were each asked to wear Shade clipped to the chest portion of their shirt for 14 days during waking hours. Shade collects the individual, time-stamped standard erythemal dose (SED), a standardized measure of UVR exposure, accumulated over the course of the day and reports readings of the SED every 6 min. The device is 1.58 inches in diameter and weighs 0.48 ounces and can be attached to clothing with a built-in magnet. The data collected by the device were synchronized using the Shade research app. Shade, which is commercially available, is accompanied by an app; however, for the purposes of our research project, we used the Shade research app. The research app did not provide participants any information on their UVR exposure, as we were focused on examining the feasibility and acceptability of wearing the device separately from the UVR feedback feature. The app was used to collect the UV data from the device and to notify participants when the device battery needed to be recharged. The participants were also instructed to avoid getting the device wet (as it is not waterproof), to synchronize the device to the Shade research app daily, and to recharge their device at least every 3 days. At the start of the 14-day study period, parents and children were asked to complete a baseline questionnaire that included items assessing demographic information. They were also asked to complete once-daily questionnaires assessing whether they had worn the device. Finally, parents and children were asked to complete an exit questionnaire assessing the feasibility and acceptability of wearing Shade. Parents and children reported on their own use of the device separately. Feasibility and acceptability were conceptually defined based on previous research [34,35]. Feasibility was defined as "Are participants capable of and willing to integrate wearing the Shade device into their daily lives?" Acceptability was defined as "To what extent wearing the Shade device was judged as suitable, satisfying, or attractive to study participants?"

Feasibility

Feasibility was assessed through four multioption quantitative items and two open-ended questions. The quantitative items included the following: (1) "During days you wore the Shade device, how much of the time between 7 am and 7 pm did you wear the device when you were outside?" (eg, "wearing it ☐ of the time" and "wearing it all of the time"); (2) "When did you wear the Shade device?" (eg, "I put it on in the morning and wore it all day [except in the shower or while swimming], and took it off again in the evening" and "I wore it most of the time but took it off at special occasions"); (3) "When you wore the Shade device, did you pay attention to it?" (eg, "Yes, I was aware that it should be clipped to my clothing, exposed to the sun, but I didn't change my behavior because of it" and "No, I didn't pay attention to it at all"); and (4) "While you wore the Shade device, did people around you notice it and ask you what it was for?" (eg, "yes, many" and "no, no one"). Open-ended feasibility questions assessed perceptions of enjoyment and usability and included the following questions: "What did you like about the Shade device?" and "What were some of the challenges of wearing the Shade device?"

Acceptability

The acceptability of using Shade was measured using a 17-item modified questionnaire that assessed the perceptions of comfort, enjoyment, privacy, and usefulness of the device [34]. The original questionnaire was modified to focus on the acceptability of wearing the device. Responses were measured on a 5-point Likert-type scale, scored 1 to 5, ranging from *strongly disagree* to *strongly agree*. For example, participants were asked to rate how much they agreed with items such as "I think the device was comfortable." All questionnaires were administered using Research Electronic Data Capture (REDCap) [36,37].

Analytic Plan

Descriptive statistics were calculated to summarize participant demographic characteristics and to report the proportions of participants' responses to quantitative feasibility and acceptability questions. Means and standard deviations were calculated to summarize the number of days the device was worn. The qualitative feasibility questions were coded using content analysis to identify common themes describing what parents and children liked about the device (eg, ease of use and awareness of their UVR exposure) and challenges they experienced when wearing the device (eg, the device falling off) [38]. The codebook was created by three research team members based on the initial coding of 10% of parents' and children's responses for each of the two open-ended feasibility questions. Overall, 50% of all parents' and children's responses were coded by two independent coders (percent agreement=95%). All discrepancies in coding were discussed and resolved by the coders before commencing the analysis.

Results

Demographic Characteristics

A total of 97 adults and 97 children (N=194 individuals) participated in this study. Among adults, 87% (83/95) were non-Hispanic white and 5% (5/95) were Hispanic and 77% (73/95) were women (Table 1). The average age of participating children was 12.7 years (SD 2.6), 85% (81/95) were non-Hispanic white and 8% (8/95) were Hispanic and 59% (56/95) were female (Table 1).

Table 1. Demographic characteristics of participants.

Characteristics	Adults (n=97)	Children (n=97)
Age (years), mean (SD)	41.6 (6.3)	12.7 (2.7)
Sex, n (%)		
Male	22 (23)	39 (41)
Female	73 (77)	56 (59)
Race, n (%)		
Non-Hispanic white	83 (87)	81 (85)
Hispanic	5 (5)	8 (8)
Asian or Asian American	5 (5)	4 (4)
Other	2 (2)	2 (2)
Marital status, n (%)		
Married or marriage-like relationship	84 (88)	N/A[a]
Divorced/separated	9 (10)	N/A
Widowed	2 (2)	N/A
Level of education, n (%)		
High school graduate or General Educational Development	8 (8)	N/A
Vocational or technical school	8 (8)	N/A
Some college, including 2-year degree	33 (35)	N/A
Bachelor's degree	25 (26)	N/A
Master's/doctoral degree	21 (22)	N/A
Family income, n (%)		
<US $50,000	23 (24)	N/A
>US $50,000	64 (67)	N/A
I would rather not report this	8 (8)	N/A
Occupation location, n (%)		
Mainly indoors	82 (86)	N/A
Mainly outdoors	9 (9)	N/A
In a motor vehicle	3 (3)	N/A

[a]N/A: not applicable (not asked of children).

Acceptability of a UV Radiation Monitoring Device

Parents and children reported moderate levels of satisfaction with wearing Shade. Parents *agreed or strongly agreed* that the device was well suited for their bodies (45/89, 51%), was comfortable (57/89, 64%), and was easy to wear (68/69, 76%; Table 2). More than 80% (73/88) of children *agreed or strongly agreed* that the device was easy to wear. Only 8% (7/89) of parents and 17% (15/88) of children *agreed or strongly agreed* that the device felt weird physically (Table 2). Only 25% (22/89) of parents *agreed or strongly agreed* that they would purchase the device.

Table 2. Parent's and children's reported acceptability of Shade, a UV radiation monitoring device.

Acceptability of Shade	Agree or strongly agree	
	Parents, n (%)	Children, n (%)
Wearing the device feels weird physically	7 (8)	15 (17)
I think the device is well suited for my body	45 (51)	39 (44)
I think the device was comfortable	57 (64)	33 (38)
I think the device was boring	57 (64)	13 (15)
I think the device was annoying	19 (21)	28 (32)
I think the device was pleasant	20 (23)	23 (26)
I think the device may threaten my privacy	3 (3)	4 (5)
If most people in my environment used the device, I would be more inclined to use it as well	24 (27)	32 (36)
If people who are influential in my life recommended that I use the device for a period of time, I would do so	43 (48)	46 (52)
I think I would wear the device only if I were forced to	14 (16)	12 (14)
If it were launched on the market at an affordable price, I would likely purchase it	22 (25)	15 (17)
If the device were available to me, I would use it	44 (49)	37 (42)
It seems tiresome to use the device	26 (29)	16 (18)
It seems easy to wear the device	68 (76)	73 (83)
The device would be incompatible with most aspects of my activities	11 (12)	26 (30)
The device limits the way in which I like to perform my activities	8 (9)	14 (16)
The device could improve the quality of my activities	15 (17)	12 (14)

Feasibility of Using a UV Radiation Monitoring Device

Parents reported wearing Shade for an average of 12.7 days (SD 2.54) out of 14 days, and children reported wearing their device for an average of 12.2 days (SD 3.03) out of 14 days. The majority of parents (65/89, 73%) and children (54/89, 61%) reported that they wore Shade whenever they were outdoors between 7 AM and 7 PM during the study period. When asked when they wore the device during the day, 80% (72/90) of parents and 71% (63/89) of children reported that they put it on in the morning and wore it all day and took it off again in the evening, indicating full compliance with the study protocol.

The vast majority of the sample (89/97, 92% of parents and 87/97, 90% of children) provided responses to the open-ended feasibility questions. The most commonly endorsed themes regarding what participants liked about Shade were the device's ease of use and compact size and that the device increased the participant's awareness about their sun-safe habits and tracked their UVR exposure (see Multimedia Appendix 1). The most commonly endorsed challenges of wearing Shade among parents and children included keeping the device's UVR sensor uncovered (eg, by clothing), remembering to wear the device, its impact on daily activities (eg, the device was in the way while doing chores and the device tugged on shirts), and the device inadvertently falling off. Another challenge mentioned by parents and children included receiving questions from others about the device (Multimedia Appendix 1).

Discussion

Principal Findings

The results of this study indicate that the use of a wearable UVR monitoring device was moderately acceptable and feasible for adults and children. In addition, parents and children were, on average, adherent to wearing the device for the vast majority of the desired monitoring days, indicating the potential for the use of monitoring devices in future melanoma prevention interventions. Although participants found wearing the device to be both acceptable and feasible, the results of this study indicated some ways in which the device could be improved for future use.

Exposure to UVR is the primary modifiable risk factor for melanoma [39]. Despite public health efforts to increase the awareness of the harmful effects of UVR through educational interventions, adults and adolescents continue to report experiencing sunburns and do not adhere to sun protection use (eg, wearing sunscreen or long sleeve shirts) [40]. The use of a feasible and acceptable UVR monitoring device, similar to the one assessed in this study, may be beneficial when combined with other health behavior strategies (eg, wearing a sunscreen and avoiding peak UVR hours) in driving behavior changes to reduce UVR exposure. Although participants were not provided with UVR exposure data in real time, 33% of adults and 9% of children reported that wearing the device made them more aware of their outdoor sun habits. More than 11% of children reported that they liked the device because it was able to track their UVR exposure. These findings suggest participants may be interested in using a wearable UVR exposure device to monitor their UVR exposure. Future studies may be helpful in identifying whether users find it feasible and acceptable to monitor their UVR exposure through the use of a monitoring device and an integrated UVR feedback system (eg, a phone app or device display). Our team is currently designing interventions to provide participants with personalized UVR feedback in real time in an effort to promote sun protection use.

Self-monitoring of health behaviors via objective measures has been shown in other populations to increase the awareness of behaviors such as sedentary periods and to counter self-reported underestimates of the time spent in sedentary activities [41]. Similarly, in the context of UVR exposure, it is likely that individuals do not have an accurate perception of the amount of UVR exposure they receive. For example, one study reported that a participant's perception of being in the sun for a *long period* could range from 30 min to an entire day, which would vastly affect the amount of UVR exposure they received [42]. Providing feedback on the amount of UVR exposure received during daily activities and accumulated throughout the course of an entire day could help individuals have a more accurate sense of their UVR exposure. Knowledge of one's daily UVR exposure will likely become increasingly important, as the overall amount of UVR that is reaching the earth's surface is increasing because of ozone depletion, which puts people at a greater risk for the harmful effects of UVR [43,44].

The results of this study also raised considerations for modifications of UVR monitoring wearable device technology for use in future research. Participants indicated wearing the device was challenging because they forgot to wear the device, it impacted their daily activities, the device fell off at times, and the device solicited questions from others. These results are similar to findings from other studies evaluating the acceptability of wearing health tracking devices. Previous studies have found that barriers to using a wearable device include remembering to put it on, the inability to wear it during certain activities, the device not being waterproof, fear of losing the device, and increased social tension resulting from peers asking about the device [45-47]. Future devices may be more acceptable to users if the device or associated mobile phone app had an alert function to remind them to put on their device each morning, if the device could be worn as a wristwatch or in another inconspicuous location so as to not attract attention from peers, and if the device was waterproof. Parents and children had differing views about some of the aspects of Shade. For example, 64% of parents and 37.5% of children *agreed or strongly agreed* that the device was comfortable, and 21.0% of parents and 31.8% of children found the device to be annoying. These differences may emphasize the need to tailor UVR wearable devices for use in adult and child populations separately.

Strengths and Limitations

The strengths of this study include the use of a commercially available wearable device, which can be accessed by the general population to track their UVR exposure. This study also included both adults and children, who could both potentially benefit from future interventions using UVR monitoring devices, given that both populations are at risk for UVR exposure. Exploring adults' and children's perceptions of the device's acceptability and feasibility separately helped to elucidate the most important challenges that parents and children may experience when using such devices. For example, remembering to wear the device was a bigger issue for children than for adults, and this information can be considered when developing future interventions and app functions. A limitation of this study was the focus on self-reported compliance to wearing the device. In the future, devices that employ accelerometers or other technologies that objectively assess whether participants were wearing the device would be better monitors for study protocol adherence. Future studies could minimize the potential for missing data due to these factors by emphasizing to participants the importance of regular synchronizing and charging their devices to prevent loss of data. Finally, this study was conducted within a single geographic area, which may reduce the generalizability of the results. Two limitations of Shade include its lack of an accelerometer (used to track compliance) and the lack of a waterproof sensor, making it impossible to be worn while swimming.

Conclusions

The findings of this study indicate that a wearable UVR monitoring device can be feasibly and acceptably used by both adults and children. The use of a wearable device to monitor UVR exposure is a unique and objective method for quantifying the amount of UVR exposure and could be used to support adults and children in reducing their UVR exposure. Ultimately, decreases in personal UVR exposure could contribute to the prevention of melanoma and other types of skin cancer in the future.

Acknowledgments

The authors appreciate Peter Kaplan and Emmanuel Dumont for their guidance on and assistance with using Shade in this study. The authors also appreciate Jared Luther for his assistance with data management. This work was supported in part by the National Cancer Institute of the National Institutes of Health (NIH; K07CA196985; YW). This work was also supported in part by a Pilot Project Award from the American Cancer Society Huntsman Cancer Institute Institutional Research Grant (129785-IRG-16-190-01-IRG) and an NIH New Innovator Award (1DP2EB022360-01; JJ). Data for this project were collected using REDCap, which is supported by the National Cancer Institute of the NIH (8UL1TR000105, formerly UL1RR025764). The content is solely the responsibility of the authors and does not necessarily represent the official views of the NIH.

References

1. Surveillance, Epidemiology, and End Results Program. Cancer Stat Facts: Melanoma of the Skin URL: http://seer.cancer.gov/statfacts/html/melan.html [accessed 2019-01-01]
2. Armstrong BK, Kricker A. How much melanoma is caused by sun exposure? Melanoma Res 1993 Dec;3(6):395-401. [doi: 10.1097/00008390-199311000-00002] [Medline: 8161879]
3. Whiteman DC, Whiteman CA, Green AC. Childhood sun exposure as a risk factor for melanoma: a systematic review of epidemiologic studies. Cancer Causes Control 2001 Jan;12(1):69-82. [doi: 10.1023/a:1008980919928] [Medline: 11227927]
4. Godar DE, Wengraitis SP, Shreffler J, Sliney DH. UV doses of Americans. Photochem Photobiol 2001 Jun;73(6):621-629. [doi: 10.1562/0031-8655(2001)073<0621:udoa>2.0.co;2] [Medline: 11421067]
5. Dobbinson S, Wakefield M, Hill D, Girgis A, Aitken JF, Beckmann K, et al. Children's sun exposure and sun protection: prevalence in Australia and related parental factors. J Am Acad Dermatol 2012 Jun;66(6):938-947. [doi: 10.1016/j.jaad.2011.06.015] [Medline: 21890234]
6. Hamilton K, Cleary C, White KM, Hawkes AL. Keeping kids sun safe: exploring parents' beliefs about their young child's sun-protective behaviours. Psychooncology 2016 Feb;25(2):158-163. [doi: 10.1002/pon.3888] [Medline: 26101815]
7. Johnson K, Davy L, Boyett T, Weathers L, Roetzheim RG. Sun protection practices for children: knowledge, attitudes, and parent behaviors. Arch Pediatr Adolesc Med 2001 Aug;155(8):891-896. [doi: 10.1001/archpedi.155.8.891] [Medline: 11483115]
8. Balk SJ, Council on Environmental Health, Section on Dermatology. Ultraviolet radiation: a hazard to children and adolescents. Pediatrics 2011 Mar;127(3):e791-e817. [doi: 10.1542/peds.2010-3502] [Medline: 21357345]
9. Geller AC, Colditz G, Oliveria S, Emmons K, Jorgensen C, Aweh GN, et al. Use of sunscreen, sunburning rates, and tanning bed use among more than 10 000 US children and adolescents. Pediatrics 2002 Jun;109(6):1009-1014. [doi: 10.1542/peds.109.6.1009] [Medline: 12042536]
10. Glanz K, Steffen AD, Schoenfeld E, Tappe KA. Randomized trial of tailored skin cancer prevention for children: the Project SCAPE family study. J Health Commun 2013;18(11):1368-1383 [FREE Full text] [doi: 10.1080/10810730.2013.778361] [Medline: 23806094]
11. Lucas RM, Valery P, van der Mei I, Dwyer T, Pender MP, Taylor B, Ausimmune Investigator Group. Sun exposure over a lifetime in Australian adults from latitudinally diverse regions. Photochem Photobiol 2013;89(3):737-744. [doi: 10.1111/php.12044] [Medline: 23311500]
12. Glenn BA, Lin T, Chang LC, Okada A, Wong WK, Glanz K, et al. Sun protection practices and sun exposure among children with a parental history of melanoma. Cancer Epidemiol Biomarkers Prev 2015 Jan;24(1):169-177 [FREE Full text] [doi: 10.1158/1055-9965.EPI-14-0650] [Medline: 25587110]
13. Stump TK, Aspinwall LG, Taber JM, Edwards R, Leachman SA. Protection-Adjusted Length of Exposure (PALE): A New Self-Report Measure of UVR Exposure That Captures Multiple Modalities of Photoprotection. In: Paper Presented at the Annual Meeting of the Melanoma Genetics Consortium. 2013 Presented at: GenoMEL'13; June 2013; Philadelphia, PA.
14. McCarty CA. Sunlight exposure assessment: can we accurately assess vitamin D exposure from sunlight questionnaires? Am J Clin Nutr 2008 Apr;87(4):1097S-1101S. [doi: 10.1093/ajcn/87.4.1097S] [Medline: 18400741]
15. O'Riordan DL, Stanton WR, Eyeson-Annan M, Gies P, Roy C. Correlations between reported and measured ultraviolet radiation exposure of mothers and young children. Photochem Photobiol 2000 Jan;71(1):60-64. [doi: 10.1562/0031-8655(2000)071<0060:cbramu>2.0.co;2] [Medline: 10649890]
16. O'Riordan DL, Lunde KB, Steffen AD, Maddock JE. Validity of beachgoers' self-report of their sun habits. Arch Dermatol 2006 Oct;142(10):1304-1311. [doi: 10.1001/archderm.142.10.1304] [Medline: 17043185]
17. Rampen FH, Fleuren BA, de Boo TM, Lemmens WA. Unreliability of self-reported burning tendency and tanning ability. Arch Dermatol 1988 Jun;124(6):885-888. [Medline: 3377517]
18. Grandahl K, Mortensen OS, Sherman DZ, Køster B, Lund P, Ibler KS, et al. Solar UV exposure among outdoor workers in Denmark measured with personal UV-B dosimeters: technical and practical feasibility. Biomed Eng Online 2017 Oct 10;16(1):119 [FREE Full text] [doi: 10.1186/s12938-017-0410-3] [Medline: 29017484]
19. Bodekær M, Petersen B, Philipsen PA, Heydenreich J, Thieden E, Wulf HC. Sun exposure patterns of urban, suburban, and rural children: a dosimetry and diary study of 150 children. Photochem Photobiol Sci 2015 Jul;14(7):1282-1289. [doi: 10.1039/c5pp00052a] [Medline: 26066309]
20. Thieden E, Agren MS, Wulf HC. Solar UVR exposures of indoor workers in a Working and a Holiday Period assessed by personal dosimeters and sun exposure diaries. Photodermatol Photoimmunol Photomed 2001 Dec;17(6):249-255. [doi: 10.1034/j.1600-0781.2001.170601.x] [Medline: 11722749]
21. Thieden E, Philipsen PA, Heydenreich J, Wulf HC. UV radiation exposure related to age, sex, occupation, and sun behavior based on time-stamped personal dosimeter readings. Arch Dermatol 2004 Feb;140(2):197-203. [doi: 10.1001/archderm.140.2.197] [Medline: 14967793]
22. Thieden E, Philipsen PA, Wulf HC. Ultraviolet radiation exposure pattern in winter compared with summer based on time-stamped personal dosimeter readings. Br J Dermatol 2006 Jan;154(1):133-138. [doi: 10.1111/j.1365-2133.2005.06961.x] [Medline: 16403106]

23. Hacker E, Horsham C, Vagenas D, Jones L, Lowe J, Janda M. A mobile technology intervention with ultraviolet radiation dosimeters and smartphone apps for skin cancer prevention in young adults: randomized controlled trial. JMIR Mhealth Uhealth 2018 Nov 28;6(11):e199 [FREE Full text] [doi: 10.2196/mhealth.9854] [Medline: 30487115]
24. King L, Xiang F, Swaminathan A, Lucas RM. Measuring sun exposure in epidemiological studies: Matching the method to the research question. J Photochem Photobiol B 2015 Dec;153:373-379. [doi: 10.1016/j.jphotobiol.2015.10.024] [Medline: 26555640]
25. Allen MW, McKenzie RL. National Institute of Water and Atmospheric Research. 2010. Electronic UV Dosimeters for Research and Education URL: https://niwa.co.nz/sites/niwa.co.nz/files/electronic_uv_dosimeters.pdf [accessed 2019-01-01]
26. Banerjee S, Hoch EG, Kaplan PD, Dumont EL. A Comparative Study of Wearable Ultraviolet Radiometers. In: Proceedings of the 2017 IEEE Life Sciences Conference. 2017 Presented at: LSC'17; December 13-15, 2017; Sydney, Australia. [doi: 10.1109/LSC.2017.8268131]
27. Webb AR. Measuring UV radiation: a discussion of dosimeter properties, uses and limitations. J Photochem Photobiol B 1995 Nov;31(1-2):9-13. [doi: 10.1016/1011-1344(95)07162-4]
28. Webb AR, Slaper H, Koepke P, Schmalwieser AW. Know your standard: clarifying the CIE erythema action spectrum. Photochem Photobiol 2011;87(2):483-486. [doi: 10.1111/j.1751-1097.2010.00871.x] [Medline: 21366601]
29. World Health Organization. Ultraviolet Radiation and Health URL: http://www.who.int/uv/uv_and_health/en/ [accessed 2019-01-01]
30. Lewis ZH, Lyons EJ, Jarvis JM, Baillargeon J. Using an electronic activity monitor system as an intervention modality: A systematic review. BMC Public Health 2015 Jun 24;15:585 [FREE Full text] [doi: 10.1186/s12889-015-1947-3] [Medline: 26104189]
31. Ridgers ND, McNarry MA, Mackintosh KA. Feasibility and effectiveness of using wearable activity trackers in youth: a systematic review. JMIR Mhealth Uhealth 2016 Nov 23;4(4):e129 [FREE Full text] [doi: 10.2196/mhealth.6540] [Medline: 27881359]
32. Køster B, Søndergaard J, Nielsen JB, Allen M, Bjerregaard M, Olsen A, et al. Feasibility of smartphone diaries and personal dosimeters to quantitatively study exposure to ultraviolet radiation in a small national sample. Photodermatol Photoimmunol Photomed 2015 Sep;31(5):252-260. [doi: 10.1111/phpp.12179] [Medline: 25850335]
33. Centers for Disease Control and Prevention. US Cancer Statistics Data Visualizations Tool URL: https://www.cdc.gov/cancer/uscs/dataviz/index.htm [accessed 2019-01-01]
34. Bowen DJ, Kreuter M, Spring B, Cofta-Woerpel L, Linnan L, Weiner D, et al. How we design feasibility studies. Am J Prev Med 2009 May;36(5):452-457 [FREE Full text] [doi: 10.1016/j.amepre.2009.02.002] [Medline: 19362699]
35. Spagnolli A, Guardigli E, Orso V, Varotto A, Gamberini L. Measuring User Acceptance of Wearable Symbiotic Devices: Validation Study Across Application Scenarios. In: Proceedings of the International Workshop on Symbiotic Interaction. 2015 Presented at: Symbiotic'15; October 7-8, 2015; Berlin, Germany p. 87-98. [doi: 10.1007/978-3-319-13500-7_7]
36. Harris PA, Taylor R, Thielke R, Payne J, Gonzalez N, Conde JG. Research electronic data capture (REDCap)--a metadata-driven methodology and workflow process for providing translational research informatics support. J Biomed Inform 2009 Apr;42(2):377-381 [FREE Full text] [doi: 10.1016/j.jbi.2008.08.010] [Medline: 18929686]
37. Harris PA, Taylor R, Minor BL, Elliott V, Fernandez M, O'Neal L, REDCap Consortium. The REDCap consortium: Building an international community of software platform partners. J Biomed Inform 2019 Jul;95:103208. [doi: 10.1016/j.jbi.2019.103208] [Medline: 31078660]
38. Elo S, Kyngäs H. The qualitative content analysis process. J Adv Nurs 2008 Apr;62(1):107-115. [doi: 10.1111/j.1365-2648.2007.04569.x] [Medline: 18352969]
39. Cancer Treatment Centers of America. Risk Factors for Skin Cancer URL: https://www.cancercenter.com/cancer-types/skin-cancer/risk-factors [accessed 2019-01-01]
40. Centers for Disease Control and Prevention. 2019. Skin Cancer: Behavior Rates: Sunburns URL: https://www.cdc.gov/cancer/skin/statistics/behavior/sunburns.htm [accessed 2019-01-01]
41. Stubbs B, Williams J, Gaughran F, Craig T. How sedentary are people with psychosis? A systematic review and meta-analysis. Schizophr Res 2016 Mar;171(1-3):103-109. [doi: 10.1016/j.schres.2016.01.034] [Medline: 26805414]
42. Shuk E, Burkhalter JE, Baguer CF, Holland SM, Pinkhasik A, Brady MS, et al. Factors associated with inconsistent sun protection in first-degree relatives of melanoma survivors. Qual Health Res 2012 Jul;22(7):934-945 [FREE Full text] [doi: 10.1177/1049732312443426] [Medline: 22645220]
43. Diffey B. Climate change, ozone depletion and the impact on ultraviolet exposure of human skin. Phys Med Biol 2004 Jan 7;49(1):R1-11. [doi: 10.1088/0031-9155/49/1/r01] [Medline: 14971768]
44. Linos E, Swetter SM, Cockburn MG, Colditz GA, Clarke CA. Increasing burden of melanoma in the United States. J Invest Dermatol 2009 Jul;129(7):1666-1674 [FREE Full text] [doi: 10.1038/jid.2008.423] [Medline: 19131946]
45. Ridgers ND, Timperio A, Brown H, Ball K, Macfarlane S, Lai SK, et al. Wearable activity tracker use among Australian adolescents: usability and acceptability study. JMIR Mhealth Uhealth 2018 Apr 11;6(4):e86 [FREE Full text] [doi: 10.2196/mhealth.9199] [Medline: 29643054]
46. Schaefer SE, Ching CC, Breen H, German JB. Wearing, thinking, and moving: testing the feasibility of fitness tracking with urban youth. Am J Health Educ 2016;47(1):8-16. [doi: 10.1080/19325037.2015.1111174]

47. Schaefer SE, van Loan M, German JB. A feasibility study of wearable activity monitors for pre-adolescent school-age children. Prev Chronic Dis 2014 May 22;11:E85 [FREE Full text] [doi: 10.5888/pcd11.130262] [Medline: 24854236]

Abbreviations

NIH: National Institutes of Health
REDCap: Research Electronic Data Capture
SED: standard erythemal dose
UVR: UV radiation

25

Assessment of Altmetrics and PlumX Metrics Scoring as Mechanisms to Evaluate the Top 100 Trending Hidradenitis Suppurativa Articles on Social Media

Chapman Wei[1], BSc; Aaron Fong[2], MD; Theodore Quan[1], BSc; Puneet Gupta[1], BSc; Adam Friedman[2], MD, FAAD

[1]George Washington University School of Medicine and Health Sciences, Washington, DC, United States

[2]Department of Dermatology, George Washington University School of Medicine and Health Sciences, Washington, DC, United States

Corresponding Author:
Adam Friedman, MD, FAAD
Department of Dermatology
George Washington University School of Medicine and Health Sciences
2150 Pennsylvania Avenue, 2B-430
Washington, DC, 20037
United States

Email: ajfriedman@mfa.gwu.edu

Abstract

Background: Dermatologists are increasingly utilizing social media platforms to disseminate scientific information. New tools, such as altmetrics and PlumX metrics, have been made available to rapidly capture the level of scientific article dissemination across social media platforms. However, no studies have been performed to assess the level of scientific article dissemination across social media regarding hidradenitis suppurativa, a disease that is still currently not well understood.

Objective: The aim of our study was to evaluate the utility of altmetrics and PlumX metrics by characterizing the top 100 "trending" hidradenitis suppurativa articles in the altmetric database by the altmetric attention score and PlumX score.

Methods: Altmetric data components of the top 100 hidradenitis suppurativa articles were extracted from the altmetric database. Article citation count was found using Web of Science. PlumX field-weighted impact scores for each article were collected from the Scopus database. Journal title, open-access status, article type, and study design of original articles were assessed. Additionally, the altmetric attention score, PlumX score, and citation count were log transformed and adjusted by +1 for linear regression, and Spearman correlation coefficients were utilized to determine correlations.

Results: Most of the top 100 "trending" hidradenitis suppurativa articles were published in *JAMA Dermatology* (n=27, 27%). The median altmetric attention score, PlumX score, and citation count were 25.5, 3.7, and 10.5, respectively. The most mentions regarding social media platforms came from Twitter. Although no correlation was observed between the citation count and altmetric attention score (r^2=0.019, P=.17), positive correlation was observed between the citation count and PlumX score (r^2=0.469, P<.001).

Conclusions: Our research demonstrated that citation count is not correlated with the altmetric attention score, but is strongly correlated with the PlumX score regarding hidradenitis suppurativa articles at this point in time. With the continual increase of social media usage by medical professionals and researchers, this study can help investigators understand the best way to captivate their audience.

KEYWORDS

altmetric; PlumX; social media; impact factor; hidradenitis suppurativa

Introduction

Dissemination of science-based peer-reviewed information is essential for increasing awareness of hidradenitis suppurativa, an inflammatory skin disease that is often underrecognized, leading to delayed diagnosis and higher severity at initial presentation [1]. Dermatologists are increasingly utilizing social media platforms to disseminate scientific information [2]. In contrast to medical journals, social media serves as a useful platform to inform the wider general public, both medical professionals and laypeople alike. New tools, including alternative metrics (altmetrics) and PlumX metrics, have been made available to evaluate the extent of an article's dissemination across social media platforms [3,4]. Provided by altmetrics, the altmetric attention score is a weighted score of the amount of "online attention" a research article has received across social media platforms. These platforms include Facebook, Twitter, Google+, blogs, and others [5]. Similarly, PlumX has a PlumX field-weighted citation impact score (PlumX score) that is also a weighted score of the level of article dissemination across similar social media metrics and includes the number of citations, linkouts, and abstract views [6]. While the citation count or "impact factor" reflects the number of citations by other articles or journals, altmetrics and PlumX metrics reflect an article's instantaneous attentiveness among news outlets, blogs, Twitter, Facebook, and other media platforms [7]. While these tools allow one to assess what kind of articles are garnering social media attention or "trending" on social media platforms, the assessment of the utility of altmetrics regarding hidradenitis suppurativa research has not been evaluated yet. Owing to the ability of these metrics to rapidly capture the level of scientific article dissemination, they have the potential of being used complementary with citation count and identifying high-impact hidradenitis suppurativa articles, since the traditional tool takes years to measure an article's impact on field advancement. To evaluate the utility of these tools, we characterized the top 100 "trending" hidradenitis suppurativa articles across social media platforms captured in the altmetric database by altmetric attention scores complemented with PlumX scores and more established markers of manuscript value. Our study aimed to assess the social media platforms that most contribute to the dissemination of literature-based hidradenitis suppurativa information. We also sought to examine how alternative metrics compare with traditional metrics, such as citation count. We hypothesized that alternative metrics will be able to better complement more traditional metrics when evaluating an article's quality.

Methods

Utilizing Altmetric Explorer, we identified articles using the PubMed search criterion "hidradenitis suppurativa." Altmetric data components of the top 100 altmetric attention score hidradenitis suppurativa articles were extracted in July 2020. The number of mentions from the following altmetric data components was extracted and examined: news mentions, blog mentions, policy mentions, Twitter mentions, Facebook mentions, Wikipedia mentions, Reddit mentions, Mendeley readers, and number of Dimension citations [6]. Mentions represent a measure of how many times a specific term, such as "hidradenitis suppurative," has been referenced on social media channels. Dimension citations include grants, publications, citations, alternative metrics, clinical trials, and patents. Data were also collected about the journal impact factor, journal title, open-access status, where the articles were published, article type, article study design, and article citation count [4,5]. PlumX field-weighted citation impact scores for each article were collected from the Scopus database. Statistical analysis was performed using Prism 8 (GraphPad software), and statistical significance was defined as a P value <.05. Spearman correlation coefficients were utilized to determine correlations [2]. Altmetric attention scores, PlumX field-weighted citation impact scores, and citation count were log transformed and adjusted by +1 for linear regression.

Results

Of the top 100 "trending" hidradenitis suppurativa articles by highest altmetric attention score, most were published in *JAMA Dermatology* (n=27, 27%), followed by *Journal of the American Academy of Dermatology* (n=16, 16%) (Table 1). The median altmetric attention score, PlumX score, and citation count were 25.5, 3.7, and 10.5, respectively. Majority of the "trending" hidradenitis suppurativa research articles were published by authors from Europe (n=47). The median journal impact factor was 6.9. The highest altmetric attention score article was a review article (altmetric attention score=352) [8]. This review article discussed the diagnosis, epidemiology, and treatment of hidradenitis suppurativa, with specific emphasis on advances in the past 5 years [8]. A total of 58 articles had an altmetric attention score above 20, a marker for the top 5% of all scientific output [4]. Of the social media platforms, the most mentions came from Twitter (2830 mentions), which was mostly used to share European-affiliated articles. The second most mentions came from news (573 mentions), which was mostly used to share North American–affiliated articles. The number of Mendeley readers and Dimension citations were 5130 and 4152, respectively. Most of the articles were original articles (53 articles). A total of 49 articles were open access. The most common study design utilized was the clinical observational design (34 articles). A correlation was observed between the altmetric attention score and journal impact factor (r^2=0.17, P<.001). Although no correlation was observed between citation count and the altmetric attention score (r^2=0.019, P=.17; Figure 1), a positive correlation was observed between citation count and the PlumX score (r^2=0.469, P<.001). The altmetric attention score was further found not to be correlated with citation count for particular article types in a chi-square analysis (P=.95). Open-access status did not affect the altmetric attention score P=.71). Out of the 100 articles, most of the articles were published in 2017 (19 articles), followed by 18 articles published in 2019 (Figure 2).

Table 1. Characteristics of the top 100 "trending" hidradenitis suppurativa articles by the altmetric score.

Characteristic	Value (N=100)
Journal, n	
JAMA Dermatology	27
Journal of the American Academy of Dermatology	16
British Journal of Dermatology	5
Journal of Investigative Dermatology	4
Other journals	48
Altmetric score, median (range)	25.5 (13-352)
PlumX field score, median (range)	3.7 (0.0-31.8)
Journal impact factor, median (range)	6.9 (0.2-70.7)
Traditional citation, median (range)	10.5 (0-389)
News mentions, total (range)	573 (0-109)
Policy mentions, total (range)	17 (0-3)
Twitter mentions, total (range)	2830 (0-706)
Facebook mentions, total (range)	190 (0-24)
Number of Mendeley readers, total (range)	5130 (0-245)
Number of Dimension citations, total (range)	4152 (0-418)
Article type, n	
Original investigation	53
Research letter/comments to the Editor/brief report	6
Review	30
Editorial	4
Viewpoint/clinical pearls	2
Guidelines/specific statement	2
Other	3
Open access	49
Study design, n	
Case report/series	6
Clinical observation	34
Clinical trial	5
Basic science	7
Region of the article's authors, n	
Europe	47
North America	37
Other	16

Figure 1. Citation count correlation with the altmetric attention score (AAS) and PlumX score.

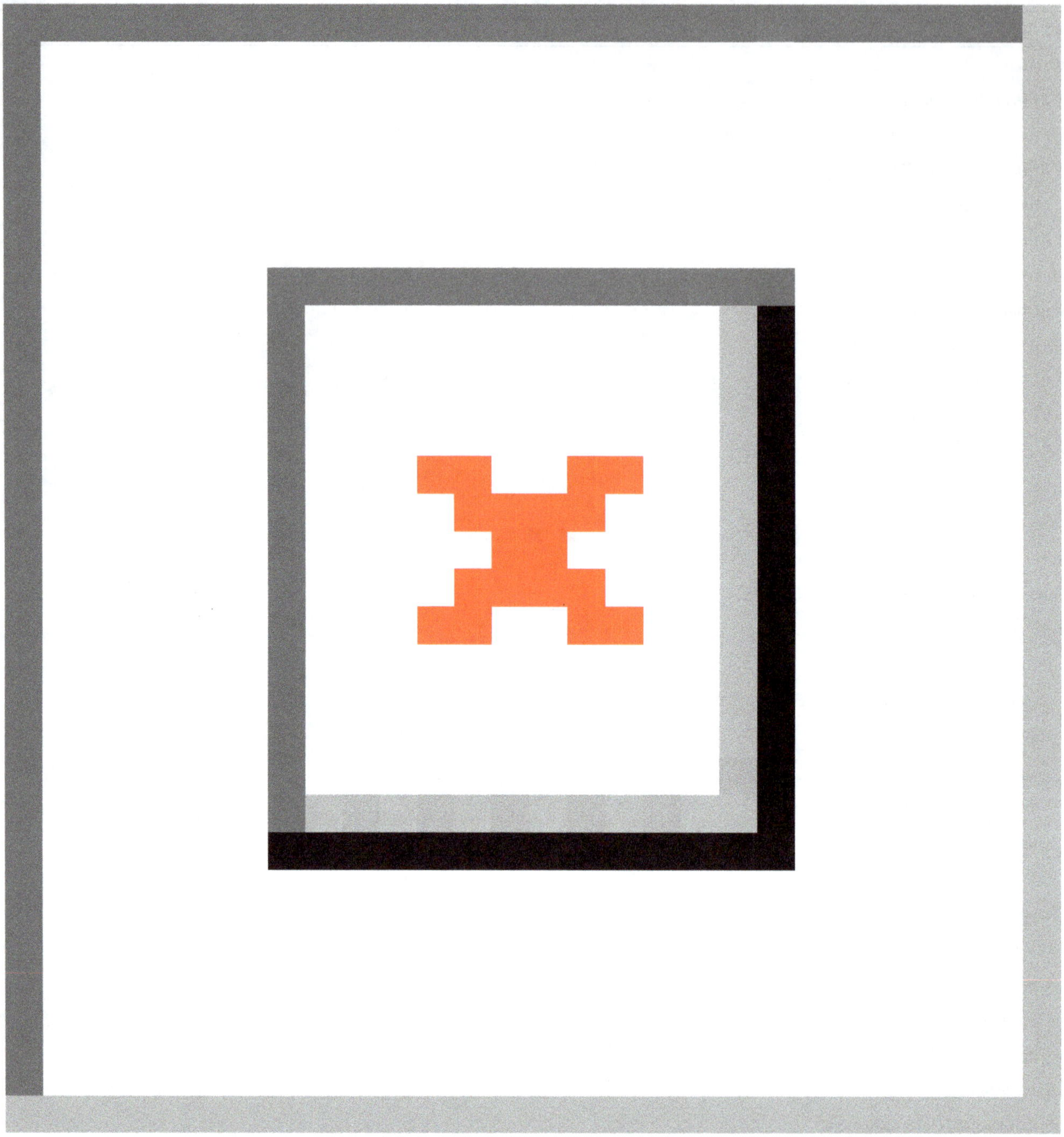

Figure 2. Year of publication for the included articles.

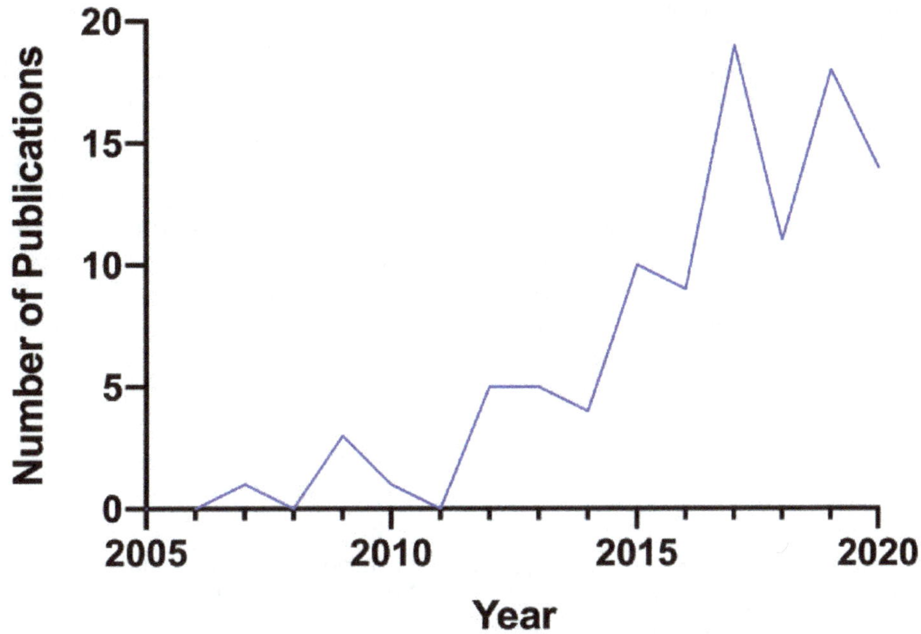

Discussion

Principal Findings

This study determined the characteristics of the top 100 "trending" hidradenitis suppurativa articles that received the greatest amount of social media attention captured in the altmetric database. Twitter was the most widely used social media platform when mentioning hidradenitis suppurativa. The article with the highest altmetric attention score, a review paper with European affiliation, achieved this high score likely because this article not only summarized the current knowledge about hidradenitis suppurativa, but also went on to provide new insights into the advances in hidradenitis suppurativa research with clear recommendations [8]. Open access, which is often an added cost to authors, did not contribute to a higher altmetric attention score. This likely occurred owing to the decline of the open-access advantage from the ease of article redistribution [9].

Comparison With Prior Work

Currently, there are no published studies evaluating the utilization of altmetrics with regard to the hidradenitis suppurativa literature. There are however multiple past altmetric studies that investigated top "trending" articles in the altmetric database regarding the correlation between traditional bibliometrics, such as citation count, and online attention, specifically the altmetric attention score. These studies included research articles about specific conditions, such as stroke and oral cancer, and also about specific medical fields, such as urology, emergency medicine, and plastic surgery [10-14]. In our study, altmetrics did not correlate with citation count in hidradenitis suppurativa literature despite its ability to rapidly assess how widely an article is disseminated, while the PlumX score did show correlation. Variable results have been reported regarding the utility of altmetrics [2,4,10-14]. While some articles reported findings similar to those in our study [10,12,13], others only showed a modest correlation at best between citation count and the altmetric attention score [2,4,11,14]. This is likely because the altmetric attention score is more dynamic than the PlumX score since the altmetric attention score focuses on tracking of real-time public interest in a particular topic. Thus, the altmetric attention score does not factor in citation count. In contrast, the PlumX score is likely a better marker because PlumX metrics factor in citation count, suggesting that PlumX metrics may be more useful in identifying high-impact hidradenitis suppurativa articles.

Limitations

There are several limitations with this study. This study was a cross-sectional study performed in July 2020, so altmetric and PlumX scores may change in the future. Altmetric and PlumX scores should be cautiously interpreted as these alternative metrics do not reflect article quality. Thus, a research article that receives a wide amount of social media attention should not be interpreted as having important results and should be examined in conjunction with in-depth article analysis to determine research quality. Additionally, since the article sample utilized in this study represented a minority of published articles on hidradenitis suppurativa, the generalizability of the findings may be limited regarding hidradenitis suppurativa literature. However, our analysis assessed all hidradenitis suppurativa articles that were in the top 5% of scientific output in the altmetrics database. More recently published hidradenitis suppurativa articles can experience a delay in their citation count compared with older articles. Lastly, our analysis did not assess the presence of journal Twitter accounts or whether the journals were active on Twitter. It is possible that journals having a larger social media presence may bolster their hidradenitis suppurativa articles with higher altmetric scores.

Future Directions

The correlation of the PlumX score and the altmetric attention score with citation count for other dermatology topics remains to be explored. Further research into identifying specific traits of hidradenitis suppurativa articles with a higher PlumX score or altmetric attention score is warranted. Given the increasing usage of social media by medical professionals and researchers, such research can be useful to investigators by helping them understand the best way to maximize their reach, including the general public. However, as is suggested by our study, it must be understood that the level of research dissemination across social media does not necessarily translate to an impact in the scientific community.

Conclusion

Since altmetrics and PlumX metrics are dynamic reflections of the general social media interest, there is still some discordance between scientific articles and social media. Although these metrics can identify the impact and dissemination to the public, they do not measure the stringent review process that articles undergo for publication in scientific journals. Despite these limitations, both metrics can be used complementary with traditional citation analysis to assess article quality. Altmetrics with PlumX may be used to rapidly capture what the general public is interested in regarding hidradenitis suppurativa, while traditional metrics can be used to assess an article's impact.

References

1. Dufour DN, Emtestam L, Jemec GB. Hidradenitis suppurativa: a common and burdensome, yet under-recognised, inflammatory skin disease. Postgrad Med J 2014 Apr;90(1062):216-21; quiz 220 [FREE Full text] [doi: 10.1136/postgradmedj-2013-131994] [Medline: 24567417]
2. Jia J, Nguyen B, Mills D, Polin DJ, Sarin KY. Comparing online engagement and academic impact of dermatology research: An Altmetric Attention Score and PlumX Metrics analysis. J Am Acad Dermatol 2020 Aug;83(2):648-650 [FREE Full text] [doi: 10.1016/j.jaad.2019.12.003] [Medline: 31836559]
3. Peters I, Kraker P, Lex E, Gumpenberger C, Gorraiz J. Research data explored: an extended analysis of citations and altmetrics. Scientometrics 2016;107:723-744 [FREE Full text] [doi: 10.1007/s11192-016-1887-4] [Medline: 27122647]
4. Patel RB, Vaduganathan M, Bhatt DL, Bonow RO. Characterizing High-Performing Articles by Altmetric Score in Major Cardiovascular Journals. JAMA Cardiol 2018 Dec 01;3(12):1249-1251 [FREE Full text] [doi: 10.1001/jamacardio.2018.3823] [Medline: 30476952]
5. Elmore SA. The Altmetric Attention Score: What Does It Mean and Why Should I Care? Toxicol Pathol 2018 Apr;46(3):252-255 [FREE Full text] [doi: 10.1177/0192623318758294] [Medline: 29448902]
6. Ortega J. Disciplinary differences of the impact of altmetric. FEMS Microbiol Lett 2018 Apr 01;365(7). [doi: 10.1093/femsle/fny049] [Medline: 29518193]
7. Patthi B, Prasad M, Gupta R, Singla A, Kumar JK, Dhama K, et al. Altmetrics - A Collated Adjunct Beyond Citations for Scholarly Impact: A Systematic Review. J Clin Diagn Res 2017 Jun;11(6):ZE16-ZE20 [FREE Full text] [doi: 10.7860/JCDR/2017/26153.10078] [Medline: 28764311]
8. Saunte DM, Jemec GB. Hidradenitis Suppurativa: Advances in Diagnosis and Treatment. JAMA 2017 Nov 28;318(20):2019-2032. [doi: 10.1001/jama.2017.16691] [Medline: 29183082]
9. Davis PM. Author-choice open-access publishing in the biological and medical literature: A citation analysis. J. Am. Soc. Inf. Sci 2009 Jan;60(1):3-8. [doi: 10.1002/asi.20965]
10. Asaad M, Howell S, Rajesh A, Meaike J, Tran NV. Altmetrics in Plastic Surgery Journals: Does It Correlate With Citation Count? Aesthet Surg J 2020 Oct 24;40(11):NP628-NP635. [doi: 10.1093/asj/sjaa158] [Medline: 32506129]
11. Nocera AP, Boyd CJ, Boudreau H, Hakim O, Rais-Bahrami S. Examining the Correlation Between Altmetric Score and Citations in the Urology Literature. Urology 2019 Dec;134:45-50. [doi: 10.1016/j.urology.2019.09.014] [Medline: 31560915]
12. Kim Y, Kim J, Kim YH, Yoon DY, Kim YJ, Bae JS. Social attention and scientific articles on stroke: Altmetric analysis of top-50 articles. Clin Neurol Neurosurg 2019 Aug;183:105386. [doi: 10.1016/j.clineuro.2019.105386] [Medline: 31207458]
13. Hassona Y, Qutachi T, Dardas L, Alrashdan MS, Sawair F. The online attention to oral cancer research: An Altmetric analysis. Oral Dis 2019 Sep;25(6):1502-1510. [doi: 10.1111/odi.13111] [Medline: 31033085]
14. Barbic D, Tubman M, Lam H, Barbic S. An Analysis of Altmetrics in Emergency Medicine. Acad Emerg Med 2016 Mar;23(3):251-268 [FREE Full text] [doi: 10.1111/acem.12898] [Medline: 26743680]

26

Performance of Artificial Intelligence Imaging Models in Detecting Dermatological Manifestations in Higher Fitzpatrick Skin Color Classifications

Pushkar Aggarwal, MBA

College of Medicine, University of Cincinnati, Cincinnati, OH, United States

Corresponding Author:
Pushkar Aggarwal, MBA
College of Medicine
University of Cincinnati
3230 Eden Ave
Cincinnati, OH, 45267
United States

Email: aggarwpr@mail.uc.edu

Abstract

Background: The performance of deep-learning image recognition models is below par when applied to images with Fitzpatrick classification skin types 4 and 5.

Objective: The objective of this research was to assess whether image recognition models perform differently when differentiating between dermatological diseases in individuals with darker skin color (Fitzpatrick skin types 4 and 5) than when differentiating between the same dermatological diseases in Caucasians (Fitzpatrick skin types 1, 2, and 3) when both models are trained on the same number of images.

Methods: Two image recognition models were trained, validated, and tested. The goal of each model was to differentiate between melanoma and basal cell carcinoma. Open-source images of melanoma and basal cell carcinoma were acquired from the Hellenic Dermatological Atlas, the Dermatology Atlas, the Interactive Dermatology Atlas, and DermNet NZ.

Results: The image recognition models trained and validated on images with light skin color had higher sensitivity, specificity, positive predictive value, negative predictive value, and F1 score than the image recognition models trained and validated on images of skin of color for differentiation between melanoma and basal cell carcinoma.

Conclusions: A higher number of images of dermatological diseases in individuals with darker skin color than images of dermatological diseases in individuals with light skin color would need to be gathered for artificial intelligence models to perform equally well.

KEYWORDS

deep learning; melanoma; basal cell carcinoma; skin of color; image recognition; dermatology; disease; convolutional neural network; specificity; prediction; artificial intelligence; skin color; skin tone

Introduction

Background

In dermatology, artificial intelligence (AI) is poised to improve the efficiency and accuracy of traditional diagnostic approaches, including visual examination, skin biopsy, and histopathologic examination [1]. Deep-learning image recognition models have had success in differentiating between dermatological diseases using images of light-skinned individuals. However, when these models are tested on images of people with skin of color, the performance drops [2]. It is thought that the primary reason for this difference is the lack of available images of dermatological diseases in individuals with darker skin color (Fitzpatrick classification of skin types 4 and 5) [3]. However, is it also possible that even when the same number of images are available, image recognition models will have a harder time differentiating between dermatological diseases in individuals with Fitzpatrick skin types 4 and 5 compared to skin types 1, 2, and 3?

Objective

The objective of this research was to assess whether image recognition models perform differently when differentiating between dermatological diseases in individuals of color (Fitzpatrick skin types 4 and 5) than when differentiating between the same dermatological diseases in Caucasians (Fitzpatrick skin types 1, 2, and 3) when both models are trained on an equal number of images.

Methods

Open-source images of melanoma and basal cell carcinoma (BCC) were acquired from the Hellenic Dermatological Atlas [4], the Dermatology Atlas [5], the Interactive Dermatology Atlas [6], and DermNet NZ [7]. Two image recognition models were trained, validated, and tested using methodology as described previously [8]. TensorFlow [9], an open-source software library by Google, was used as a deep-learning framework and was used to retrain Inception, version 3 (v3). Inception v3 is a deep convolutional neural network. This neural network consists of a hierarchy of multiple computational layers that each have an input and output. All layers except the final layer of this neural network are pretrained with more than 1.2 million images. The final layer of the neural network was retrained with the gathered dermatological images. During the retraining process, the neural network underwent both a training and validation step. In the training step, the inputted images were used to train the neural network. In the validation step, inputted naïve images were used to iteratively assess training accuracy [10].

After the model had been retrained (trained and validated), a user-inputted testing/assessment step was performed in which test images were inputted and the results were statistically analyzed. The program assessment output is expressed in terms of percentages of the probability of each of the dermatological manifestations for each testing image inputted. R software (R Foundation for Statistical Computing) [11] was used to perform the statistical analysis. Sensitivity, specificity, positive predictive value (PPV), negative predictive value (NPV), and F1 score were calculated for each dermatological manifestation. The F1 score is the harmonic average of the sensitivity and PPV (mean of the recall and precision).

The goal of each model was to differentiate between melanoma and BCC.

The first model was:

- Trained on 150 images of individuals with light skin color (Fitzpatrick skin types 1, 2, and 3), 75 melanoma and 75 BCC images;
- Validated on 38 images of individuals with light skin color (Fitzpatrick skin types 1, 2, and 3), 19 melanoma and 19 BCC images;
- Tested on 30 images of individuals with light skin color (Fitzpatrick skin types 1, 2, and 3), 15 melanoma and 15 BCC images.

The second model was:

- Trained on 150 images of individuals with skin of color (Fitzpatrick skin types 4 and 5), 75 melanoma and 75 BCC images;
- Validated on 38 images of individuals with skin of color (Fitzpatrick skin types 4 and 5), 19 melanoma and 19 BCC images;
- Tested on 30 images of individuals with skin of color (Fitzpatrick skin types 4 and 5), 15 melanoma and 15 BCC images.

Area under the receiver operating characteristic (AUC) curves for melanoma and BCC were calculated to determine the performance of the two models.

Results

When asked to differentiate between melanoma and BCC, the image recognition model trained and validated on images of light skin color had higher sensitivity, specificity, PPV, NPV, and F1 score than the image recognition model trained and validated on images of skin of color (Table 1).

In predicting melanoma, the image recognition model trained and validated on images of light skin color had a sensitivity of 0.60, specificity of 0.53, PPV of 0.56, NPV of 0.57, and F1 score of 0.58. On the other hand, in predicting melanoma, the same image recognition model trained and validated on images of skin of color had a sensitivity of 0.53, specificity of 0.47, PPV of 0.50, NPV of 0.50, and F1 score of 0.52.

In predicting BCC, the image recognition model trained and validated on images of light skin color had a sensitivity of 0.53, specificity of 0.60, PPV of 0.57, NPV of 0.56, and F1 score of 0.55. On the other hand, for prediction of BCC, the same image recognition model trained and validated on images of skin of color had a sensitivity of 0.47, specificity of 0.53, PPV of 0.50, NPV of 0.50, and F1 score of 0.48.

The average AUC for the two light skin color image recognition models was 0.598, compared to 0.500 (values point out the difference) for the skin of color image recognition models (Table 1 and Figure 1).

Table 1. Statistical measures of the deep-learning model trained, validated, and tested on different Fitzpatrick skin type classifications (types 1, 2, and 3 vs types 4 and 5) for evaluating melanoma and basal cell carcinoma.

Measure	Melanoma model		Basal cell carcinoma model	
	Skin types 1, 2, and 3	Skin types 4 and 5	Skin types 1, 2, and 3	Skin types 4 and 5
Sensitivity	0.60	0.53	0.53	0.47
Specificity	0.53	0.47	0.60	0.53
Positive predictive value	0.56	0.50	0.57	0.50
Negative predictive value	0.57	0.50	0.56	0.50
F1 score	0.58	0.52	0.55	0.48
Area under the receiver operating characteristic curve	0.59	0.57	0.60	0.53

Figure 1. Receiver operating characteristic curves for melanoma and basal cell carcinoma (BCC) in each of the two models for different skin types. FC: Fitzpatrick classification.

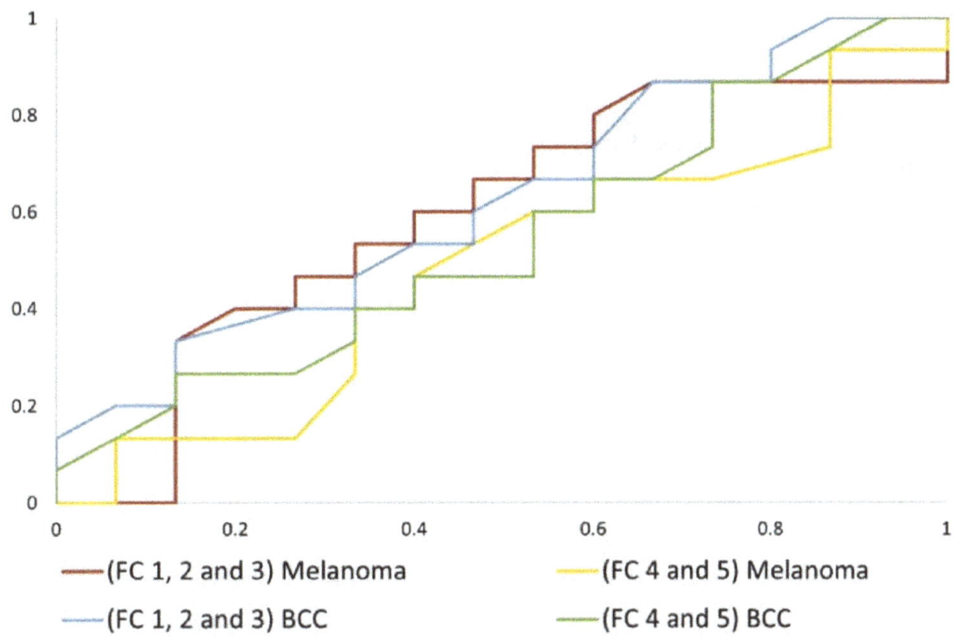

Discussion

Limitations

The number of images available was limited for Fitzpatrick skin types 4 and 5; as such, both the light skin color and skin of color models were investigated with this constraint for the number of images used during training. A larger sample size would have been better to test if the results recur consistently.

Conclusion

When the same number of images is used for training, validation, and testing, the AI model that was provided images of melanoma and BCC belonging to Fitzpatrick classification skin types 1, 2, and 3 performed better than the AI model that was provided with images of melanoma and BCC in skin types 4 and 5. This may be because dermatological diseases can have more variability in presentation in individuals with darker skin; additionally, cutaneous manifestations may not be as easily distinguished from the surrounding skin in darker-skinned individuals. As such, a higher number of images of skin of color with dermatological diseases than images of light skin color with dermatological diseases would need to be gathered for the AI models to perform equally well.

References

1. Patel S, Wang JV, Motaparthi K, Lee JB. Artificial intelligence in dermatology for the clinician. Clinics in Dermatology 2021 Mar;21(8):e208 [FREE Full text] [doi: 10.1016/j.clindermatol.2021.03.012] [Medline: 34237259]
2. Kamulegeya LH, Okello M, Bwanika JM, MusinguziD D, Lubega W, Rusoke D, et al. Using artificial intelligence on dermatology conditions in Uganda: A case for diversity in training data sets for machine learning. bioRxiv. Preprint posted online October 31, 2019 [FREE Full text] [doi: 10.1101/826057]

3. Adamson AS, Smith A. Machine Learning and Health Care Disparities in Dermatology. JAMA Dermatol 2018 Nov 01;154(11):1247-1248. [doi: 10.1001/jamadermatol.2018.2348] [Medline: 30073260]
4. Verros CD. Hellenic Dermatological Atlas. 2011. URL: http://www.hellenicdermatlas.com/en/ [accessed 2021-09-02]
5. da Silva SF. Dermatology Atlas. 2021. URL: http://www.atlasdermatologico.com.br/ [accessed 2021-09-02]
6. Usatine RP, Madden BD. Interactive Dermatology Atlas. 2019. URL: https://www.dermatlas.net/ [accessed 2021-09-02]
7. Oakley A, Suhonen R, Ashton R, Waikato District Health Board, New Zealand Dermatological Society Inc. DermNet NZ. URL: https://dermnetnz.org/ [accessed 2021-09-02]
8. Aggarwal P. Data augmentation in dermatology image recognition using machine learning. Skin Res Technol 2019 Nov;25(6):815-820. [doi: 10.1111/srt.12726] [Medline: 31140653]
9. Abadi M, Barham P, Chen J, Chen Z, Davis A, Dean J, et al. TensorFlow: A system for large-scale machine learning. arXiv. Preprint posted online May 27, 2016 [FREE Full text]
10. Zhang YC, Kagen AC. Machine Learning Interface for Medical Image Analysis. J Digit Imaging 2017 Oct;30(5):615-621 [FREE Full text] [doi: 10.1007/s10278-016-9910-0] [Medline: 27730415]
11. R Core Team. R: A language and environment for statistical computing. Vienna, Austria: R Foundation for Statistical Computing URL: http://www.R-project.org/ [accessed 2021-09-02]

Abbreviations

AI: artificial intelligence
AUC: area under the receiver operating characteristic
BCC: basal cell carcinoma
NPV: negative predictive value
PPV: positive predictive value

Permissions

All chapters in this book were first published by JMIR Publications; hereby published with permission under the Creative Commons Attribution License or equivalent. Every chapter published in this book has been scrutinized by our experts. Their significance has been extensively debated. The topics covered herein carry significant findings which will fuel the growth of the discipline. They may even be implemented as practical applications or may be referred to as a beginning point for another development.

The contributors of this book come from diverse backgrounds, making this book a truly international effort. This book will bring forth new frontiers with its revolutionizing research information and detailed analysis of the nascent developments around the world.

We would like to thank all the contributing authors for lending their expertise to make the book truly unique. They have played a crucial role in the development of this book. Without their invaluable contributions this book wouldn't have been possible. They have made vital efforts to compile up to date information on the varied aspects of this subject to make this book a valuable addition to the collection of many professionals and students.

This book was conceptualized with the vision of imparting up-to-date information and advanced data in this field. To ensure the same, a matchless editorial board was set up. Every individual on the board went through rigorous rounds of assessment to prove their worth. After which they invested a large part of their time researching and compiling the most relevant data for our readers.

The editorial board has been involved in producing this book since its inception. They have spent rigorous hours researching and exploring the diverse topics which have resulted in the successful publishing of this book. They have passed on their knowledge of decades through this book. To expedite this challenging task, the publisher supported the team at every step. A small team of assistant editors was also appointed to further simplify the editing procedure and attain best results for the readers.

Apart from the editorial board, the designing team has also invested a significant amount of their time in understanding the subject and creating the most relevant covers. They scrutinized every image to scout for the most suitable representation of the subject and create an appropriate cover for the book.

The publishing team has been an ardent support to the editorial, designing and production team. Their endless efforts to recruit the best for this project, has resulted in the accomplishment of this book. They are a veteran in the field of academics and their pool of knowledge is as vast as their experience in printing. Their expertise and guidance has proved useful at every step. Their uncompromising quality standards have made this book an exceptional effort. Their encouragement from time to time has been an inspiration for everyone.

The publisher and the editorial board hope that this book will prove to be a valuable piece of knowledge for researchers, students, practitioners and scholars across the globe.

List of Contributors

Nishita Maganty, Muneeb Ilyas, Zachary Ginsberg and Amit Sharma
Department of Dermatology, Mayo Clinic Arizona, Scottsdale, AZ, United States

Elliot J Coups and Sharon L Manne
Rutgers Cancer Institute of New Jersey, Rutgers, The State University of New Jersey, New Brunswick, NJ, United States
Department of Medicine, Rutgers Robert Wood Johnson Medical School, Rutgers, The State University of New Jersey, New Brunswick, NJ, United States

Kevin R Criswell
Rutgers Cancer Institute of New Jersey, Rutgers, The State University of New Jersey, New Brunswick, NJ, United States

Sherry L Pagoto
Department of Allied Health Sciences, College of Agriculture, Health and Natural Resources, University of Connecticut, Storrs, CT, United States

James S Goydos
Rutgers Cancer Institute of New Jersey, Rutgers, The State University of New Jersey, New Brunswick, NJ, United States
Department of Surgery, Rutgers Robert Wood Johnson Medical School, Rutgers, The State University of New Jersey, New Brunswick, NJ, United States

Angela M Rodrigues, Falko F Sniehotta, Mark A Birch-Machin, Patrick Olivier and Vera Araújo-Soares
Newcastle University, Newcastle, United Kingdom

Tiago M de Carvalho, Eline Noels, Marlies Wakkee and Tamar Nijsten
Department of Dermatology, Erasmus Medical Center, Rotterdam, Netherlands

Andreea Udrea
Department of Automatic Control and System Engineering, Polytechnic University of Bucharest, Bucharest, Romania

Anne K Julian, Jessica Welch, Sarah Shahid and Frank M Perna
Behavioral Research Program, Division of Cancer Control and Population Sciences, National Cancer Institute, Rockville, MD, United States

Maddison M Bean
College of Public Health and Human Sciences, Oregon State University, Corvallis, OR, United States

Sau Huu Nguyen and Thu Hoai Thi Le
National Hospital of Dermatology and Venereology, Hanoi, Vietnam
Department of Dermatology and Venereology, Hanoi Medical University, Hanoi, Vietnam

Giang Thu Vu
Center of Excellence in Evidence-based Medicine, Nguyen Tat Thanh University, Ho Chi Minh City, Vietnam

Long Hoang Nguyen
Center of Excellence in Behavioral Medicine, Nguyen Tat Thanh University, Ho Chi Minh City, Vietnam

Cuong Tat Nguyen
Institute for Global Health Innovations, Duy Tan University, Da Nang, Vietnam
Faculty of Medicine, Duy Tan University, Da Nang, Vietnam

Tung Hoang Tran
Institute of Orthopaedic and Trauma Surgery, Vietnam-Germany Hospital, Hanoi, Vietnam

Bach Xuan Tran
Institute for Preventive Medicine and Public Health, Hanoi Medical University, Hanoi, Vietnam
Bloomberg School of Public Health, Johns Hopkins University, Baltimore, MD, United States

Carl A Latkin
Bloomberg School of Public Health, Johns Hopkins University, Baltimore, MD, United States

Wilson W S Tam
Center of Excellence in Evidence-based Medicine, Nguyen Tat Thanh University, Ho Chi Minh City, Vietnam
Alice Lee Centre for Nursing Studies, Yong Loo Lin School of Medicine, National University of Singapore, Singapore

Cyrus S H Ho
Department of Psychological Medicine, National University Hospital, Singapore

Roger C M Ho
Center of Excellence in Behavioral Medicine, Nguyen Tat Thanh University, Ho Chi Minh City, Vietnam
Department of Psychological Medicine, Yong Loo Lin School of Medicine, National University of Singapore, Singapore
Institute for Health Innovation and Technology (iHealthtech), National University of Singapore

Teevit Dunnsiri, Takumi Kawashita, Sharon C Lee and Aaron Kumar Monga
Western University of Health Sciences, Pomona, CA, United States

Jessica Fitts Willoughby and Stephanie Gibbons
The Edward R Murrow College of Communication, Washington State University, Pullman, WA, United States

Jessica Gall Myrick
Donald P Bellisario College of Communications, Pennsylvania State University, University Park, PA, United States

Clark Kogan
Center for Interdisciplinary Statistical Education and Research, Washington State University, Pullman, WA, United States

Megan Andreas Moreno and Marina C Jenkins
Department of Pediatrics, University of Wisconsin-Madison, Madison, WI, United States

DeAnn Lazovich
Department of Epidemiology and Community Health, University of Minnesota, Minneapolis, MN, United States

Andrina Mamo
Department of Dermatology, University of Colorado Anschutz Medical Campus, Aurora, CO, United States

Roya Mirhossaini
Department of Medicine, Riverside Community Hospital, Riverside, CA, United States

Andrew Fortugno
Department of Medicine, University of Tennessee Health Sciences Center, Memphis, TN, United States

Christie Jaime
Department of Public Health, William Paterson University, Wayne, NJ, United States

Priscila E Laforet
Division of Hematology/Oncology, Department of Medicine, Columbia University Irving Medical Center, New York, NY, United States

Grace C Hillyer
Department of Epidemiology, Mailman School of Public Health, Columbia University, New York, NY, United States

Erica J Seidel
Department of Student Life/Counseling Center, Borough of Manhattan Community College, New York, NY, United States

William Kim, Sophia M Wolfe and Caterina Zagona-Prizio
University of Colorado School of Medicine, Aurora, CO, United States

Robert P Dellavalle
Dermatology Service, Rocky Mountain Regional VA Medical Center, Eastern Colorado Health Care System, Aurora, CO, United States
Colorado School of Public Health, Aurora, CO, United States
Department of Dermatology, University of Colorado Anschutz Medical Campus, Aurora, CO, United States

Torunn Elise Sivesind and Mindy D Szeto
Department of Dermatology, University of Colorado School of Medicine, Aurora, CO, United States

Robert Paul Dellavalle
Department of Dermatology, University of Colorado School of Medicine, Aurora, CO, United States
Dermatology Service, Rocky Mountain Regional VA Medical Center, Aurora, CO, United States

Monique A Sager and Mila Tamminga
Perelman School of Medicine, University of Pennsylvania, Philadelphia, PA, United States

Aditya M Kashyap, Sadhana Ravoori and Christopher Callison-Burch
Department of Computer Science, University of Pennsylvania, Philadelphia, PA, United States

Jules B Lipoff
Department of Dermatology, University of Pennsylvania, Philadelphia, PA, United States

Benjamin K P Woo
Department of Psychiatry, Olive View Medical Center, University of California Los Angeles Medical Center, Sylmar, CA, United States

Ashley Payton
Department of Psychiatry, Olive View Medical Center, University of California Los Angeles Medical Center, Sylmar, CA, United States
College of Osteopathic Medicine of the Pacific, Western University of Health Sciences, Pomona, CA, United States

Moshe Y Bressler
New York Institute of Technology College of Osteopathic Medicine, Old Westbury, NY, United States
Department of Dermatology, Jamaica Hospital Medical Center, Richmond Hill, NY, United States

Yaakov Bressler and Rebecca Tamez
Department of Dermatology, Jamaica Hospital Medical Center, Richmond Hill, NY, United States

Eugene Grudnikoff
Department of Psychiatry, South Oaks Hospital, Amityville, NY, United States

John G Zampella
Ronald O Perelman Department of Dermatology, New York University, New York, NY, United States

Ryan Ottwell, Micah Hartwell, Taylor Calli Rogers and Matt Vassar
Oklahoma State University Center for Health Sciences, Tulsa, OK, United States

Tracy Beswick
Center for Dermatology, Tulsa, OK, United States

Heather Ivy
Philadelphia College of Osteopathic Medicine, Roswell, GA, United States

Marcus Goodman
Goodman Dermatology, Roswell, GA, United States

Connor Heapy and Kerry Montgomery
Department of Psychology, University of Sheffield, Sheffield, United Kingdom

Steven Ersser
Department of Nursing, University of Bournemouth, Bournemouth, United Kingdom

Matt Gass and Nina Goad
British Association of Dermatologists, London, United Kingdom

Andrew R Thompson
Cardiff and Vale University Health Board / Cardiff University, South Wales Clinical Psychology Training, Cardiff, United Kingdom

Bettina Trettin
Department of Dermatology and Allergy Centre, Odense University Hospital, Odense, Denmark
Faculty of Health Science, Institute of Clinical Research, University of Southern Denmark, Odense, Denmark
Centre for Innovative Medical Technology, Odense University Hospital, Odense, Denmark

Dorthe Boe Danbjørg
Faculty of Health Science, Institute of Clinical Research, University of Southern Denmark, Odense, Denmark
Department of Dermatology, Aalborg University Hospital, Aalborg, Denmark
Private Hospital Molholm, Vejle, Denmark

Hanne Agerskov
Faculty of Health Science, Institute of Clinical Research, University of Southern Denmark, Odense, Denmark
Department of Nephrology, Odense University Hospital, Odense, Denmark

Corey H Basch and Rachelle-Ann Romero
William Paterson University, Department of Public Health, Wayne, NJ, United States

Sarah A MacLean
The Icahn School of Medicine at Mount Sinai, New York, NY, United States

Danna Ethan
Lehman College, CUNY, New York, NY, United States

Flemming Andersen
Private Hospital Molholm, Vejle, Denmark
Department of Dermatology, Aalborg University Hospital, Aalborg, Denmark
Faculty of Health Science, Institute of Clinical Research, University of Southern Denmark, Odense, Denmark

Steven Feldman
Center for Dermatology Research, Wake Forest School of Medicine, Winston-Salem, NC, United States

Japbani K Nanda and Michael A Marchetti
Dermatology Service, Department of Medicine, Memorial Sloan Kettering Cancer Center, New York, NY, United States

Jennifer L Hay
Department of Psychiatry and Behavioral Sciences, Memorial Sloan Kettering Cancer Center, New York, NY, United States

Bell Raj Eapen and Norm Archer
Information Systems, McMaster University, Hamilton, ON, Canada

Kamran Sartipi
Department of Computer Science, East Carolina University, Greenville, NC, United States

Elizabeth Sela Nagelhout
Department of Family and Preventive Medicine, University of Utah, Salt Lake City, UT, United States

Riley Lensink, Angela Zhu and Bridget G Parsons
Huntsman Cancer Institute, Salt Lake City, UT, United States

Jakob D Jensen
Department of Communications, University of Utah, Salt Lake City, UT, United States

Yelena P Wu
Huntsman Cancer Institute, Salt Lake City, UT, United States
Department of Dermatology, University of Utah, Salt Lake City, UT, United States

Chapman Wei, Theodore Quan and Puneet Gupta
George Washington University School of Medicine and Health Sciences, Washington, DC, United States

Aaron Fong and Adam Friedman
Department of Dermatology, George Washington University School of Medicine and Health Sciences, Washington, DC, United States

Pushkar Aggarwal
College of Medicine, University of Cincinnati, Cincinnati, OH, United States

Index

T

W

www.ingramcontent.com/pod-product-compliance
Lightning Source LLC
LaVergne TN
LVHW082225200926
848484LV00008B/2304